Advances in the
Management of Cleft Palate

Advances in the Management of Cleft Palate

Edited by

M Edwards M Phil LCST
Area Speech Therapist, Notts Area Health Authority.

A C H Watson FRCS(Ed)
Consultant Plastic Surgeon, Lothian Health Board;
Senior Lecturer, Department of Clinical Surgery, University of Edinburgh.

Foreword by
D R Millard Jr MD FACS

CHURCHILL LIVINGSTONE
EDINBURGH LONDON MELBOURNE AND NEW YORK 1980

CHURCHILL LIVINGSTONE
Medical Division of Longman Group Limited

Distributed in the United States of America by
Churchill Livingstone Inc., 19 West 44th Street, New York,
N.Y. 10036, and by associated companies,
branches and representatives throughout
the world.

First published 1980

ISBN 0 443 01601 1

British Library Cataloguing in Publication Data
Advances in the management of cleft palate.
  1. Cleft palate
  I. Edwards, Margaret   II. Watson, A C H
  617'.522   RD525   80–40099

Printed in Great Britain by
Butler & Tanner Ltd, Frome and London

Foreword

Facial clefts are not dissimilar in many aspects to blow-out wounds, which cripple speech and ravage facial expression. As these anomalies usually occur in the otherwise happily normal infant, the contrast is the more pathetic. A pair of normal eyes, often strikingly beautiful, emphasize the accompanying disparities and in their haunting expression, cry out for relief. It is little wonder that surgeons, dentists and speech physiologists through the years have been challenged to devote so much thought and energy toward facial cleft correction and rehabilitation. So enthusiastic are those involved that a multitude of articles and books have been inspired throughout the world on this subject, far outnumbering what would be expected considering their relatively low incidence in the overall population.

This book *Advances in the Management of Cleft Palate* has evolved from two educational centers, one in England and one in Scotland. Co-edited by Margaret Edwards, a Nottingham speech therapist, and A. C. H. Watson, an Edinburgh plastic surgeon with both Scots and American surgical training, there has been a blending of both specialities. They have chosen an outstanding group of authors to cover all aspects expertly. This extends the popular cleft palate team approach and brings out the importance of the intricate interrelationship of specialists and the influence and assistance that each renders the other in guiding the patient toward the common goal of 'look well, eat well and speak well'.

This is a complete, concise, updated textbook with a major emphasis on cleft palate. Clear, diagrammatic drawings outline the modern popular surgical techniques being used in unilateral and bilateral cleft lip, cleft alveolus and clefts of the hard and soft palate. No attempt is made to present photographic records of 'before' conditions and 'after' results of specific cases. A strong aspect of this work is the thorough handling of speech physiology, assessment and therapy. Also included are succinct chapters on the other important facets, psychosocial aspects, orthodontia and prosthodontia. In conclusion, a concise review of future prospects in this field is made with a plea for the team approach, better parent counseling, continual research, carefully controlled recording with increased standardization among major centers, but with care not to smother the progress in individual inspiration.

This is indeed an excellently condensed, modern guide for anyone involved in the field of cleft lip and palate research and rehabilitation.

1980   D.R.M.

Preface

Muriel Morley's book, *Cleft Palate and Speech*, first published in 1945 has become one of the internationally established texts on this subject. The seventh edition published in 1970 continues to find a steady sale.

This present book owes its existence to the recognition by both Dr Morley and the publishers that in the light of so much knowledge which has accrued in the intervening years, there is now a need for an updated review of the subject.

The decision to produce a multi-author book has been determined to a great extent by two factors; the first factor being that the disability of cleft palate is now regarded as having implications which extend well beyond those directly attributable to the structural condition, and the second, relating to the sheer impossibility of any one author being able to do justice to the burgeoning literature by writing authoritatively on all facets of such a wide subject.

It is the hope and belief of the editors that by inviting contributions from authors of acknowledged experience and repute, this book will reflect, as objectively as is possible, the important trends which have influenced the management of cleft palate over the past ten years.

The concept of the team approach is one which, in this field, has gained increasing favour. Such a fruitful co-operation is only brought about when each member of the team can have some insight into the particular problems faced by his colleagues and into the ways in which these may impinge upon his own strategies of management. For this reason, the book seeks to offer an account of aspects which may enhance such an insight.

Broadly speaking, it is intended for all those concerned with the care of children with cleft lip and palate. A certain degree of selectivity is advocated on the part of the reader. Not every member of the team will need to study each chapter with the same attention to detail. But by attempting to offer a comprehensive account of current thought on the subject the editors consider that the reader will be brought to a better understanding and thus to make a more effective contribution to the wellbeing of those who suffer from this condition.

A considerable debt of gratitude is acknowledged to Muriel Morley and to Ralph Millard, who have stimulated and fostered our interest in the subject over many years.

We also gratefully extend thanks to Catherine Renfrew and to Alistair Bachelor, who offered us much sound help and advice. And finally we say thank you to Anne Watson, Margaret Hamilton and Elizabeth Jennings for so valiantly battling with editorial idiosyncrasies in the preparation of the manuscripts.

1980   M. E.
                                                                A. C. H. W.

Contributors

J K F Anthony
Department of Linguistics, University of Edinburgh, Adam Ferguson Building, 40 George Square, Edinburgh, UK.

Muriel L Campbell
Nursing Officer, The Royal Hospital for Sick Children, Sciennes Road, Edinburgh, UK.

Margaret Edwards
Area Speech Therapist, 17 Clarendon Street, Nottingham, UK

P Fogh-Andersen
16 Carl Feilbergs Vej, DK-2000 Copenhagen F, Denmark.

T D Foster
Professor of Children's Dentistry, Dental School, University of Birmingham, Birmingham, UK.

B Fritzell
Professor of Phoniatrics, Huddinge University Hospital, Huddinge S 141 86, Sweden.

G B Hopkin
Orthodontic Department, The Edinburgh Dental Hospital, 31 Chambers Street, Edinburgh, UK.

Ruth M Lencione
Professor of Language and Speech, School of Medicine, 23–33 Rehab Center, The Center for the Health Sciences, 1000 Veteran Avenue, Los Angeles, USA.

D Ralph Millard Jr
The Plastic Surgery Centre, 1444 NW 14th Avenue, Miami, USA.

Muriel Morley
Beechroyd, Hillside Road, Rothbury, Northumberland, UK.

R W Pigott
Consultant Plastic Surgeon, Frenchay Hospital, Bristol, UK.

Peter Randall
Hospital of the University of Pennsylvania, 1000 I S Ravdin Institute, 3400 Spruce Street, Philadelphia, USA.

A C H Watson
Consultant Plastic Surgeon, The Royal Hospital for Sick Children, Sciennes Road, Edinburgh, UK.

Mary-Anne Witzel
Speech Pathologist, Facial Research and Treatment Centre, Hospital for Sick Children, Toronto, Canada.

George A Zarb
Professor and Chairman of Prosthodontics, Facial Research and Treatment Centre, Hospital for Sick Children, Toronto, Canada.

Contents

1

Introduction

Children born with clefts of the lip and palate constitute only a minority of those suffering congenital deformity of one sort or another. Yet this condition engages the continuing interest of many workers from a variety of disciplines, not only in the quest for improved techniques of remediation, but also in relation to questions of aetiology, of epidemiology and to far-reaching implications of its effect upon the individual. Why should this be so? There are many reasons, but one of the most immediate explanations may lie with the impact of the facial disfiguration in the unoperated state. Those concerned with the obstetric and neonatal care of babies born with clefts of the lip and palate will testify to the traumatic effect the sight of their newborn has on the parents. Present-day society sets considerable store by physical appearance and it is undoubtedly a potent factor in the initial formation of human relationships. In the chapter on Psychosocial Aspects reference is made to studies which describe the unconscious reaction of teachers to cosmetically unattractive children even to the extent of an underrating of their intellectual ability.

The infant with cleft palate is also potentially at a disadvantage in his ability to communicate. In the past, patterns of speech traditionally associated with this condition carried with them a stigma of ridicule. A paper presented by Catherine Renfrew to the Royal Society of Medicine in 1976 states: 'Many of the children who come for therapy are apathetic or aggressive, some are rejected by their families, most are teased by their schoolfellows.'

Of course there is a need to guard against overdramatization of the plight of such children. It must be borne in mind that, for many, successful surgery is followed by normal development in all parameters including speech and language. In a high percentage of cases the skills of surgeons produce results which are cosmetically satisfactory and there is then little cause for embarrassment. Nevertheless a small percentage of children do not react in this satisfactory manner and indeed it is one of the aims of the ensuing chapters to discuss the factors which may be contributory to this failure.

Cleft palate also brings with it many directly or indirectly associated problems. Thus many disciplines participate in the management programme.

Perhaps more so in this condition than in many others, the cliché of team participation is relevant and it is a truism to say that any single member of that team who pursues his speciality unilaterally, without recourse to other members of the team, is liable to face failure in adequate management of at least a proportion of cases. It is therefore in a spirit of joint and equal participation that this book is produced.

Many questions about cleft still remain unanswered. For example, there seems no clearcut reason for the reported increase in incidence to which reference is made, and the manner of inheritance is still not entirely understood.

Other considerations still generate sound and fury, most notably the timing and method of surgical intervention. Whichever regime is favoured by one, there will be others who advance cogent arguments to repudiate it in preference to another type of programme. The surgeon is thus faced with a choice between developing and refining skill in a particular method or adapting techniques in the face of a somewhat arbitrary judgement as to what may be best for the patient in question. Neither course allows for the presence of an x factor which decrees that some patients achieve remarkably good standards of speech in the presence of poor anatomical structure while others remain defective speakers despite a more favourable prognosis.

Both orthodontist and prosthodontist are crucially involved in cases of cleft lip and palate because involvement of primary and secondary palates rarely escapes dental and occlusal complications. Initially the role may be more concerned with facilitation of feeding and with preliminary realignment of maxillary segments, but it is more than likely that such children will remain in their care often through to adolescence and perhaps even later.

The pattern of intervention here is doubly complicated by the possible co-existence of structural anomalies common to the non-cleft palate population together with those more characteristic of facial clefts. Attention is also increasingly focused upon oral neurophysiology as it relates to muscle balance and to tongue movement and their influence on growth and dentition.

The high incidence of hearing loss has received much attention over the past few years and the early intervention of the otologist has become increasingly important. It seems that by the far the most prevalent form of hearing impairment is of the conductive type. Again there is controversy about the exact cause underlying the pathology, exactly in what way the Eustachian tube fails to fulfil its function, and also arguments continue about appropriate types of remediation.

What does appear to be established, however, is the fact that even a minor degree of hearing loss may well have a profoundly deleterious effect upon developing speech. For the child to be able to discriminate accurately the contrasting features of the sounds which combine to create speech, a high level of auditory sense is critical. Later on, there are contextual cues to guide him, but in this time of emerging language the primacy of hearing is beyond dispute.

Improved surgery has brought about a modification in the role of the speech therapist. That is not to say that disorders of resonance traditionally associated with incompetent velopharyngeal function are not still of concern, but on the whole they feature less frequently. As a corollary with the decrease in hypernasality has come an increased attention on other types of speech disorder. Deviant articulation not the direct result of the structural condition gives rise to questions of a more generalized neuromuscular impairment. Disorders of voice resulting in hoarseness are associated with abnormalities of structure and positioning of laryngeal cartilages. These are all aspects of speech production which have received scant attention until recently.

Developments in modern electronics have enabled physiologists to produce much more precise information about the timing and sequence of movement so that features of speech disorder which might formerly have been thought to have an anatomical basis may now be regarded as examples of asynchrony of movement.

Evidence about the pattern of language development in children with cleft palates is conflicting and at present there are few studies utilizing the tremendous upsurge of knowledge of normal language acquisition which came about in the 1960s. Monitoring of language development is the concern of speech therapists working in this field. Here there will be close co-operation with psychologists and possibly with social workers.

The reports on levels of intelligence appear to indicate a tendency towards a slightly lower level of intellectual ability. But these conclusions must be qualified. Of significance is the fact that it is in measures involving verbal ability that the cleft palate group is less able; on performance tasks there is no detriment. Then there is the fact that where cleft palate appears as one feature of a syndrome, mental retardation may appear as another. Therefore a direct correlation is not possible.

Traditional patterns of speech therapy have produced disappointing results because they offered little opportunity for reinforcement and generalization of newly learned skills. The move towards provision of specialized intensive therapy through summer camps in the United States and in a somewhat different form in the United Kingdom at Bristol and in Glasgow, must surely offer a better prognosis.

The paediatric nurse is the person with whom parents and baby are likely to have the closest contact in the early stages. Herein lies the responsibility for advice on welfare, for the cushioning of initial trauma, and for the instillation of hope and the bestowing of comfort, although subsequently this is a role assumed by all those concerned with cleft palate.

The chapters devoted to a review of current technology serve to emphasize the way in which these developments have proved such valuable adjuncts in the process of diagnosis. The advantages of objective information are manifold and certainly advances in the field of optics have provided much-needed information formerly unobtainable on velopharyngeal function. Now there are indications that the development of ultrasound may herald the coming of even more precise methods of assessment. Similarly improved techniques for assessment of air flow have enabled more exact data to be collated on ratios of nasal and oral resonance.

The following chapters seek to describe some of these changes which have been brought about over the past few years. They do not aspire to provide a comprehensive text, but rather aim to alert the reader to ways in which thought on the subject of cleft palate is developing. Almost without exception each contributor pleads for further research in all aspects of the condition. It is hoped that the book will serve as a stimulus for such research, for, as William James wrote: 'Without continuing enquiry there is no progress.'

REFERENCE

Renfrew C E 1976 The Role of the speech therapist with cleft palate patients. Proceedings of the Royal Society of Medicine 69 (1): 31–32

Cleft palate—an historical perspective

EARLY HISTORY

References to disorders of speech due to cleft palate have been found in the writings of Ancient Egypt, and the condition is thought to have been not uncommon among primitive peoples. The French surgeon Paré described the making of obturators to 'fill the cavity of the palate' in 1561. There are records of attempts to repair a hare lip as early as AD 1000, but one of the first operations to repair a cleft of the palate surgically was by Le Monnier, a French dentist, in 1764, mainly to facilitate eating and drinking (Eldridge 1968).

BEFORE 1925—ANATOMICAL CLOSURE OF THE CLEFT

During the nineteenth century various European countries opened centres for the treatment of cleft palate, and many differing methods were devised to repair the cleft using (1) median suture, (2) various types of flaps to cover or occlude the cleft, and (3) compression methods to narrow the cleft before suture. Many of these procedures were ingenious, but were, in general, means of covering or closing the cleft with no consideration as to the normal anatomy and function of the palate, nor the restoration of normal muscle activity in either the palate or nasopharynx (Morley 1970).

From early in the nineteenth century surgeons had attempted to close the cleft by median suture after treating the edges of the cleft so that they might unite after suture. As the tension produced in the palate usually caused a failure of union, attention was directed towards relieving this tension by means of various types of relaxation incisions. In 1826, Dieffenbach first suggested separation of the soft tissues of the palate from the underlying bone, when attempting to repair the hard palate. Fergusson (1844) and von Langenbeck (1862), using median suture, were among those surgeons who contributed notably to the advancement of cleft palate surgery at that time. Other surgeons devised operations using flaps of tissue taken from some other part of the body and grafted these to close the cleft. Flaps removed from the tongue, the neck, upper arm, forehead, and even the implantation of a little finger, were all tried during the latter half of the nineteenth century. However, such techniques made no attempt to reconstruct a functioning soft palate. A tense and fibrous septum between the mouth and nasal passages was the usual result.

Other surgeons, notably Brophy in 1923, suggested that mid-line suture would be simplified if the palatal gap were first narrowed by compression. Continuous pressure was applied over the cheeks and maxilla by a mechanical device as early after birth as possible and retained until suture could be achieved with less tension. However, as the two halves of the palate do not equal one normal palate, due to limited growth resulting from arrested development, such closure, where there is a deficiency of palatal tissue, could only result in gross deformities with breakdown of the palatal tissues as growth proceeded.

Probably the first to consider the postoperative speech was Passavant, who, in 1861, attempted various surgical methods directly designed to assist speech. The following year, he described a cushion, or ridge, which appeared on the posterior pharyngeal wall during phonation, visible in a patient with a cleft palate, but at a level above the posterior margin of the velum in the normal. He thereafter devised several types of pharyngoplasty to assist speech. However, these operations produced little improvement in speech, and by the early part of the twentieth century some form of speech therapy was being provided for some cleft palate patients in a few hospital clinics.

It was during World War I that plastic surgery was developed by certain surgeons to deal with the numbers of gunshot wounds causing facial and other deformities. Some of these surgeons thereafter directed their skills to the repair of clefts of the palate. Names which are remembered are Harold Gillies and Pomfret Kilner in London, Victor Veau in Paris, William Wardill in Newcastle upon Tyne, England, Gänzer, Halle and Ernst in Germany, and Dorrance in the United States of America.

Noting the many postoperative deformities of the maxilla, Harold Gillies pointed out in 1921 that closure of the cleft of the hard palate by such methods as compression and various types of flaps, or even the Langenbeck operation of median suture, tended to cause a collapsed and narrowed upper jaw with malocclusion of the teeth, narrowed nasal passages, and a failure of subsequent development towards the normal. Working with Kelsey Fry, a dental surgeon, he therefore advised closure of the soft palate only, leaving the defect in the hard palate to be closed by a dental plate.

Gillies argued that in unoperated cases involving a cleft of the hard palate the occlusion of the teeth was usually normal, and that most of these patients needed to wear a denture whether the hard palate had been operated upon or not. He therefore recommended that the soft palate should be detached from the hard palate and sutured as far back as possible in the pharynx, thus increasing the defect in the hard palate. He also advised that the operation on the lip should be carried out as soon after birth as possible, and surgery on the palate before the development of speech. Postoperatively, a dental plate was then fitted to assist in feeding, to maintain the soft palate in its posteriorly displaced position, to enable it to make contact with the posterior pharyngeal wall, and to prevent the escape of oral air into the nasal cavities. A permanent prosthetic appliance was thereafter used to compensate for the deficiency in the hard palate, and, if necessary, the anterior part of the soft palate.

THE NEXT 25 YEARS.

Physiological requirements for speech

It was early in the 1920s that William Wardill had become interested in the causes of the postoperative persistance of abnormal speech. With the aid of simple tests he first proved that absolute closure in the nasopharynx was possible, occurred during swallowing to prevent regurgitation, and, although normally a reflex action, could be controlled at will at some point above the posterior border of the soft palate. He also showed that normal articulation was dependent upon the ability to obtain complete closure and control of the airstream through the nasopharyngeal airway.

With the co-operation of a colleague in the Department of Anatomy, James Whillis (Whillis 1930), dissections were carried out on the palate and pharynx which demonstrated that certain muscle fibres in the posterior pharyngeal wall, possibly responsible for the ridge of Passavant, passed through the lateral pharyngeal walls to be inserted into the tissues of the soft palate. Thus, in conjunction with the levators of the palate, they formed a sphincter, contraction of which made possible complete closure of the nasopharyngeal airway, comparable to closure of the lips on contraction of the orbicularis oris. Thus the basic anatomical and physiological requirements to improve the speech result were described and the findings presented to the Royal College of Surgeons, London, in a Hunterian Lecture in 1928 (Wardill 1928).

At that time there were no techniques by which such closure could be confirmed visually, but direct visual observations of the movements of the upper surface of the velum became possible in 1935 in an elderly lady in whom the eye and part of the surrounding face had been removed for treatment of carcinoma. Careful observations showed that, at the commencement of speech, the soft palate was raised from the resting position into a position almost in contact with the posterior pharyngeal wall, described as the 'ready' position, from which position the mucosa of the palate and pharynx was capable of small, rapid movements at extremely high speed during continuous speech. These findings were fully described and published in 1936 (Wardill & Whillis 1936). However, it was not until another 20 years had elapsed that such movements of the palatal and pharyngeal muscles could be adequately demonstrated using lateral X-rays.

Now that the essential mechanism for speech had been described, with increasing appreciation of the anatomical and physiological requirements for normal speech, varying operative procedures were devised and described by many surgeons during the 1930s and 1940s. Veau, Wardill and Dorrance used various methods to elongate the soft palate, sometimes described as push-back operations. Differing types of pharyngoplasties were described, designed to compensate for a short soft palate, by Wardill, Browne and Hynes. The pharyngeal flap was described and used, either inferiorly or superiorly based, but while this sometimes improved speech it produced an abnormal situation anatomically in the pharynx, and was not always functionally successful.

Veau modified the Langenbeck technique by carrying the lateral incisions further forward, just within the alveolar margin, freeing the flaps completely anteriorly, and allowing them to be displaced posteriorly, thus increasing the length of the soft palate. He also sutured the palate in three layers, the mucous membrane of the nasal surface, to avoid formation of scar tissue on the upper surface, suture of the muscles of the palate, and of the oral mucous membrane.

Wardill devised an operation on the pharyngeal wall, a pharyngoplasty, designed to reduce the increased dimensions of the nasopharynx and produce a forward prominence at the level of the ridge of Passavant. At first he combined this with procedures on the palate similar to those of Veau, but later devised a four-flap operation, used with the pharyngoplasty, producing a V–Y advancement, and lengthening the velum as far as possible. Wardill and Veau both repaired the lip and anterior part of the hard palate as early in life as possible, and found that the repaired lip helped to mould the dental arch of the maxilla prior to surgery on the palate.

Dorrance used a two-stage operation on the palate. The two halves of the palate were first united, and later, lateral and anterior incisions were made. The whole of the united palatal tissue was then displaced posteriorly, with a skin graft on the upper, nasal surface of the palate. Hynes developed a pharyngoplasty involving a muscle transplant by means of which the size of the pharynx was reduced, and an actively contractile sphincter was produced in the nasopharynx.

Bone grafting was tried by some surgeons in an attempt to obviate the limited development of the hard palate. These bone inlays, taken from various sites, were implanted into the hard palate to help to bridge the anterior part of the cleft, and, as a result of further bone development and growth, prevent the inward displacement of the maxilla and give support to the alveolar arch.

It was increasingly recognized that surgery designed to improve the speech of the patient must include freeing of the muscles so that the palate could be sutured without tension. Many surgeons fractured the hamular processes to relieve tension in the tensor palati muscles, a procedure first advocated by Billroth in 1889. Otherwise, they believed, there would be interference with the mobility of the palate, breakdown in the suture line and the formation of tension fistulae. Suturing was carefully carried out to minimize the formation of scar tissue, as fibrosed tissue would hinder, or even prevent, further growth and development of the palate and the attainment of velopharyngeal closure.

Increasingly about this time, surgeons were becoming interested in the post-operative results, particularly speech and subsequent growth and development. There was also discussion as to the existence and importance of the ridge of Passavant for speech. It was suggested that it was possibly related to nasopharyngeal closure during swallowing and was not important for speech. Or, it was suggested, that when present in the cleft palate patient it could represent hypertrophy of the muscles involved when attempting to compensate for an open nasopharynx. However, towards the end of this period, in the 1950s, radiographic studies were then developing sufficiently to demonstrate that the ridge of Passavant might be involved in speech in both the individual with a normal palate and in the cleft palate patient. Whether or not a ridge of Passavant was present, it became increasingly obvious that the ability to obtain adequate closure in the nasopharynx was essential for normal speech, and that this ability was associated with contraction and bunching of the mucosa resulting from the activity of the underlying muscles.

Thus, while the first period in the history of the treatment of cleft palate was mainly concerned with anatomical closure of the cleft, the second period from 1925 to 1950 was notable for emphasis on methods to improve the speech result, based on the increasing knowledge of the anatomical and functional requirements for normal speech.

Team work

This second period was also marked by an increasing awareness on the part of the surgeon that even adequate surgery did not necessarily produce normal speech in the older child or adult, especially when defective speech had been fully stabilized before surgery. Hence the development of team work, the surgeon relying on the speech therapist to assess the postoperative speech condition and to complete the work he had initiated.

It was also found that members of the various branches of the dental profession were needed to contribute to treatment. Orthodontists pointed out that alveolar alignment might be good in spite of an alveolar cleft, but that malalignment could occur, either due to tongue pressure not balanced by lip pressures, or following certain methods of surgical repair of the lip. Appliances were therefore designed to control the growth of the dental arch, to improve the alignment of the alveolar segments in the unilateral cleft, or to assist the more normal positioning of the premaxilla in the bilateral cleft. Obturators to close the palatal cleft, frequently with a bulb fitted into the nasopharynx, were being used, and where there was a deficiency of tissue, insufficient to close the cleft without sacrificing the length of the soft palate, a small fistula sometimes remained. To prevent the lack of air pressure for articulation as the result of the air escaping through the fistula a dental plate was required to cover the defect in the hard palate. Many of these small fistulae tended to close spontaneously with growth. Dentition also required observation and treatment.

While surgery, speech pathology and therapy, and the various branches of the dental profession, including orthodontics and prosthodontics, provided the three main members of the team, it was recognized that advice was also required from paediatricians, nurses, psychologists, otolaryngologists, audiologists and radiologists. All had a contribution to make to the treatment of the patient with cleft lip and palate.

Because this was increasingly realized in the early 1940s, the American Cleft Palate Association was formed in 1943. The aim of this association was to bring together members of all the various professions that contribute to the knowledge of cleft palate and its treatment. Conferences have been held each year in the United States of America, and today membership extends to at least 24 other countries. In 1969, the first International Congress was held in Houston, Texas, to be followed in 1973 by the second in Copenhagen, and in 1977 in Toronto. It is the policy of the Association to hold such a congress once every four years.

THE YEARS 1950 TO 1965.

Further advancement in knowledge of the condition and of treatment

During this period surgical techniques continued to develop, and there were investigations into the aetiology of the condition, and much discussion as to the age at which the cleft palate should be repaired.

Aetiology

The possible causes of cleft lip and palate were summarized by Fenton Braithwaite in 1963 under four headings: (1) Maternal infection and toxicity; (2) Maternal dietary imbalance; (3) Maternal hormone activity; and (4) Genetic interferences. Cortisone, insulin, and also aspirin have been implicated. Braithwaite described how the fetus normally inherits an orderly pattern of development in which a series of active outbursts of cellular multiplication follow one another at different sites. The overall pattern of this sequence is laid down by inheritance, and is probably ultimately governed by chemical processes inherent in the genes. Requiring a free and adequate supply of oxygen, these cellular processes are susceptible to changes in the maternal environment and metabolism. It has been shown by others that the toxic effects of rubella in the first three months of pregnancy may have certain teratogenic effects, and that drugs which are cytotoxic to the growth of tumours result in congenital deformities in animals. A diet deficient in folic acid and excessive doses of vitamin A may produce a wide range of deformities, while members of the vitamin B complex afford some measure of protection. Interference with normal processes at the appropriate time can undoubtedly lead to deformity of the corresponding site. Fogh-Anderson (1942) made extensive and careful studies of genetic patterns and found two different hereditary genes, one was for hare lip with or without cleft palate, more common in boys, and one for isolated cleft palate, more common in girls.

The optimum age for surgery

There was always considerable divergence of opinion among surgeons as to the best time to operate. Some operated during the baby's first few months of life, or even during the first weeks, while others preferred to defer surgical treatment until later childhood or adult life. Three factors were considered in making this decision, namely, mortality, speech development and growth.

Some surgeons, notably Veau and Wardill, in the 1930s and 1940s, preferred to operate on the palate at about the end of the first year of life, the lip cleft, if any, being repaired earlier. The results obtained seemed to justify this procedure. However, much depended upon the skill of the surgeon. From the middle of the nineteenth century surgeons had found that closure of the cleft under tension, and with residual raw areas on the upper surface of the palate, as in the Langenbeck operation, led to gross scarring and marked contractures of the palatal tissues. The blood supply was often inadequate postoperatively, and growth was thereby severely impeded, resulting in marked deformities of the maxilla and hard palate. Veau and Wardill were among the first to appreciate this and always carefully sutured the upper surface as well as the lower mucosa of the palate, including suture of the muscles, especially the levators of the palate.

Growth
In the late 1940s some surgical procedures were producing such gross palatal and facial deformities that it was suggested that surgery too early in life was responsible, causing damage to the blood supply and to the growing points of the maxilla, so that subsequent growth was thereby seriously impeded. As a result, many surgeons abandoned early surgery and waited until the child was at least 4 years of age, or even 7 or 8 years, when the greater part of palatal growth would have occurred. The most rapid growth is known to take place before 4 years of age, by which time five-sixths of the total growth is probably completed. It was again suggested by some that the soft palate could be repaired, leaving the hard palate to be closed at a later date. (Also suggested by Gillies and Fry in the 1920s.)

But the most serious effect of this delay was on the developing speech. Abnormal patterns of speech developed and became stabilized, and such faulty development of speech became increasingly difficult to eradicate, and frequently resulted in emotional trauma in the growing child which might never be completely overcome.

Jolleys (1954) studied the results in a series of children who had been operated upon in infancy, and from his findings he considered that the muscle fibres of the cleft velum failed to grow at the normal rate because they lacked the pull of the muscles on the opposite side.

Wardill (1928) had also shown, from measurements of cleft palate skulls, that the dimensions of the pharynx were increased, especially from side to side, in unrepaired clefts when compared with the normal. These findings were confirmed in cleft palate patients by Peyton (1931) and Subtelny (1955). This increase is especially apparent in adults with unrepaired clefts, or where surgery has failed to close the cleft. It was left to further surgery to demonstrate that *early* repair did not necessarily cause interference with growth, and could produce a functional palate with good speech results.

Speech
The advantages of early surgery so far as speech is concerned are related to the processes by which a child develops speech. As understanding of these processes developed, the need for early surgical treatment became increasingly imperative. During the 1950s, with increasing knowledge of the processes involved in the *normal* development of speech, comparisons could be made with the speech development in the child with an unrepaired cleft of the palate. The reasons for the persistence of defective articulation postoperatively then became increasingly apparent, leading to the realization of the importance of early surgery so far as speech development was concerned.

Speech development
Speech develops in early childhood as the result of direct imitation of the speech heard in the environment. The severely deaf child does not hear the sounds

of speech and so cannot imitate them, although he may develop some understanding for language through lip reading. The movements for the articulate
sounds of speech are based on functions such as respiration, sucking and swallowing. Normal speech development is therefore dependent upon both adequate
anatomical conditions and normal functioning neurological processes.

Writing in 1959, Sheridan stated: 'It is difficult to appreciate that these developmental processes in early childhood, which so seldom fail and are so effortless, are so exceedingly complicated. We are still only at the beginning of understanding the biological, otological, neurological, psychological, emotional and
educational implications. Intelligence, auditory capacity, visual localization,
kinaesthetic awareness, motor control and personality are all important.' (Sheridan, 1959.) Teuber (1960) again stressed our ignorance of the neural basis of
speech: 'We simply do not know how the listener manages to analyse the stream
of speech, structure it into phonemes and morphemes and comprehend strings
of sentences according to syntactic rules.'

While in cleft palate we were concerned with the effect of an anatomical condition which determined the ability to articulate normally and clearly the
actual phonetic sounds used in speaking, the many other conditions which influenced the development and intelligibility of spoken language could not be
ignored. To summarize thinking at that time: speech develops from the reflex
behaviour involved in crying, sucking, swallowing and respiration; on this basis,
sounds develop to indicate hunger, reactions to comfort or to pain. Such sounds
involve co-ordinations and motor activity associated with sensory feedback, lay-
ing the foundations for the use of voice in speech.

The child progresses from these primitive reflex movements and sounds to
more spontaneous behaviour, such as vocalizing and babbling, with an increasing awareness of and response to environmental sounds, leading to imitative
verbal behaviour, and the ability to use words, series of words, and eventually
fully developed speech.

Such behaviour involves sensorimotor experience through which a monitoring system evolves, forming an automatic control system in a closed loop circuit.
Mysak (1966) described the speech mechanism as a complex multiple closed-
loop system, and suggested that such activities of the human organism were
the basis of learned skills which became stabilized through experience, leaving
the higher brain centres to engage in more intellectual pursuits. Use of articulation in speaking would therefore be a learned sensorimotor skill, and could be
compared to any other learned skill such as walking, swimming, playing a
musical instrument, driving a car, writing or using a typewriter.

Because speech is a learned skill, few children develop a complete phonological system without some use of incorrect articulation. It was found (Morley
1972) that, at 4 years of age, only 42 per cent of children seen in an investigation
into the speech development of a sample group of 1142 children were using
all articulate sounds normally. Eleven per cent were not intelligible except perhaps to the mother or to other children. At 5 years of age, 4 per cent were still
using so many incorrect sounds that speech was still not fully intelligible. In
a few children these defects might have persisted longer but for speech therapy.
It was also found that although there was considerable variation in the growth

of vocabulary, and the use of words in sentences, the most rapid period of development occurred probably between 2.5 and 3 years of age. This is therefore an argument against the postponement of operative treatment on the palate until after the second year of life.

Speech development in the child with a cleft palate
Such development was then considered as it was modified and affected in the child with a cleft palate. A child with a cleft of the palate and/or lip differs from the normal child from about the 7th week of intrauterine existence, by which time the lip and palate are normally complete, or by the 10th week, when the palatal plates should normally be fused, followed by the growth of the soft palate, thought to be complete by the 12th week. Faulty basic co-ordinations of respiratory, tongue and lip movements occur, therefore, even before birth, and are further developed during sucking, swallowing and breathing and crying in infancy, and subsequently during the early stages of speech development and of spoken language in the first, second and third years of life. With increasing fluency, these complex developing patterns become stabilized through experience, and increasingly automatic through repeated experience, the intellectual faculties becoming more and more concerned with the thought expressed, and not with the means by which it is accomplished. Thereafter such patterns of activity become ever more difficult to change. It then becomes necessary to return to the early stages of speech development in order to change these basic patterns, and thereafter to incorporate these changed patterns of articulation into spoken language.

At that time it was fully accepted that the basic cause of the development of defective articulation in these children was the lack of adequate intra-oral air pressure when the nasopharyngeal sphincter was incompetent. The expiratory airstream used for articulation is normally controlled at three positions. The first of these is the larynx. The airstream can be interrupted by closure of the vocal cords, or the ventricular bands, but, once past this point, the expiratory air has two alternative outlets, either through the nasopharynx and nostrils, as in quiet breathing, and controllable by the nasopharyngeal sphincter, or through the mouth and lips, controlled by the tongue, orbicularis oris and other facial muscles, as in blowing, whistling and speech. These two outlets are used as alternatives, are rarely used simulateneously and never in speech. Normal speech requires primarily the adaptation, co-ordination and control of the muscles concerned in the activities of these three muscle groups, laryngeal, pharyngeal and oral.

For articulation, air is momentarily held in the mouth under slight pressure between the cheeks, tongue and palate, or lips, with the nasopharyngeal airway closed by the sphincter muscles. The air is then released through the mouth producing a plosive sound, or pressure is released more gradually through a narrowed outlet between the tongue and teeth, or palate, as for fricative consonants. In cleft palate it is the consonant sounds which are mainly affected, and even between these there is some variation in the degree of oral pressure required. Vowel sounds offer little or no interference to the passage of oral air and are, therefore, usually recognizable, although there may be some distortion of vocal tone. Only three consonants, /m/, /n/ and /ng/, are normally produced with some air and resonance passing through the nasal airways with the oral airway closed at the lips, tongue tip and anterior palate contact, and mid-tongue and mid-palate contacts respectively.

It was found that the child with a cleft palate acquired various compensations in attempting to reproduce the sounds he heard, and he therefore developed a form of phonemic usage which, although it might be unintelliglble to others, he identified completely with the speech he heard from others around him. Such a child will accept a recording of his speech as abnormal but will fail to recognize it as his own speech, and is unaware that his speech differs from that which he hears around him. He is then perplexed and worried as to why people fail to understand him. The strength of the habit factor relates to the inability of individuals to hear their own speech as others hear it. We have all been surprised when first hearing our own speech on a recording, and manner of speaking is as recognizable and personal to an individual as is his facial appearance. It is a common experience to recognize a speaker by his speech over the telephone. Such firmly established patterns of speech are correspondingly resistant to change. While there are many individual variations in ability to mimic speech heard, to learn to speak a foreign language, or to respond to speech therapy, a local dialect may be retained throughout life.

The strength of this habit factor was well demonstrated in certain patients who, having had a repair of the palate, had subsequent inability to control the nasopharyngeal airway adequately. A pharyngeal obturator was fitted to assist closure for improved consonant articulation (Blakely 1960). It was then found that the patient attempted to maintain his accustomed nasalized speech and resonance by relaxing the pharyngeal muscles around the obturator bulb, and, initially, it was found essential to use an obturator bulb large enough to completely occlude the nasopharyngeal airway both for speech and for respiration. It was necessary for speech to be completely denasalized and remain so until such time as the patient had become accustomed to, and accepted, the changed sensory feedback. Speech therapy was then required until the patient had acquired acceptable articulation, when an obturator reduction programme was begun and continued until compensatory muscle activity was optimal.

With this awareness of the basic problems involved, it was becoming apparent that the longer the abnormal speech co-ordinations persisted the more difficult they were to change. Not all surgeons were interested in the subsequent speech development of their patients, but those who were interested in the functional, as well as the anatomical result, increasingly realized that surgery before the development of speech was an advantage to the child. Observations by surgeons and speech therapists suggested that, as described, once the developing stages of speech were completed at 4 to 5 years of age, with phonemic usage stabilized and automatically incorporated into fluent language, there was stronger resistance to change. Following surgery during the earlier stages of speech development, changes were found to occur spontaneously within a few months of successful surgery or were easily made with minimal guidance. When operation was successfully performed during the first or even the second year of life, when speech in its early stages was still unstable, it was usual for speech to develop normally, other conditions being within the normal range.

Thus certain surgeons always operated whenever possible on children at, or around the end of the first year, in order to avoid the stabilization of abnormal speech with the inherent disadvantages, if not distress, which this could cause to a young child. That this change is possible has been proved by some surgeons who were operating at this age during the 1950s and subsequently.

The development of speech after early surgery

Developing speech was observed over many years following early surgery in a series of approximately 400 children operated upon for clefts of the palate by Fenton Braithwaite in Newcastle upon Tyne, between 1950 and 1965. Braithwaite devoted much of his career to the study of the causes and nature of clefts of the lip and palate as his major interest, and applied a scientific approach and skilful hands to the treatment of this condition.

For Braithwaite, however, surgery was not the end of treatment but the beginning, as, following repair of the palate at 10 to 18 months, the children returned at six-monthly intervals until they were at least 15 years of age. At these clinical follow-up sessions the surgeon assessed the surgical result, the orthodontist the dental development, and the speech therapist the developing speech. Only by such regular assessments over a considerable period of time can the results be adequately determined and the wisdom or otherwise of the procedures confirmed. Careful observations, regularly recorded, indicated not only that the type of surgery performed did not appear to interfere with growth, but that growth was actively stimulated at the normal growth periods.

Utilization of growth—results of treatment

This work marked the third period in the development of the treatment for clefts of the lip and palate, demonstrating the utilization of normal growth processes following surgery in infancy and at the optimum time. Because of the carefully documented information through the long and regular postoperative observations, the work and results of Fenton Braithwaite will be described as demonstrating what was being achieved by repair of the cleft palate in infancy at that time.

However, Braithwaite was not alone in this work. McCollum in the United States, among other surgeons, was also operating on young children and he also carried out postoperative study of his patients and published his results (McCollum et al 1956). He operated on the lip when the child was 6 pounds in weight, and on the palate at 20 pounds weight. The mortality was nil. Speech results showed, in a selected group, that of 108 children operated upon between 1942 and 1952, 70 per cent developed normal, non-nasal speech. In a consecutive series of 75 children, operated upon between 1946 and 1947, 50 per cent were found to have normal speech when seen in 1956. In addition, 13 per cent and 21 per cent respectively had non-nasal speech with faulty articulation. Seventeen per cent, and 15 per cent respectively had slight degrees of nasality. The total number of 'non-nasal cases' was respectively 83 per cent and 71 per cent.

It was also found, using cephalometric evaluation, that although facial patterns differed from the *ideal* normal pattern, they did not differ appreciably from those of a random sample of the normal population. Early operation had not, in these children, therefore, contributed towards deformity of the maxilla, nor seriously affected dental occlusion.

Braithwaite did not normally operate on the pharyngeal wall, as he preferred not to disturb normal tissue, so he did not use any type of pharyngoplasty, nor a pharyngeal flap, as a standard primary procedure. He chose to operate on the lip when the child was about 10 pounds weight, with no loss of life in a series of 485 children. If the cleft lip extended through the alveolus into the palate, the anterior primary palate was repaired at the same time as the lip. The developing lip then helped to realign the united alveolar arch, and growth was assisted through normal muscle activity. Braithwaite has described his surgical procedures (Braithwaite 1963, 1964), which basically involved wide freeing of the facial musculature from its bony attachments laterally until the margins of the cleft approached each other and could be sutured without tension. It was his aim to produce a short, full upper lip, a baby's lip, and not one artificially lengthened to resemble an adult lip. To ensure adequate muscular function, he carefully united the mucosa and the muscles of the separate elements of the lip, thus producing a functioning orbicularis oris. He aimed to unite the tissues as nature had intended, and to leave growth, stimulated by muscle activity, to complete the process of further development. It was found that the earlier in life this process of union was achieved, other factors also considered, the better for growth and subsequent appearance. Regular observation over many years confirmed the value of this procedure.

When repairing the palate the same principles were considered, extensive freeing of the tissues, muscle transplantation and careful suturing of the mucosal surfaces and the muscles of the palate without tension. Braithwaite was the first to stress the importance of complete mobilization of the muscles which are abnormally inserted, and their transposition and suture across the mid-line.

Braithwaite was interested in the theory put forward by Podvinec (1952), and from his own observations of muscle movements and attachments suggested that closure of the nasopharyngeal airway was probably achieved by the resultant interaction of the levators, superior constrictor and palatopharyngeus, and he stressed the importance of the inward movement of the lateral pharyngeal walls (10.36). He described (1963) the action of the levators and palatopharyngeus muscles as two interacting slings, the levator sling elevating the soft palate in a backward and upward direction, and the palatopharyngeus approximating the lateral walls and narrowing the pharynx. Acting together they have a common insertion for their activity, each muscle loop affording counter purchase for the other. On contraction, the U shape of each sling is converted into a V. Hence the need for careful suture of the divided muscles when repairing the cleft (Figs 2.1 to 2.6). (Current views on palatopharyngeal function are described in Chapter 6.)

Braithwaite's operation is still widely practised and the technical details are described in Chapter 9.

Because Braithwaite considered it most important to produce an intact velum, he sometimes sacrificed complete closure of the hard palate when there was a deficiency of tissue due to arrest of development in the early stages. This resulted in some children having a small residual fistula in the anterior or medial part of the hard palate which could be occluded by a small dental plate. With subsequent growth many of these defects closed spontaneously.

Following surgery based on the principles described, it was observed that such a repair of the lip and palate, accomplished with minimal scarring and tension, tended to produce increasing muscle activity, not possible until the muscles had been united. Such muscle activity apparently stimulated growth, with improving function.

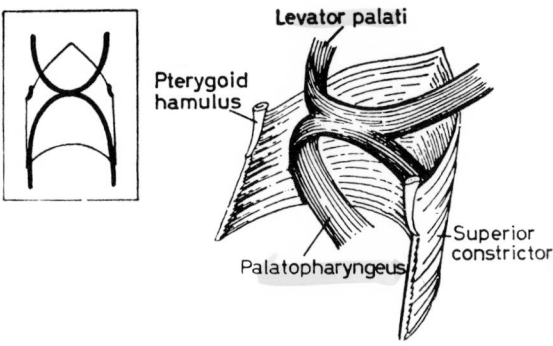

Fig. 2.1 The levator palati and the palatopharyngeus muscles illustrated as an 'x'-shaped muscle

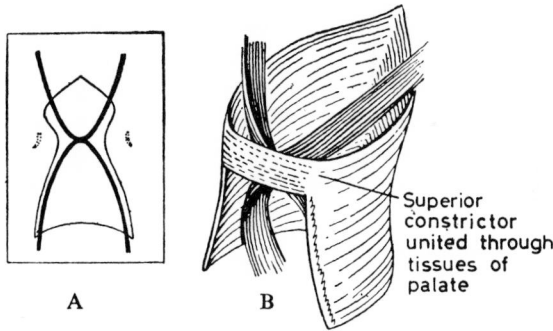

Fig. 2.2 (a), the 'scissors' effect of contracture of the 'x' shaped muscle. (b) The sphincter effect produced when the superior constrictor is freed from the medial pterygoid lamella and the hamulus, with the palate united

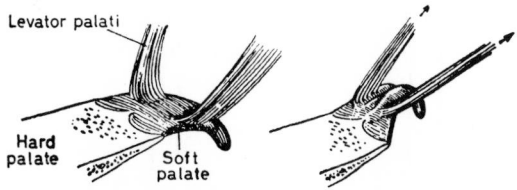

Fig. 2.3 The effect of the contracting arms of the two levator palati muscles. (From Modern trends in plastic surgery, vol 1, Butterworth 1963)

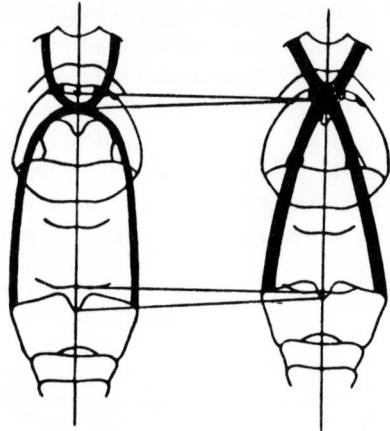

Fig. 2.4 Diagram representing the slings of the levator and palatopharyngeus muscles when relaxed and when contracted

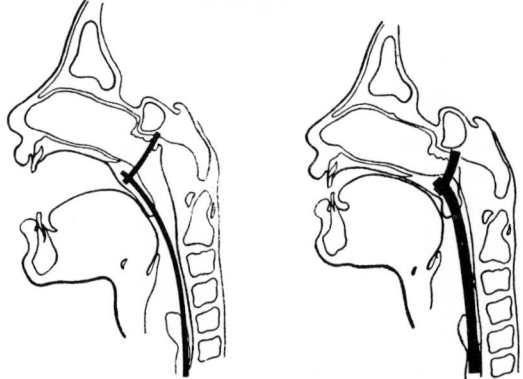

Fig. 2.5 Lateral view showing the effect of interaction of the levator and palatopharyngeus muscles on the movement of the soft palate

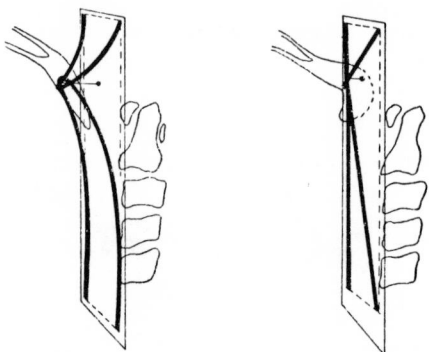

Fig. 2.6 Diagrammatic view of the muscle action in Fig. 2.5

While it was interesting and informative for the surgeon to observe and assess his results, it was also of great interest to the speech therapist to be able to observe development of speech in so many children with cleft palate, over such a long period of time, extending from 1948 to 1963.

The analysis and assessment of the results

There are now many technological devices for assessing the degree of surgical success in achieving the requirements for normal speech, but in 1950 the aids were limited. The speech therapist therefore relied on the use of tests for blowing to indicate ability to blow without nasal escape of air, to sustain intra-oral air pressure with lips closed, and to release the air either through the lips or through the nasopharyngeal sphincter. Use of a manometer to test and to measure breath pressure was introduced in the early 1960s, but the degree of air pressure registered tended merely to show the extent of the lung capacity and muscular strength of the patient on blowing. Like other blowing tests it did not demonstrate whether or not the nasopharyngeal sphincter was competent to maintain and control the oral air pressure for articulation. Lateral radiographs were also improving and could demonstrate the ability of the velum to make contact or not with the posterior pharyngeal wall, but they did not always show clearly whether or not there was full competence of the nasopharyngeal sphincter.

Also assessed was the ability to articulate consonant sounds in continuous speech, dependent upon the trained ear of the therapist, and ability to analyse rapidly the sounds being used. In spite of modern technology, which is now so useful in providing objective evidence of the success of the surgical result, the ultimate analysis and assessment must be based on the use of actual conversational speech to the trained ear. It must also be recognized that normal articulation is not so much proportional to the *degree* of nasopharyngeal closure, nor to the *size* of the velopharyngeal aperture, as on the child's ability to achieve a degree of nasopharyngeal closure which is sufficient to maintain momentarily the requisite intra-oral air pressure and mobility for the adequate articulation of each of the rapidly occurring sequences of the articulate sounds used in speech. Thus the first assessment was that of the degree of the intra-oral air pressure.

The second assessment was of vocal tone and resonance balance. This normally varies between individuals due to day-to-day infections of the nasal and pharyngeal mucous membranes, sinus conditions, growth of adenoids, and so forth. There are also modifications in boys during the change of voice at puberty. Again, it is the trained ear which must assess what is within the acceptable range, and what is associated with the cleft palate defect.

The third factor to be assessed was the use of articulate sounds in speech, and it may be some considerable time postoperatively before speech has developed sufficiently for a full assessment. There is always a wide age range for the onset of speech, and some children with cleft palate may develop speech later than the normal. This may or may not be related to general mental retardation, but to emotional problems, hospitalization and other factors. In any ongoing survey of a series of patients, such as this, there will always be some who are too young for a full assessment of articulation, or in whom operation is too recent for the final speech result to have been achieved.

It was noticed that, following the production of a competent sphincter in early life, some children passed through a period when, as in the normal, articulation was at first inaccurate. In the child with a cleft palate, especially, the basic co-ordinations related to sucking and swallowing have not been normal, and adjustments of these reflex processes follow closure of the cleft. It was found that many of these children began to speak using defective articulation, but that normal speech developed spontaneously without any specialized help, and within a reasonable time, once the means for normal speech had been created surgically. Such phonemic difficulties may persist for a longer period in the cleft palate child, or may relate to delayed surgical treatment, especially if speech is developing early with faulty co-ordinations before surgery. Also, they seemed to be more marked and persistent in children with the more severe type of cleft, such as unilateral and bilateral clefts.

It was also necessary to consider other relevant conditions such as a hearing loss, even if only intermittent, mental retardation, and the possibility of a speech disorder irrespective of and unrelated to the cleft palate.

The assessments were first made of nasopharyngeal control and of articulate sounds in the child's first words, such as 'bye bye', 'ta ta', 'da da', 'up', 'car' and so forth; and later in single words, short phrases, rhymes and finally in conversational speech. Judgements were always made on phonemic adequacy during spontaneous speech, however limited, and not on the ability to repeat test words or phrases.

Assessments were therefore based on an analysis of speech at the stage of development reached. At any one time there were: (a) those who had not acquired normal phonemic usage with no trace of articulatory defect due to the cleft palate or any other condition; (b) those with fluent speech and no defect attributable to insufficient intra-oral air pressure, but with some resolving defects of articulation; these could be minimal, such as a slight distortion of /s/, or there might be more defective use of articulation, but not due to lack of adequate intra-oral air pressure; (c) there were also those who had insufficient linguistic development for a complete analysis; and (d) there were those with defective articulation due to surgical failure to provide a competent sphincter, or who had a residual anterior fistula when the sphincter was fully competent.

The first assessments made on the speech of the children operated upon by Braithwaite was in 1955, on children operated upon between 1949 and 1955. After five years the surgeon wished to evaluate his operative procedures by the functional results being obtained. During this period 117 children had had a repair of the palate. The age at operation varied considerably in this first period: 81 children were under 2 years of age, four being under 1 year; 36 were over 2 years, nine being over 4 years, including two who were aged 27 and 30 years respectively. Braithwaite first came to Newcastle in 1948 and, owing to unavoidable delays, the proportion of older patients in this first series was high, 30 per cent being over 2 years at the time of operation on the palate. The detailed results are shown in Table 2.1.

Although at the time of this first survey it was found that only 34 (29 per cent) of the children had fully normal speech, 107 (92 per cent) had been provided with a competent nasopharyngeal sphincter, the essential requirement for normal speech. Seventy-three children (63 per cent) were still too young for speech to have developed fully, or were in a transitional stage of progression towards acquiring good speech but had resolving defects of articulation and an incomplete phonological system.

When the results were analysed according to type of cleft it was found that a competent nasopharyngeal sphincter had been provided in 83 per cent of those children with bilateral clefts, in 92 per cent with a unilateral cleft, in 92 per cent of those with a postalveolar cleft, and in 100 per cent in both the two children with submucous clefts.

The results analysed according to the age of the child at operation showed that of the 81 children who were under 2 years of age at the time of operation 75 (92.5 per cent) had adequate nasopharyngeal closure postoperatively. Of the remaining 36 patients, operated upon when over 2 years of age, nine being over

Table 2.1 Results of operation carried out between 1949 and 1955

Type of cleft	Bilateral (12)	Unilateral (39)	Postalveolar (64)	Submucous (2)	Total (117)
Anatomical result					
Competent nasopharyngeal sphincter	10	36	59	2	107 (92%)
Incompetent sphincter	2	3	5	0	10 (8%)
Speech result					
Normal	1	11	22	0	34 (29%)
Resolving defects of articulation	6	21	23	2	52 (45%)
Too young for assessment	3	4	14	0	21 (18%)
Defects of articulation due to lack of intra-oral air pressure	2	3	5	0	10 (8%)

4 years, 32 (88.9 per cent) had a successful anatomical result with the essential requirements for normal speech. These results were considered by the surgeon to be sufficiently encouraging for him to continue, and to further develop his operative procedures.

The second survey was made five years later in 1960. The total number of patients assessed then was 360, this number including the 117 patients previously assessed, still under review, and described in Table 2.1. In this survey 237 children (66 per cent) were under 2 years of age, and only 44 children (12 per cent) were over the age of 3 years.

Anatomical results. Of the 360 children, 345 (95.5 per cent) achieved normal speech, while eight children (2.5 per cent) also had nasopharyngeal competence but there was some inco-ordination at times in its control for speech: for example, two of these children could maintain full oral air pressure for blowing but had some slight degree of nasal escape at times during speech; two other children had normal speech except when nervous or excited, when there was a similar inco-ordination; another child had adequate intra-oral air pressure on single words which was not always maintained fully in continuous speech. The speech of these eight children was fully intelligible, and to the casual listener, would have been accepted as normal. Many of these children gain full control later with further growth and development, and without any need for further surgery. Therefore 353 children (98 per cent) had been provided with a functioning nasopharyngeal sphincter, while only seven children (2 per cent) had an incompetent sphincter with obvious uncontrollable nasal escape of air on blowing and during speech.

Speech analysis. Thirty-one children (9 per cent) had not developed sufficient speech for a full assessment of their use of articulation; 23 of these were under 4 years of age, seven were mentally retarded and had limited speech development, and one had a severe congenital hearing defect of inner ear type, preventing both understanding for and the development of speech. Eighty-two children (23 per cent) still had resolving defects of articulation, 50 being under 6 years of age at that time, and with no trace of any nasal escape of air, or any other typical cleft palate defect during speech. There were 16 children (4 per cent) who each had a small residual fistula in the anterior part of the hard palate and were waiting for provision of a small dental plate to give them adequate oral air pressure for speech, seven of them being under 2 years of age. As previously described, where there is a marked limitation of palatal development and of tissue for repair, the hard palate may be sacrificed in order to produce a useful soft palate. Many of these fistulae close spontaneously with growth, but until such time as full closure is obtained speech can be helped by the closing of the fistula by a dental plate. Each of these children had a competent nasopharyngeal sphincter, and has been grouped with those children who had resolving defects of articulation. The remaining 199 children (64 per cent) had fully developed normal conversational speech, many having passed through stages postoperatively when they had varying degrees of defective articulation, unrelated to insufficient intra-oral air pressure for speech, although probably resulting from basic reflex inco-ordinations and early attempts to speak before surgery, when normal use of articulate sounds was not possible. Each had a fully competent nasopharyngeal sphincter.

Therefore, of this group of 360 children, only seven (2 per cent) had an incompetent sphincter and could be classed as surgical failures. Speech was, of course, defective with typical cleft palate defects due to inadequate intra-oral air pressure for normal articulation.

It was sometimes suggested that a child might acquire normal speech, but that later, due to possible anomalies of palatal or other growth processes, competent nasopharyngeal closure might be lost, and that normal speech, once acquired, might not persist.

A further survey was carried out in 1968. As many as possible of those patients included in the 1955 and 1960 surveys were recalled for a further assessment. It was found that, in general, spontaneous development of speech had continued, and that speech was normal in 255 children (71 per cent of those seen). The majority of the remaining children required only minimal speech therapy or guidance for the mother, while 36 (10 per cent) required more intensive help, although intra-oral air pressure was adequate and there was no excessive nasal resonance. In most, the residual defect was only slight, frequently a somewhat distorted articulation of /s/ only. However, the more extensive difficulties were not necessarily the result of the cleft palate, since intra-oral air pressure remained adequate with a competent nasopharyngeal sphincter. Delay in receiving surgical treatment until after the stabilization of defective articulation, sometimes due to unavoidable circumstances, could have been the cause in some cases, but, as previously described, in the normal population there are always some children who fail to develop normal phonemic usage without help. A comparison of the results of the three surveys in 1955, 1960 and 1968 is shown in Table 2.2. The spontaneous resolution of defects of articulation is shown by the reduction of the number of children in this category from 45 per cent to 26 per cent, and the increase in normal speech from 29 per cent of the children in 1955 to 71 per cent in 1968. Defects due to inco-ordination also decreased from 2.5 per cent to 1 per cent.

Hearing. Many surgeons find that hearing is affected more frequently in children with cleft palate than in the normal population. Causes suggested were

Table 2.2 Comparison of results in 1955, 1960 and 1968

	1955	1960	1968
Competent nasopharyngeal sphincter	92%	98%	98%
Speech			
Too young for assessment	18%	9%	0
Resolving defects of articulation	45%	28.5%	26%
Normal speech	29%	58%	71%
Defects of articulation due to an incompetent sphincter	8%	2%	2%
Defects due to inco-ordination	0	2.5%	1%

abnormal functioning in the nasopharynx when surgical procedures were delayed, or abnormal conditions and tensions due to pharyngoplasties or pharyngeal flaps. It was thought possible that early surgery might have assisted middle ear drainage and helped to avoid more serious interference with hearing. Three hundred and two children seen (84 per cent) had no hearing disability. Four children in the series had a congenital hearing loss of inner ear type, one so severe as to necessitate education in a school for the deaf. Forty children had some middle ear hearing loss with otorrhoea and otalgia. This was intermittent and associated with nasal infections. Four children had a more persistent middle ear loss, but not sufficient to affect speech development. Removal of adenoids was essential in nine children. This condition is sometimes responsible for the inco-ordination noticed in a few children, or may result in temporary incompetence of the nasopharyngeal sphincter, full competence usually being regained within a short period of time.

McWilliams & Musgrave (1971) also stressed that speech is more than directing the expiratory airstream appropriately for articulation, and discussed some of the problems encountered in the assessment of cleft palate children. They emphasized that children with clefts experienced retardation in the early stages of expressive language, and that there is a need to consider intelligence, hearing, emotional factors, dental anomalies and neuromotor ability, in addition to velopharyngeal control, and the adequacy of language development in relation to chronological and mental age.

Over the years it was noticed that typical defects of articulation due to cleft palate were gradually modified, apparently related to changes in surgical procedures and results. The most common defects in the 1930s and 1940s were the substitution of a plosive glottal sound—the glottal stop—for many or even all plosive consonant sounds, and the use of a pharyngeal fricative sound as a substitution for consonant sounds such as /s/—the 'pharyngeal /s/', While the child with a normal palate may have difficulty in the normal articulation of /s/, the substitutions used are not the pharyngeal or nasal sounds frequently used by the patient with a cleft palate.

During the period of time from 1930 to 1965 the glottal stop and pharyngeal substitutions became increasingly rare. This was thought to be due to improving surgical techniques resulting in less postoperative tension in the pharynx and velum, with better control of the nasopharyngeal airway.

A comparison of the substitutions used for /s/ in four groups of children is shown in Table 2.3: (a) cleft palate patients seen in the 1930s; (b) cleft palate patients seen in the 1950s and 1960s; (c) children with normal palates but defective articulation including (s); and (d) children in a sample group of 1142 children, representing the normal population, seen in 1951. Substitutions for /s/ were finally classed as posterior (pharyngeal), medial, and anterior. It will be seen that the cleft palate patients have many more posterior substitutions for /s/ than those with normal palates, and that there is also a marked difference between groups (a) and (b), cleft palate patients, in this respect (10.204–209).

It would probably be a mistake to imply that the results descibed were universal during the period described. Any surgery in the small cavity of a baby's mouth presents many problems. Probably several factors contributed to the results as described: early surgery, before 2 years of age; the simplicity of the design of the surgical method, based on a study of the development, anatomy and function of the normal palate; and in addition the manipulative skill of a particular surgeon. However, these results did show that surgery in infancy could successfully provide a competent nasopharyngeal sphincter, that maxillary growth was thereby assisted rather than impeded, and that normal speech could develop spontaneously postoperatively. There could at first be minimal, transient defects of articulation when surgery was completed before speech developed, probably related to early inco-ordinations in sucking, swallowing and babbling in infancy, but these rapidly resolved. However, the longer such abnormal phonemic patterns persisted before surgery, the more firmly did they become established. They then became incorporated into the developing speech, until once speech was fully automatic there was ever-increasing resistance to change. The argument for early successful surgery, so far as speech was concerned, could no longer be gainsaid. It was therefore concluded that whenever possible, early surgery, producing a competent sphincter, allowing for stimulation of growth with subsequent development towards the normal, should be the aim for every child with a cleft palate.

This review of the history of the development of the treatment of cleft palate up to 1965 has shown how surgical procedures changed over the years, has de-

Table 2.3 Defective articulation of /s/ in children with clefts of the palate and children with normal palates

Consonant substitutions for /s/	Cleft palate		Normal palate	
	60 children with repaired cleft palates 1930–40	88 children with repaired cleft palates seen during 1950–68	88 children with normal palates and defective articulation of /s/ 1951	58 children with defective /s/ from a group of 1142 children, 162 of whom had defective articulation 1951
Not attempted	10	5	8	3
Anterior				
w	—	—	—	1
f	—	—	1	1
θ [th]	—	2	8	3
ts	—	—	1	—
t	1	3	43	33
weak attempt	—	9	—	—
slight defect	—	8	—	—
Medial				
l	—	—	—	1
ʃ [sh]	—	17	5	6
lateral /s/	—	11	13	6
ç fricative in k position	2	18	3	1
Posterior				
s (nasal)	20	5	2	—
Nasopharyngeal h	—	2	—	1
	—	—	4	2
Pharyngeal	27	8	—	—
Total	60	88	88	58
Anterior substitutions	1.6%	25%	60%	65%
Medial substitutions	3.3%	52%	24%	24%
Posterior substitutions	78%	17%	7%	5%

scribed how techniques improved with increasing knowledge of the anatomy and function of the palatopharyngeal muscles used in speech and has mentioned the advantages of early surgery in relation to speech and to growth processes. With developing chemotherapy, increasing use of antibiotics, modern methods of anaesthesia and increasing knowledge of the principles of plastic surgery and nursing care, the mortality rate was reduced so as to be no longer an important factor when considering the age for operation. The development of team work in the 1940s has been described, and the increasing knowledge of speech development and of the defects especially related to cleft palate, with the need for close co-operation of all those concerned in the care and treatment of these children.

Since the beginning of the 1960s, during the last 15 to 20 years there have been many new developments, particularly technological devices for the assessment of the surgical and speech results. These will be described in this book to which this chapter forms an introductory historical survey.

REFERENCES

Blakely R W 1960 Temporary speech prosthesis as an aid in speech training. Cleft Palate Bulletin 10:63

Braithwaite F 1963 Cleft lip and palate. In: Gibson T (ed) Modern trends in plastic surgery. Butterworth, London, vol 1

Braithwaite F 1964 Cleft lip and palate. In: Rob C, Smith R (eds) Clinical surgery. Butterworth, London, ch 5

Braithwaite F, Morley M E 1963 Cleft lip and palate. Speech Pathology and Therapy 6:1, 2

Eldridge M 1968 A history of the treatment of speech disorders. Livingstone, Edinburgh

Fogh-Anderson P 1942 Inheritance of harelip and cleft palate. Busak, Copenhagen

Jolleys A 1954 A review of results of operation for cleft palate with reference to maxillary growth and speech. British Journal of Plastic Surgery 7: 229

McCollum D W, Richardson S O, Swanson L T 1956 Habilitation of the cleft palate patient. New England Journal of Medicine 254: 299

McWilliams B J, Musgrave A H 1971 Diagnosis of speech problems in patients with cleft palate. British Journal of Disorders of Communication 6: 26

Morley M E 1970 Cleft palate and speech, 7th edn. Churchill Livingstone, Edinburgh

Morley M E 1972 The development and disorders of speech in childhood, 3rd edn. Churchill Livingstone, Edinburgh

Mysak E E 1966 Speech pathology and feedback theory. Thomas, Springfield, Illinois

Peyton W T 1931 Dimensions and growth of the palate in the normal infant or in the infant with gross maldevelopment of the upper lip and palate. Archives of Surgery 22: 704

Podvinec S 1952 The physiology and pathology of the soft palate. Journal of Laryngology 66: 452

Sheridan M D 1959 The development of speech and hearing in young children. Medical Press Aug 19 147

Subtelny J D 1955 Width of the nasopharynx and related anatomied structures in normal and un-operated cleft palate children. American Journal of Orthodontics 41: 889

Teuber H L 1960 Perception. In: Field J, Magoun H W, Hall V R Handbook of physiology, sect 1 Neuro-physiology, American Physiological Society, Washington DC, vol 1

Wardill W E M 1928 Cleft palate. British Journal of Surgery 26: 6

Wardill W E M, Whillis J 1936 Movements of the soft palate. Surgery, Gynaecology and Obstetrics 62: 836-839

Whillis J 1930 A note on the muscles of the palate and the superior constrictor. Journal of Anatomy 65 (1): 92–95

3

Embryology of cleft lip and palate

Knowledge of the main steps in the development of the face is an invaluable aid to the understanding of the various abnormalities which make up the cleft palate deformity. It is also important to appreciate that clefting of the palate is so intimately related to cleft lip that the development of the one cannot be considered without the other. The changes in appearance of the embryo face have been established for over a century but the timing of the changes, which is usually given so confidently, is largely a matter of conjecture and there is still argument as to what is actually happening to produce them. This is not so strange as it seems at first when one realizes that only 12 human embryos with cleft lip and palate have ever been examined and reported in the world literature. Millard (1976), with characteristic pithiness, has described the problem as like trying to recreate an intricate movie from a few random frames. As a result, much of what we believe to be happening in the human embryo is based on observations of animal development, which in many respects differs from species to species. The descriptions and timing of events which follow must, therefore, be regarded as provisional.

It is between the 5th and 9th weeks of pregnancy that the most important alterations are taking place in the developing face. At the end of the 4th week the embryo, which is only about 3.5 mm long, has nothing resembling a head or face, while by the end of the 8th week it is 30 mm long and the face is fully formed. The palate is not completed for another three weeks.

In the early embryo the foregut, which is lined by entoderm, ends blindly and is separated from a shallow surface depression called the *Stomodaeum* or *oral pit* (lined by ectoderm) by the *buccopharyngeal membrane* (Fig. 3.1a). The breakdown of this membrane during the 4th week allows the foregut to communicate with the oral pit. At this stage the oral pit is very shallow but the subsequent forward growth and development of the tissues around it results in the site of the buccopharyngeal membrane (i.e. the junction between entoderm and ectoderm) eventually lying in the region of the tonsil. This forward growth is the result of the migration and proliferation of mesoderm—which is the name given to the primitive cells and the gelatinous ground substance which supports them, which fill the space between the entoderm and ectoderm.

At 4 weeks a *frontal prominence* is present in the mid-line, forming the upper or cephalic boundary of the oral pit. On each side of this is a flattened area known as the *olfactory placode* which will eventually form the organs of smell

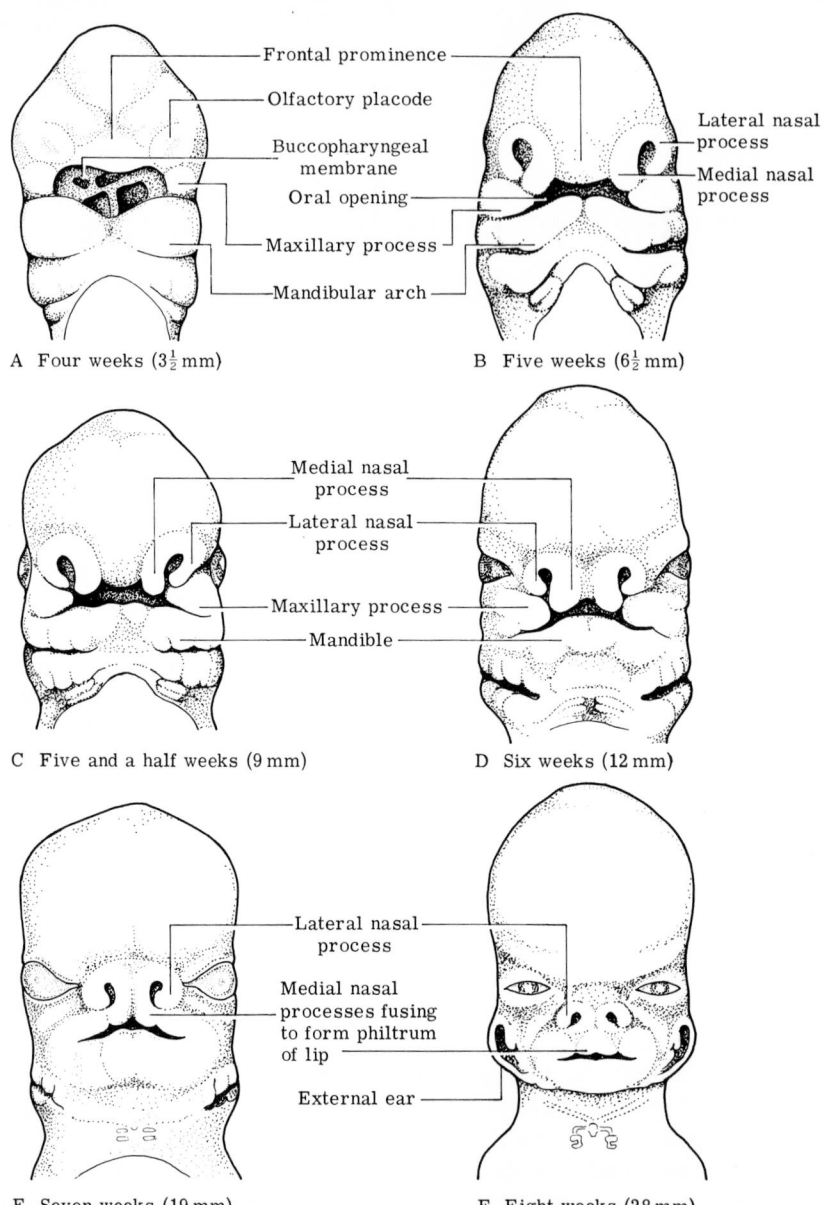

Fig. 3.1 The classical description of the development of the face. (Redrawn after Patten 1968: Human embryology, 3rd edn. Used by permission of McGraw-Hill Book Company)

high in the roof of the nose. During the 5th and 6th weeks horseshoe-shaped elevations develop around these and grow rapidly so that the placodes become recessed at the bottom of olfactory pits. The medial and lateral halves of these elevations are known respectively as *medial* and *lateral nasal processes* (Fig. 3.1b and c). The medial nasal processes grow more rapidly than the lateral and approach one another in the mid-line. They eventually give rise to the central part of the upper lip, alveolus and teeth and the small area of anterior palate lying in front of the incisive foramen. The lateral nasal processes develop into the alae of the nose and the opening of the nasal pits into the nostrils. Meanwhile the lower or caudal margin of the oral pit is becoming thickened and projects forward to form the *mandibular arch* from which the lower lip and jaw develop (Fig. 3.1c). The mandibular arch is the first of the *branchial arches* and arises as paired swellings on each side of the mid-line which, as they develop, coalesce to form the continuous arch.

THE CLASSICAL THEORY OF THE DEVELOPMENT OF UPPER LIP AND JAW

There is controversy regarding the further development of the upper lip and jaw. The classical theory of His (1874), which is still subscribed to by some eminent authorities such as Patten (1971), describes the development of *maxillary processes* which grow forwards towards the mid-line from the superolateral margins of the oral pit. They grow beneath the lateral nasal processes and abut against the medial nasal processes (Fig. 3.1d). These processes are free finger-like projections and, when they meet, the epithelial coverings fuse to form an epithelial plate. This subsequently breaks down to allow the mesoderm to become continuous and to complete the formation of the upper lip. This fusion takes place towards the end of the 6th week and the beginning of the 7th (Fig. 3.1e and f), and if it fails in any way a complete or incomplete cleft of lip, alveolus and anterior palate may occur.

THE THEORY OF MESODERMAL REINFORCEMENT OF EPITHELIAL MEMBRANES

The classical theory of facial development outlined above, particularly the concept of free finger-like processes advancing across a gap and fusing with each other, has been subjected to much criticism. Victor Veau, a pioneer of modern surgical correction of cleft lip and palate, became dissatisfied with the way the classical theory explained the clinical deformity. He was the first (Veau & Politzer 1936) to publicize an alternative theory based on the study of 145 normal embryos, but he gave the credit for the concept to Fleischmann, Professor of Zoology at Erlangen. This theory has since been developed by Stark (1954, 1977; Stark & Ehrmann 1958).

In essence, the theory suggests that the upper lip and jaw are formed by the penetration of mesoderm between the layers of a pre-existing epithelial membrane formed by the invagination of the oral pit (Fig. 3.2). The mesoderm (or, more properly, mesenchyme) may originate from neuroectoderm at the neural crest and migrate from the back of the head by three routes. The first route is over the top of the developing head and down into the central part of the face—that is, the region of the frontal prominence. The other routes are around the sides of the head into the areas of the developing cheeks (Fig. 3.3). As the mesoderm penetrates between the layers of epithelium it gives rise to the surface swellings already described as the medial and lateral nasal processes and the

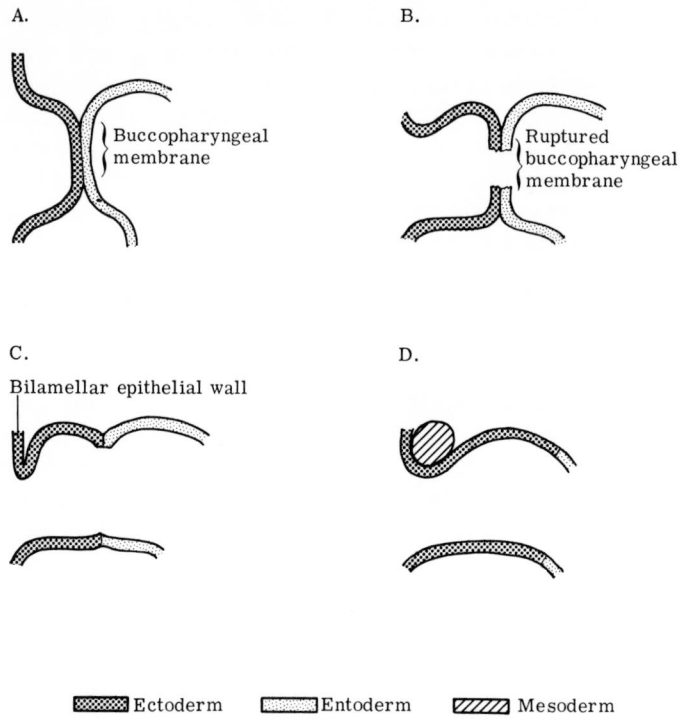

Fig. 3.2 Diagrammatic representation of the development of the upper lip by mesodermal penetration of an epithelial membrane. Sagittal section. (a) Oral pit with buccopharyngeal membrane. (b) Invagination and breakdown of oral pit, with (c) production of bilamellar epithelial wall. (d) Penetration of wall by mesoderm to produce upper lip

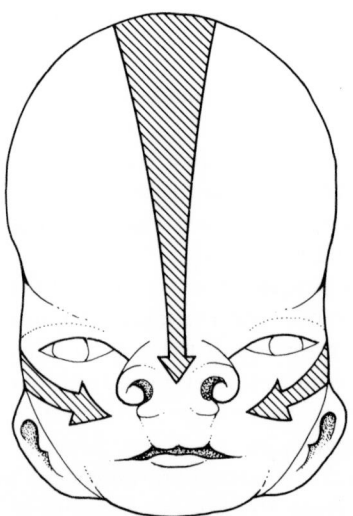

Fig. 3.3 The migration of mesoderm into the face. (After Stark 1977, in: Converse (ed) Reconstructive plastic surgery 2nd edn. Used by permission of W B Saunders Co)

maxillary processes. A congenital cleft of the lip, alveolus or anterior palate is due to failure of penetration of mesoderm and the subsequent breakdown of the unsupported epithelial membrane, and not to the failure of fusion of separate processes. However, even if these processes exist only as ridges and the apparent fissures between them are only furrows, their names are generally accepted and remain useful in description.

FURTHER DEVELOPMENT OF THE LIP

The first mesoderm to arrive in the region of the upper lip comes from above into the area which will lie just anterior to the *incisive foramen* (i.e. the anterior or *primary palate*). It flows thence into the nostril floor and upper lip from above downwards to the vermilion. The mesoderm migrating from each side then piles up on each side of the mid-line of the lip to produce the philtral ridges.

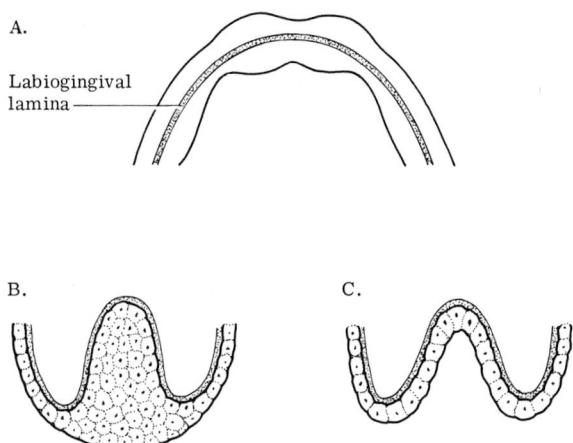

Fig. 3.4 The separation of lip from alveolus. (a) The situation of the labiogingival lamina. (b) The labiogingival lamina in cross-section. (c) The epithelial cells farthest from the basement membrane breakdown, so forming the labiogingival sulcus. (Adapted from Stark 1977, in: Converse (ed) Reconstructive plastic surgery, 2nd edn. Used by permission of W B Saunders Co)

Along the free margin of the primitive lip a ridge of epithelial cells develops and penetrates into the mesoderm. It is called the *labiogingival lamina* (Fig. 3.4). The cells in the centre of this ridge break down, creating a cleft which becomes the buccal sulcus, separating the lip anteriorly from the gum or alveolus which arises from the posterior part. The teeth are formed from another similar epithelial ridge (*the dental lamina*) which develops along the margin of the gum. That part of the lip formed from the nasomedial process is called the *prolabium* and the alveolus arising from this area is the *premaxilla*.

If mesodermal migration is inadequate or delayed the degree of clefting will depend on the extent of the deficiency. The mildest cleft will occur at the last place at which mesoderm arrives—the vermilion—and if there is no mesodermal penetration at all, or if its arrival is greatly delayed, the cleft will involve lip, alveolus and palate as far back as the incisive foramen. If the cleft in the lip is complete, then no mesoderm can pass across from the lateral elements and no philtral ridge can be formed—a deficiency very noticeable in the complete bilateral cleft. Other features of the bilateral cleft lip—the absence of muscle in the prolabium and the absence of a buccal sulcus between prolabium and premaxilla—suggest that muscle and labiogingival lamina also are derived from the lateral mesoderm. The reason for the absence of columella is still an unresolved problem, but the prolabium, which was at one time thought to be the misplaced columella, is now generally accepted as being in its proper place in the centre of the lip.

DEVELOPMENT OF THE NOSE

During the early part of the 6th week the two nasal pits are moving closer together, and as the mesoderm flows around them they become deeper. Anteriorly their openings become the nostrils. At their deep end they are separated from the oral cavity by an epithelial membrane, the *oronasal membrane*, which ruptures by the end of the 6th week to form the primitive posterior nares. The block of tissue lying in front of these openings and separating the nose and mouth is the primary palate, to which we have already referred.

As the two medial nasal processes or ridges move closer together, they merge and the furrow between them becomes filled in. From the part of this mass of mesoderm above the developing lip arise the columella (between the nostrils), the nasal bridge and the nasal septum. The lateral nasal processes give rise to the alae of the nose.

DEVELOPMENT OF THE SECONDARY PALATE

To summarize, by the beginning of the 7th week the primitive lip is formed, although the buccal sulcus has yet to appear. The primary palate lies immediately behind the, as yet fused, premaxilla and prolabium and separates the anterior part of the nasal cavities from the mouth. Behind the primary palate there is a common cavity for both nose and mouth. However, from the inner aspect of the maxillary processes on each side are already developing a pair of shelves which are destined to fuse in the mid-line to complete the palate. Because this part of the palate forms after the anterior part it is known as the *secondary palate* (Fig. 3.5).

At first the tongue, which is also developing at this time, lies between the two palatal shelves which hang vertically down on either side (Fig. 3.6a), but as the neck begins to extend during the 8th week the tongue moves downwards and the palatal shelves spring upwards above it to the horizontal position where they can grow towards each other (Fig. 3.6b). There is no argument about the secondary palate being formed from freely projecting processes or shelves, but the mechanism of descent of the tongue and the horizontal movement of the shelves is still a matter of speculation.

By the end of the 8th week the shelves have made contact with each other and with the primary palate anteriorly and the free margins fuse together. The incisive foramen comes to lie at the junction of the primary and secondary palate in the mid-line. Fusion proceeds from front to back, but is not completed until the 11th week. It seems to occur slightly earlier in males than females, which may account for the greater frequency of clefts of the secondary palate in the female. At the same time as the secondary palate is fusing, the nasal septum is growing downwards and fuses with it in the mid-line, completing the separation of the two nasal cavities.

Recent research suggests that the mechanism of fusion is similar to that described in the classical theory of fusion of the facial processes. The edges of

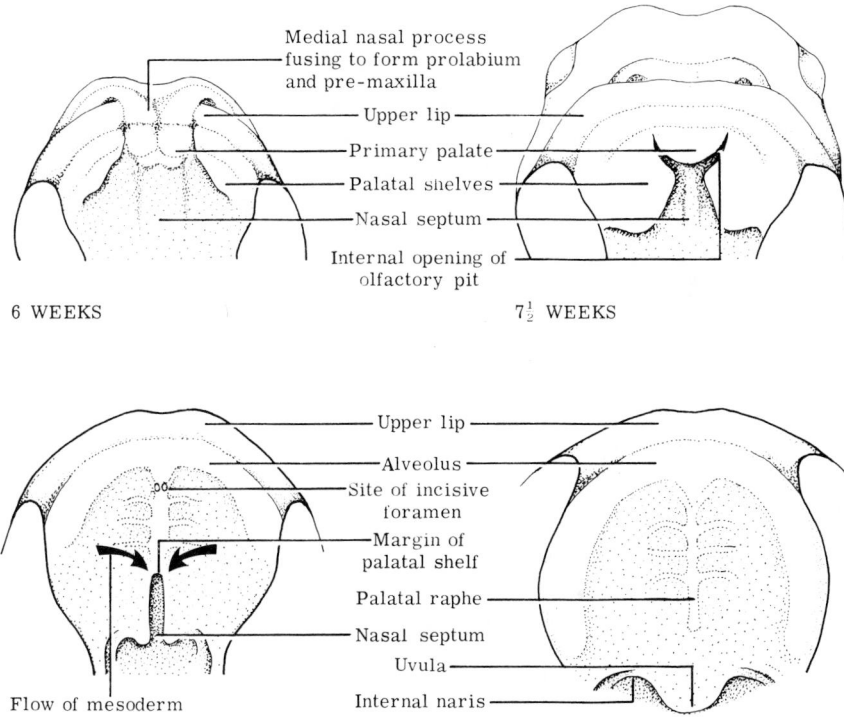

Medial nasal process fusing to form prolabium and pre-maxilla

Upper lip

Primary palate

Palatal shelves

Nasal septum

Internal opening of olfactory pit

6 WEEKS

$7\frac{1}{2}$ WEEKS

Upper lip

Alveolus

Site of incisive foramen

Margin of palatal shelf

Palatal raphe

Nasal septum

Uvula

Flow of mesoderm

Internal naris

$8\frac{1}{2}$ WEEKS

11 WEEKS

Fig. 3.5 Development of the palate. (Adapted from Patten 1968: Human embryology, 3rd edn. Used with permission of McGraw-Hill Book Company)

the advancing palatal shelves become sticky either shortly before they are due to fuse or when they come into contact with the opposite shelf, and electron microscopic studies show histological changes in the epithelial cells suggesting that they may be 'programmed' to fuse. The epithelial layers adhere to one another and persist as a distinct lamina for some time, and then they break up and disappear. However, nests of epithelial cells can commonly be found at the site of fusion even in adult life. There is some evidence that the soft palate may not fuse, but develop by the inflow of mesoderm from the hard palate and merging of the two halves, as in the face.

In the weeks after fusion has taken place, the mesoderm in the anterior half of the secondary palate develops centres of ossification and gives rise to the hard

palate, while posteriorly it differentiates into the muscles of the soft palate, forming a sling across the mid-line. This mesoderm has been shown to migrate from
the pharyngeal wall and the palatal and pharyngeal muscles therefore have very
close embryological links.

A cleft of the secondary palate can occur if for any reason fusion does not
take place. This may be due to failure of descent of the tongue, keeping the
two palatal shelves apart. It may be due to the failure of mesodermal migration
into the palatal shelves so that they fail to reach the mid-line, resulting in a wide

7 WEEKS

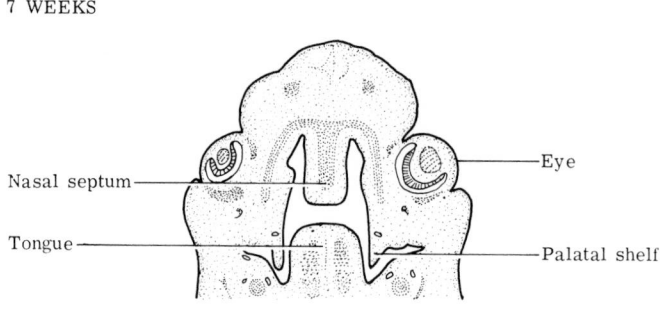

8½ WEEKS

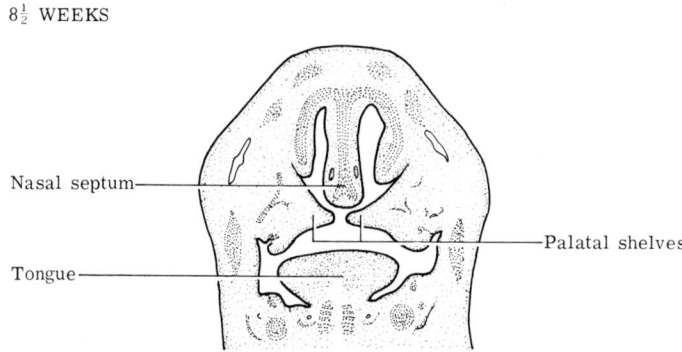

Fig. 3.6 Downward movement of the tongue and horizontal movement of palatal shelves during
the 8th week. (Adapted from Patten 1968: Human embryology, 3rd edn. Used with permission
of McGraw-Hill Book Company)

cleft with a deficiency of tissue, or it may be due to a delay in migration; so
that the developing face is too wide for closure to occur by the time the mesoderm has arrived in place. This will produce a cleft with much less lack of tissue.
Alternatively, the cleft may be the result of a disturbance in the changes which
bring about fusion in the free edges of the shelves. Each cause will produce
a cleft of different configuration. If the causative factor occurs early it will
result in a complete cleft of the secondary palate, and if late in an
incomplete cleft of the soft palate only or in a *submucous cleft*. The latter
presents an interesting problem for the embryologist, but Poswillo (1974) has
induced a similar deformity in the mouse and has shown in this animal that,

while the palatal shelves fuse normally, the ingrowth of mesoderm is defective, and it fails to meet in the mid-line. Subsequent ossification of the hard palate is incomplete and the developing muscles of the soft palate do not meet across the mid-line but form bundles running forwards to the back of the hard palate with a double layer of epithelium between them. Why this unsupported epithelial lamina should behave in a different way from the others described by Stark, and fail to break down, remains, at the moment, another of the many unsolved mysteries of orofacial development.

DISTORTIONS DUE TO DISTURBED INTRAUTERINE GROWTH

Although the cleft deformity is established in the first trimester of pregnancy, by the time the baby is born a number of other distortions have been superimposed on the primary deformity. Latham (1969, 1973) has made detailed studies of the nature of the skeletal deformities. They are partly due to the disturbance of the normal attachments between structures which are actively growing. For example, the nasal septum appears to be a very important growth centre in embryonic and early fetal life. It is attached to the premaxilla by a well-defined ligament and its forward growth draws the premaxilla forward. Normally the forward movement of the premaxilla is restrained by its attachment to the maxillary processes, but when there is a cleft between premaxilla and maxillary process this constraint is lost. As a result, the premaxilla in a bilateral cleft lies too far forward, suspended from the tip of the septum, and the maxillary segments, deprived of the forward pull of the premaxilla, lie too far back. In the unilateral cleft the attachments on the non-cleft side restrain forward growth, so that the anterior septum and premaxilla deviate towards the normal side. This in turn leads to the septum bulging into the cleft side of the nose more posteriorly. The maxillary process on the cleft side, lacking support from the premaxilla, may collapse in behind it.

Soft tissues can also play a part in producing secondary deformities *in utero*. The interruption of the normal rings of muscle in the cleft lip and soft palate can allow the two halves of a completely cleft maxilla to drift apart. The action of the tongue pushing up between the cleft palatal shelves can contribute to this deformity, and in addition may push the shelves into a more vertical position than normal.

An intriguing aspect of the cleft lip and palate deformity is the great variation in the extent and configuration of the deformity at birth. For all cases with a given type of cleft (e.g. a complete unilateral cleft), the intrauterine growth of normal structures around the cleft should exert the same influence on the eventual distortion, as the altered attachments and constraints are the same in all cases. The influence of disturbed muscular action may vary to some extent, but the most important factor is the difference between clefts established at the time they first appear. A relationship can be assumed between the extent of the primary mesodermal deficiency and the disturbance of growth potential in the tissues adjacent to the cleft. Unfortunately at the present time this disturbance cannot be predicted, and this enormously complicates studies of postnatal development. These problems are discussed in greater detail in Chapter 7.

REFERENCES

His W 1874 Unsere Koerperform und des Physiologische Problem ihrer Entstehung, p 87 Vogel, Leipzig

Latham R A 1969 The pathogenesis of the skeletal deformity associated with unilateral cleft lip and palate. Cleft Palate Journal 6: 404

Latham R A 1973 Development and structure of the premaxillary deformity in bilateral cleft lip and palate. British Journal of Plastic Surgery 26: 51

Millard D R 1976 Cleft craft. Little Brown, Boston, vol 1

Patten B M 1971 Embryology of the palate and the maxillofacial region. In: Grabb W C, Rosenstein S W Bzoch K R (eds) Cleft lip and palate. Little Brown, Boston, p 21

Poswillo D 1974 The pathogenesis of submucous cleft lip and palate. Scandinavian Journal of Plastic and Reconstructive Surgery 8 (1–2): 34–41

Stark R B 1954 The pathogenesis of harelip and cleft palate. Plastic and Reconstructive Surgery 13: 20

Stark R B 1977 Embryology of cleft lip and palate. In Converse J M (ed) Reconstructive plastic surgery. Saunders, Philadelphia, p 1941

Stark R B, Ehrmann N A 1958 The development of the centre of the face with particular reference to surgical correction of bilateral cleft lip. Plastic and Reconstructive Surgery 21: 177.

Veau V, Politzer J 1936 Embryologie du bec-de-lievre. Annales d'Anatomie Pathologique 13: 275

4

Classification of cleft palate

In this chapter we can give only a brief review of the history of classification, and outline those methods which are widely used at the present time or those which seem to have particular advantages.

DEVELOPMENT OF CLASSIFICATION

In America, Davis & Ritchie presented their classification in 1922, and some people may still use it (Table 4.1). Certainly the classification introduced by Veau in 1931 (Table 4.2) is still widely used in Europe: referral to a 'Veau 1 cleft' clearly identifies to many people a cleft restricted to the soft palate. Unfortunately, these systems were not sufficiently comprehensive and failed to include some common variants of the deformity. Veau's classification, for example, ignored clefts of the lip or of the lip and alveolus alone.

Table 4.1 Davis & Ritchie's classification of clefts (1922)

Group 1	Prealveolar cleft
	Lip clefts only, with subdivisions for unilateral, median and bilateral
Group 2	Postalveolar cleft
	Degrees of involvement of the soft and hard palates could be specified, up to the alveolar ridge; submucous clefts could also be included
Group 3	Alveolar clefts
	Complete clefts of the palate, alveolar ridge and lip, with subdivisions for unilateral, median and bilateral

Table 4.2 Veau's classification of clefts (1931)

Group I	Cleft of the soft palate only
Group II	Cleft of the hard and soft palate to the incisive foramen
Group III	Complete unilateral cleft of the soft and hard palate, and the lip and alveolar ridge on one side
Group IV	Complete bilateral cleft of the soft and hard palate, and the lip and alveolar ridge on both sides

In Britain, Wardill, Kilner and others distinguished, as had Davis and Ritchie, between prealveolar clefts, alveolar clefts associated with cleft of lip and/or palate, and postalveolar clefts. These systems placed too much emphasis on the alveolar ridge. Embryologically it is the incisive foramen, and not the alveolus, which marks the boundary between two differently derived structures, i.e. those we have called the primary and secondary palates (see Chapter 3), and this is reflected in the types of cleft that are found clinically.

CLASSIFICATIONS BASED ON EMBRYOLOGY

In 1942 Fogh-Andersen published the results of his study of the incidence of cleft lip and palate in Denmark (see Chapter 5). He classified clefts into (a) harelip (including alveolus and as far back as the incisive foramen), (b) harelip and cleft palate and (c) isolated clefts of the palate as far forward as the incisive foramen. He showed that types (a) and (b) were quite distinct in their aetiology from type (c), and this classification, with its sound foundation on embryological and aetiological differences, is the basis of the variety of systems of nomenclature which are in use today.

Table 4.3 Kernahan & Stark's classification of clefts (1958)

Clefts of primary palate only
  Unilateral (right or left)
    Complete
    Incomplete
  Median
    Complete (premaxilla absent)
    Incomplete (premaxilla rudimentary)
  Bilateral
    Complete
    Incomplete

Clefts of secondary palate only
  Complete
  Incomplete
  Submucous

Clefts of primary and secondary palates
  Unilateral (right or left)
    Complete
    Incomplete
  Median
    Complete
    Incomplete
  Bilateral
    Complete
    Incomplete

The names introduced by Kernahan and Stark (1958) (Table 4.3) are probably those most commonly used at the present time, and are those which we use in this book. They called the lip, alveolar ridge and triangle of palate anterior to the incisive foramen the *primary palate* and the rest of the palate (derived from the palatal shelves of the embryo) the *secondary palate*. Clefts of the primary palate may be complete or incomplete, and they may be unilateral, bilateral or median. Clefts of the secondary palate may be complete, incomplete or submucous.

Unfortunately this simple and straightforward system has two significant disadvantages. The first is the possible confusion caused by calling the lip part of the primary palate. To call a cleft of the lip alone an incomplete cleft of the primary palate is obviously not ideal, but it is widely accepted. In an attempt to resolve this confusion, the American Cleft Palate Association (Harkins et al 1960) recommended 'prepalate' and 'palate' for primary and secondary palates as an alternative, and the International Confederation for Plastic and Reconstructive Surgery (1968) suggested 'anterior palate' for primary palate. This seems to have no advantage. Spina (1974) referred to pre-incisive foramen clefts, trans-incisive foramen clefts and post-incisive foramen clefts, terms which are precise but rather ponderous.

Table 4.4 American Cleft Palate Association's classification (1962)

Clefts of prepalate		
Cleft lip	—Unilateral	—right, left
		—extent in thirds ($\frac{1}{3}$, $\frac{2}{3}$, $\frac{3}{3}$)
	—Bilateral	—right, left
		—extent in thirds
	—Median	—extent in thirds
	—Prolabium	—small, medium, large
	—Congenital scar	—right, left, median
		—extent in thirds
Cleft of alveolar process	—Unilateral	—right, left
		—extent in thirds
	—Bilateral	—right, left
		—extent in thirds
	—Median	—extent in thirds
		—submucous right, left, median
Cleft of prepalate	—Any combination of foregoing types	
	—Prepalate protrusion	
	—Prepalate rotation	
	—Prepalate arrest (median cleft)	
Clefts of palate		
Cleft soft palate	—Extent	—posteroanterior in thirds
		—width (maximum in mm)
	—Palatal shortness	—none, slight, moderate, marked
	—Submucous cleft	—extent in thirds
Cleft hard palate	—Extent	—posteroanterior in thirds
		—width (maximum in mm)
	—Vomer attachment	—right, left, absent
	—Submucous cleft	—extent in thirds
Cleft of soft and hard palate		
Clefts of prepalate and palate	—Any combination of clefts described under clefts of prepalate and clefts of palate.	

The other disadvantage of Kernahan and Stark's classification is that, in its simplicity, it makes recording of fine detail difficult and cumbersome. For example, it has no subdivision between soft and hard palate, nor of lip and alveolus, and it does not offer an easy way of recording the degree of displacement of parts or of tissue deficiency. It was for this reason that the American Cleft Palate Association introduced their much more complex classification (Table 4.4). Berlin (1971) subjected such attempts to produce a comprehensive system to detailed and constructive criticism. He included McCabe's immensely detailed computer coding manual, which must have been only one of many efforts to record and store the information on computer. These systems are all daunting in their complexity.

GRAPHIC METHODS OF RECORDING CLEFTS

In an attempt to simplify recording of data, Pfeifer (1964) proposed a symbolic method which was attractive in its simplicity (Fig. 4.1a). Kernahan (1971) proposed a striped Y classification (Fig. 4.1b), and in search for a way to identify more detail this has since been modified by Elsahy and again by Millard (1976) (Fig. 4.1c). Millard used his modification throughout his book, and although

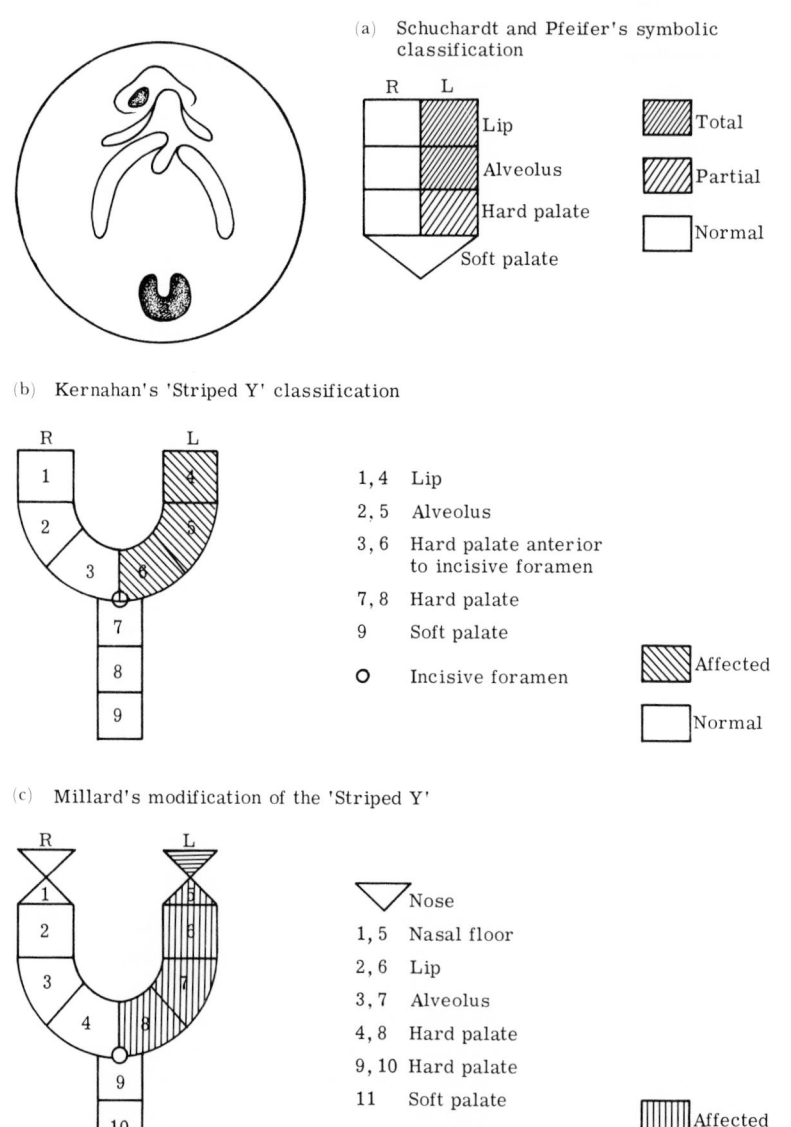

Fig. 4.1 Symbolic methods of classifying cleft lip and palate. All can be reproduced by a rubber stamp. Complete left-sided cleft of primary palate used as an example

it has lost some of the simplicity of Kernahan's original, it remains a fairly easily assimilated graphic representation of the cleft. It is concise and infinitely less intimidating than the lengthy tables needed to record the same details in words, and the numbering would allow simple storage and retrieval of information. (Elsahy's modification, quoted by Millard (1976), is not shown here to avoid confusion. It is much more complex and therefore more comprehensive in what it can record, and those who feel a need to use such a detailed method are referred to Millard's book.)

DISCUSSION

In deciding on a way of describing clefts it is important to distinguish between two quite separate requirements: there is the need in clinical practice to describe a particular cleft concisely and clearly to one's colleagues, and there is the different need to record the precise details of the deformity to allow later comparison of the progress of different groups of patients either within one unit or between different centres.

To fulfil the first requirement the Kernahan and Stark classification is excellent, although it may often be best to use terminology which everyone understands; for example, 'an incomplete left-sided cleft of the lip with notching of the alveolus' or 'a cleft of the soft palate and posterior third of the hard palate'.

However, this classification is not adequate for recording or reporting a series of cases, since for these purposes there is the need to compare one group or series with another. In some circumstances a very simple grouping is adequate. For example, in references to the two genetically distinct groups of cleft patient we often find the abbreviations $CL + P$ or $CL(P)$ and CP. In context the meaning is clear in spite of the brevity. It is when more detail is required that the problems arise, and at the present time each cleft palate centre will have to choose the system which seems best to fulfil its own needs. We must hope that in the near future a satisfactory compromise will achieve general acceptance, even though we recognize that this is not very likely. In the meantime, our choice of classification should be one which can be compared without too much difficulty with others in common use.

REFERENCES

Berlin J 1971 In: Grabb W C, Rosenstein S W Bzoch K R (eds) Cleft lip and palate. Little Brown, Boston, p 68–80

Davis J S, Ritchie H P 1922 Classification of congenital clefts of the lip and palate. Journal of the American Medical Association 79: 1323

Fogh-Anderson P 1942 Inheritance of harelip and cleft palate. Busck, Copenhagen

Harkins C S, Berlin A, Harding R, Longacre J J, Snodgrasse R 1960 Report of the nomenclature committee of the American Cleft Palate Association. Cleft Palate Bulletin 10:11

International Confederation for Plastic and Reconstructive Surgery 1968 Cleft lip and palate nomenclature. Newsletter (March)

Kernahan D A 1971 The striped Y—a symbolic classification for cleft lips and palates. Plastic and Reconstructive Surgery 47: 469

Kernahan D A, Stark R B 1958 A new classification for cleft lip and cleft palate. Plastic and Reconstructive Surgery 22: 435

Millard D R 1976 Cleft craft: The evolution of its surgery. Little Brown, Boston, vol 1, p 49–52

Pfeifer G 1964 In: Schuchardt Treatment of patients with clefts of lip, alveolus and palate. Thieme, Stuttgart, p 225–226

Spina V 1974 A proposed modification for the classification of cleft lip and cleft palate. Cleft Palate Journal 10: 251

Veau V 1931 Division palatine. Masson, Paris

5

Incidence and aetiology

INCIDENCE

Cleft lip and palate belong to the most common of all congenital deformities. They seem to occur among all peoples of the world and were known before the time of Christ. Reports from various countries suggest that the incidence at birth has been rising, from 1 per 1000 in the first third of this century, to between 1.5 and 2 per 1000 during the last few decades. Exact figures from birth certificates are not easy to obtain because of unreliable reporting, especially of isolated cleft palate. It is difficult, therefore, to compare figures from different times in different countries, but due to centralized registration and treatment, in Denmark we have accurate data for the past 35 years, demonstrating a significant increase of incidence during most of the period.

All Danish-born patients with cleft lip and palate are reported to the National Institute for Defects of Speech, and the surgical treatment is completely centralized in Copenhagen. The number of patients operated on rose steadily from 1.3 per 1000 of total live-births in the country during the first five-year period to 1.8 per 1000 in the last five years, corresponding to an increase of the incidence at birth from 1.45 per 1000 to about 2 per 1000 (Fogh-Andersen 1967, 1971). Similar increasing figures of incidence have been reported from other Scandinavian countries: Finland 1.8 per 1000 (1962) (Gylling & Soivio 1962), Iceland 1.94 (1965) (Moller 1965) and quite recently from Norway 2.08 (1978) (Åbyholm 1978). The increasing incidence is difficult to explain; it might be apparent due to better reporting or diagnosing of minor clefts, particularly submucous cleft palate. More likely, however, we are also dealing with a true, slight increase of the incidence at birth, genetically or environmentally determined.

A lower incidence of cleft deformities among Negroes than in the white population has been reported by American writers, which indicates a racial difference (Sesgin & Stark 1961). An observation of interest in this connection regards the relative incidence of cleft palate alone (isolated cleft palate) in different populations (Fogh-Andersen 1961). Morphologically three main types exist: cleft lip, cleft lip with cleft palate, and cleft palate alone. In Denmark as a whole, we have fairly consistently found cleft palate alone (CP) to be 25 per cent and 75 per cent for cleft lip with or without cleft palate (CL(P)) whereas the distribution in the geographically isolated Danish territories of Faroe Islands and Greenland is just the reverse, with a relative incidence of CP about 70 to 80 per cent. This finding might be due to a racial difference, the Eskimo population of Greenland, especially, differing widely from the rest of the Danish population. Most European and American statistics show a relative distribution of CP between 25 and 40 per cent, with a tendency to higher figures in the northern part of Scandinavia, i.e. Finland 48 per cent (1957) and northern Sweden 41 per cent (1972) (Soivio 1957; Beckman & Myrberg 1972).

AETIOLOGY

Most likely, the majority of congenital deformities in humans are due to a combination of exogenous factors and a gene pattern predisposing to malformations, i.e. a 'multifactorial' basis. Today, all agree that heredity is an important factor—probably the most important—in the aetiology of facial clefts.

Heredity

The influence of heredity has been presumed for more than 200 years. A statistical analysis of 703 families (1942) (Fogh-Andersen 1942) showed that cleft lip, CL, and cleft lip with associated cleft palate, CLP, both conditions being more common in males, apparently belong to one genetic group, CL(P), with a positive family history of clefts in about two-fifths of the cases; whereas cleft palate alone, CP, more frequent in females, is genetically independent and in only one-fifth of cases has there been a history of clefts, indicating a presumably greater influence of exogenous factors in this type of cleft. In atypical, rare clefts the heredity factor seems to be very unusual.

In general, evidence that CP is genetically distinct from CL(P) has been confirmed in various countries, based on statistical family analyses and presentation of pedigrees (Fraser 1970). Figure 5.1 shows the code used in some typical pedigrees taken from the original Danish material.

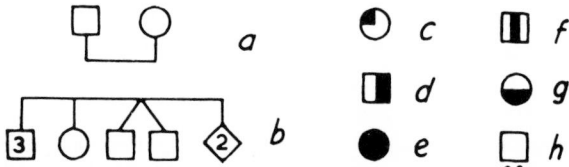

Fig. 5.1 Meaning of symbols used in the pedigrees: a, married couple (male and female without malformations); b, series of sibs (3 males, 1 female, pair of male twins, 2 of unknown sex); c, left cleft lip (CL); d, right cleft lip and palate (CLP); e, double CLP; f, CLP, side unknown; g, cleft palate alone (CP); h, fistula of lower lip

Investigations of twins in Denmark and other countries have been of great value for the study of heredity in facial clefts (Fogh-Andersen 1942). A review of unselected series of twins with clefts has shown concordance in one-third to one-half of the monozygotic twins. All degrees of concordance are found, from symmetrical or identical cleft in both twins, to a severe, combined cleft lip and palate in one and a small, simple cleft lip in the other (Fig. 5.2). However, no single example of one twin partner having CL(P) and the other CP has yet turned up, a fact that strongly supports the theory of the genetic independence of the two cleft groups (Shields, Bixler and Fogh-Andersen 1979).

One apparent exception to this rule of genetic independence of the two cleft groups is in the case of accompanying fistula of the lower lip (Fogh-Andersen 1967), i.e. that cleft lip and cleft palate alone are found in the same family in which the rare congenital lip fistula* (Fig. 5.3) is a typical dominant character

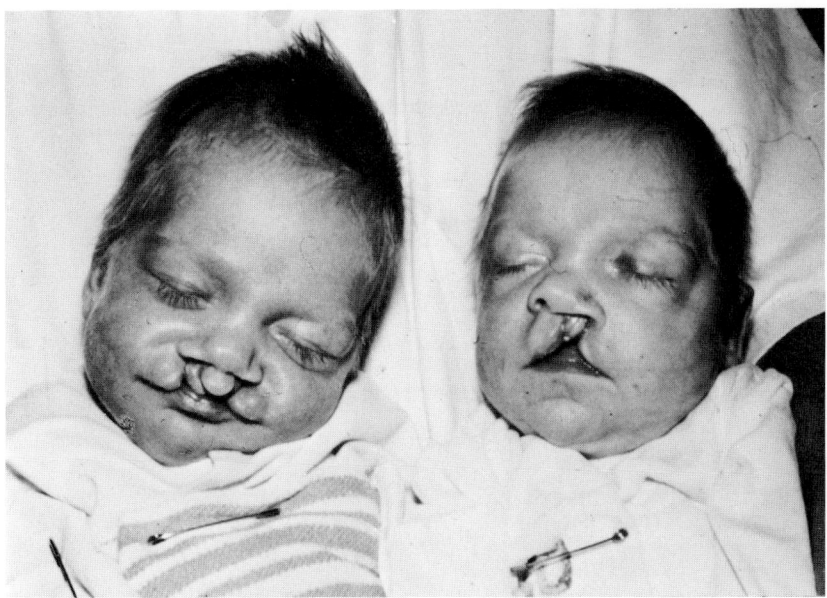

Fig. 5.2 Pair of monozygotic twins, one twin with bilateral the other with unilateral cleft lip and palate, at age of 2 months

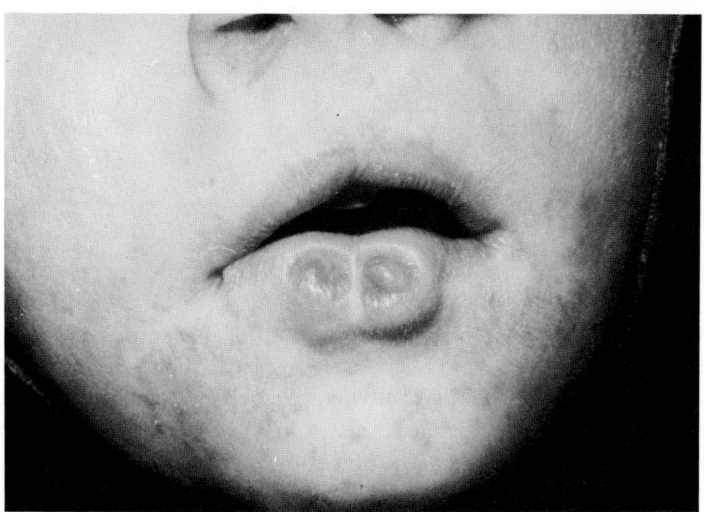

Fig. 5.3 Bilateral fistula of lower lip in a patient previously operated on for bilateral cleft lip and palate

* Sometimes called 'lip pits'.

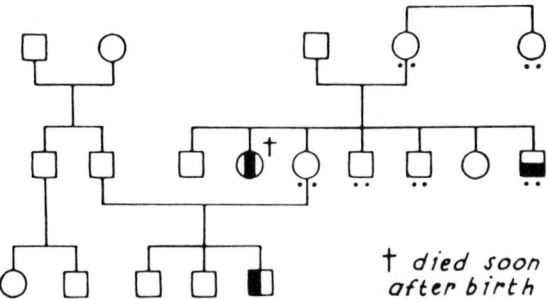

Fig. 5.4 Pedigree of a 'lip fistula family' in which cleft lip with cleft palate and cleft palate alone both occur

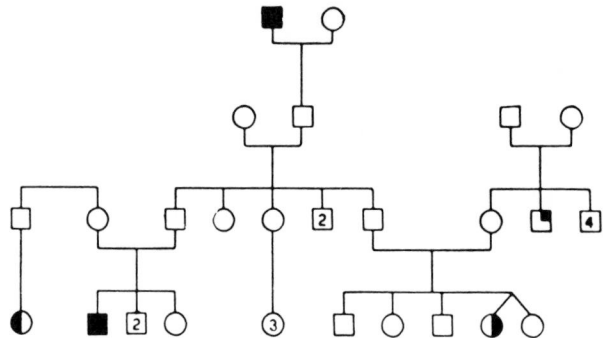

Fig. 5.5 Pedigree of a CL(P) family

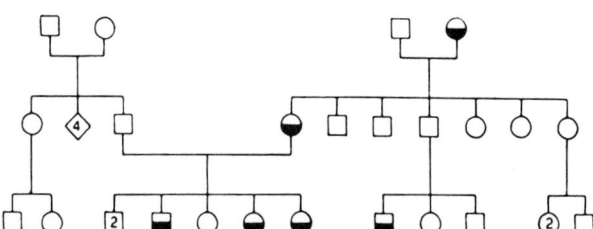

Fig. 5.6 Pedigree of a CP family

(so-called Van der Woude's syndrome) (Fig. 5.4). A few reports indicate the possibility of other exceptions, but further investigations are still needed.

The mode of inheritance is still not clear. For CL(P) the pedigrees may show a recessive character (Fig. 5.5), but apparently dominance occurs: probably the genetic basis of CL(P) is generally 'polygenic'. In the case of CP, the few pedigrees mostly show simple dominance (Fig. 5.6) with more or less reduced penetrance, but a polygenic concept also seems to be possible. Evidence that several genes are probably contributing appear from investigations of the frequency among near relatives of patients in combined series from several sources (Copenhagen, London, Montreal) (Carter 1969; Fraser 1970), showing a higher frequency among sibs when the patient is more severely affected. Frequency figures for offspring of cleft patients in the different groups are still based on series too small to be reliable (Bixler et al 1971), but interesting findings are to be expected in this field in the future.

Irrespective of adequate hypotheses of genetic mechanism, some empiric risk figures are of greatest practical value for counselling. The most important figures, based on combined analyses from various countries (Fogh-Andersen 1971), are the following: when both parents are unaffected and have one child with a cleft, the recurrence risk is about 4–5 per cent, possibly rising to about 9 per cent after two affected; when one parent and one child are affected the risk is about three times as great (13–14 per cent).

Chromosome anomalies are interesting and have, during the last few decades, proved to be responsible for some rare atypical clefts mostly as part of multiple deformities (Gorlin et al 1976), but numerically they are of minor practical importance, and most of the children die very early.

Exogenous factors

Whereas there is no doubt whatever about the role of heredity in the formation of facial clefts, it remains a fact that at least three-fifths of the CL(P) and four-fifths of the CP are so-called 'solitary' cases. A certain proportion of these are presumably also 'hereditary' and sometimes appear to be so later when sibs or children with similar afflictions are born; but not all. We just do not know how many of the cases are due to 'exogenous' factors.

Regarding geographic, seasonal and social distribution, parental age, birth order and other exogenous factors, no convincing results in favour of environmental influences have been reported, except for a slightly increased parental age noted in some of the published materials (Fraser & Calnan 1961; Meskin & Pruzansky 1968).

A few exogenous factors have been proved to be causative in human clefts, e.g. aminopterin (Warkany et al 1959) and thalidomide (Fogh-Andersen 1966); neither drug, however, is of any practical importance today.

With our present knowledge, we still must consider heredity to be the most important aetiological factor in typical cleft deformities—for CL(P) probably in 40–50 per cent, and in CP in 20–25 per cent. In atypical, rare clefts (Fogh-Andersen 1965), however, and in clefts associated with other malformations (Gorlin et al 1971), it is rather unusual to find a history of cleft deformities in several generations except in the families with lower lip fistula and in cases of some other very rare cleft syndromes.

REFERENCES

Åbyholm F E 1978 Cleft lip and palate in Norway I. Registration, incidence and early mortality of infants with CLP. Scandinavian Journal of Plastic and Reconstructive Surgery 12: 29.
Beckman L, Myrberg N 1972 The incidence of cleft lip and palate in northern Sweden. Human Heredity 22: 417
Bixler D, Fogh-Andersen P, Conneally P M 1971 Incidence of cleft lip and palate in the offspring of cleft parents. Clinical Genetics 2: 155
Carter C O 1969 The inheritance of common congenital malformations. In Steinberg, Bearn (eds) Progress in Medical Genetics, vol 4, p 54. Grune and Stratton, New York

Fogh-Andersen P 1942 Inheritance of Harelip and Cleft Palate. Thesis. Busck, Copenhagen

Fogh-Andersen P 1961 Incidence of cleft lip and palate—constant or increasing? Acta chirurgica scandinavica 122: 106

Fogh-Andersen P 1965 Rare clefts of the face. Acta chirurgica scandinavica 129: 275

Fogh-Andersen P 1966 Thalidomide and congenital cleft deformities. Acta chirurgica scandinavica 131: 197

Fogh-Andersen P 1967 Genetic and non-genetic factors in the etiology of facial clefts. Scandinavian Journal of Plastic and Reconstructive Surgery 1: 22

Fogh-Andersen P 1971 Epidemiology and etiology of clefts. In: Bergsma D (ed) Birth defects: original article series, vol 7, no 7, p 50. Williams and Wilkins, Baltimore

Fraser F C 1970 The genetics of cleft lip and cleft palate. American Journal of Human Genetics 22: 336

Fraser G R, Calnan J S 1961 Cleft lip and palate: seasonal incidence, birth weight, birth rank, sex, site, associated malformations and parental age. Archives of Disease in Childhood 36: 420

Gorlin R J, Červenka J, Pruzansky S 1971 Facial clefting and its syndromes. In: Bergsma D (ed) Birth defects: original article series, vol 7, no 7, p 3. Williams and Wilkins, Baltimore

Gorlin R J, Pindborg J J, Cohen M M 1976 Syndromes of the Head and Neck, 2nd edn. McGraw-Hill, New York

Gylling U, Soivio A 1962 Frequency, morphology and operative mortality in cleft lip and palate in Finland. Acta chirurgica scandinavica 123: 1

Meskin L H, Pruzansky S 1968 Epidemiologic relationship of age of parents to type and extent of facial clefts. Acta chirurgica plasticae 10: 249

Moller P 1965 Cleft lip and cleft palate in Iceland. Archives Oral Biology 10: 407

Sesgin M Z, Stark R B 1961 The incidence of congenital defects. Plastic and Reconstructive Surgery 27: 262

Shields E D, Bixler D, Fogh-Andersen P 1979 Facial clefts in Danish twins. Cleft Palate Journal 16: 1

Soivio A 1957 The treatment of harelips and cleft palates in Finland. In: Transactions of the International Society Plastic Surgeons. First Congress, Williams and Wilkins, Baltimore, p 185

Warkany J, Beaudry P H, Bornstein S 1959 Attempted abortion with aminopterin (4-amino-pteryol-glutamic acid). American Journal of Diseases of Children 97: 274

6

Anatomical and physiological considerations

Cleft lip and palate seriously affects the structures and functions of the nose and mouth. In this chapter, relevant features of the normal anatomy and physiology of the region will be reviewed and some anatomical and physiological problems associated with clefts will be pointed out.

NOSE

The function of the external nose is to keep the entrance to the airways open. The supportive tissues are formed by bone in the upper part, and cartilage in the lower part (Fig. 6.1). The nostrils are separated by the *columella* in the mid-line, and the lateral boundaries are the nasal wings (alae nasi) (Fig. 6.3).

The nasal cavities are separated by the septum, in the mid-line. The nasal septum, formed partly by cartilage and partly by bone, often deviates more or less to one side, even in normal subjects. The space of the nasal cavities is to

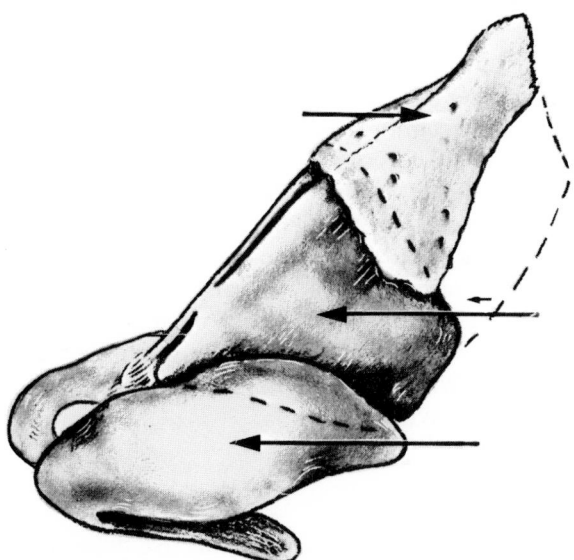

Fig. 6.1 Supportive tissues of the external nose. Arrows indicate nasal bone (top), upper lateral cartilage, and lower lateral cartilage (bottom). (From Hinderer 1971: Fundamentals of anatomy and surgery of the nose. Published by courtesy of the Aesculapius Publishing Company)

a large extent taken up by the nasal conchae, which force the air to spread and pass between narrow walls (Fig. 6.2). The mucous membrane of the nasal cavities is lined by ciliated columnar epithelium, and is rich in blood vessels. Variations in blood flow may cause the mucous membrane to swell or shrink, which allows the nose to be effective in filtering, warming and moistening the inspiratory air.

The nasal cavities also serve as resonators in speech. By opening the velopharyngeal port we give nasal quality to the sound produced by the larynx. Because of the many narrow passages of the nasal cavities which make the sound-absorbing area large, and because of the thick ciliated mucosal lining, sounds produced through the nose are more damped than sounds passing through the mouth.

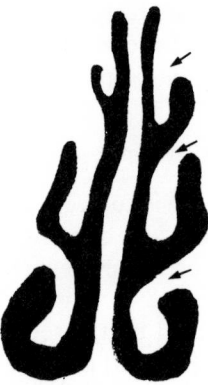

Fig. 6.2 The nasal cavities as seen in a frontal section through the posterior part. Arrows indicate the upper, middle and lower conchae

In patients with cleft lip and palate, asymmetries of the nostrils are almost always present, even after the most successful surgical repair. In some patients, and with some surgical techniques, the nostril on the cleft side is too narrow for a normal passage of air. Gross septal deviations are not uncommon. It has also been demonstrated that, in unilateral clefts, the nasal cavity on the cleft side is narrower than the corresponding nasal cavity on the normal side. Furthermore, in some patients with gross velopharyngeal incompetency, posterior rhinoscopy may reveal a large bluish swelling of the posterior end of the inferior concha, which almost occludes the posterior opening of the nasal cavity, the choana. Thus patients with cleft lip and palate often have a reduced passage of air through the nose, which impairs nasal respiration; it also influences the nasal resonance, causing hyponasality.

UPPER LIP

The body of the lips is formed by muscle, connective tissue and glands. Externally the lips are covered by skin, and internally by mucous membrane with non-keratinized stratified squamous epithelium. The borderline between the skin and the red zone of the lips is slightly elevated, and this is called the mucocu-

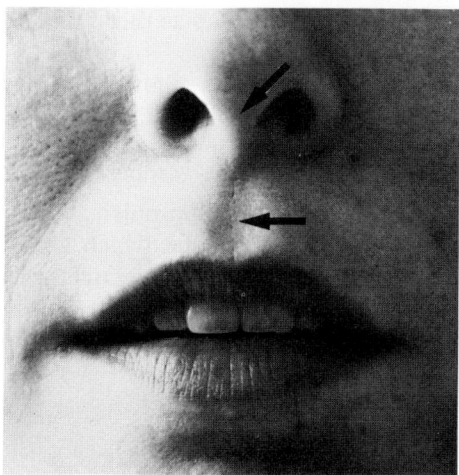

Fig. 6.3 Columella (upper arrow) and philtrum (lower arrow)

taneous ridge. In the middle of the upper lip, this mucocutaneous ridge forms the *Cupid's bow*. In the mid-line of the upper lip, between the columella of the nose and the Cupid's bow, there is a vertical furrow called the *philtrum* (Fig. 6.3).

On the inside, between the lips and the alveolar ridge, there is a deep but narrow space called the vestibulum oris. In the mid-line, there is a band between the lip and the alveolar ridge called the *frenulum*.

The primary *muscle* of the lips is the *orbicularis oris*, which encircles the mouth, directly under the skin (Fig. 6.4). The orbicularis muscle closes the lips, e.g. for bilabial consonants, and is responsible for the rounding of the lips in speech, notably for the 'oo' sound. Other muscles, coming from neighbouring structures, insert into the lips and the angles of the mouth. These muscles are

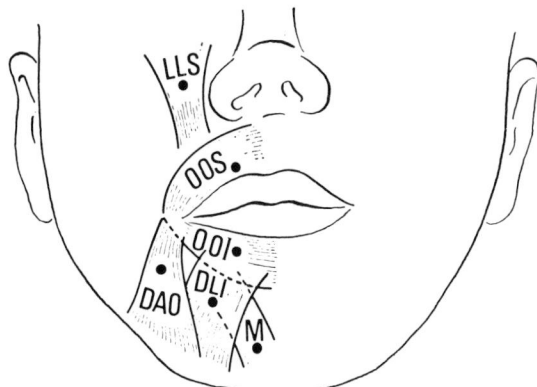

Fig. 6.4 The labial muscles most important in speech; LLS, m. levator labii superioris; OOS and OOI, m. orbicularis oris superior and inferior, respectively; DAO, m. depressor anguli oris; DLI, m. depressor labii inferioris; M, m. mentalis (From Leandersson 1972. Published by courtesy of the author)

responsible for other lip movements, such as the spreading of the lips for the 'ee' sounds (Leanderson et al 1971).

The lips serve very basic functions. It might be claimed that they are the baby's most important means of contact with the environment during the first months of life. And, in fact, all through life the lips are important for sucking, blowing, kissing and speech.

Clefts of the lip only, usually present no problems. The surgical repair successfully restores normal function. In clefts which also involve the maxilla, especially if bilateral, the upper lip may be defective in various ways. It may be too short, it may adhere to the alveolar ridge, or its motility may be impaired. Abnormal lip function may influence the growth and development of the maxilla and the upper teeth.

UPPER JAW

The upper jaw is formed by the alveolar ridge of the maxilla, the gingiva—which is the mucous membrane of the alveolar ridge—and the teeth. The primary functions of the jaws are biting and chewing. The newborn baby makes chewing movements with the toothless jaws during feeding to empty the lactiferous sinuses of the breast. The upper jaw is also important in speech. A number of consonants are produced by the lower lip or the tip or the tongue articulating against the upper teeth and the alveolar ridge.

In clefts involving the jaw, there are always problems with dentition. Teeth are missing or malpositioned. The upper jaw is often too narrow after surgery, and the growth of the mid-face may be impaired, so that various forms of malocclusion are very common. There may remain fistulas after surgery. These structural deviations often give rise to articulatory problems.

HARD PALATE

The bony structure of the hard palate is formed by the maxillary bones in the anterior three-quarters, and by the palatine bones posteriorly (Fig. 6.5). The most anterior part of the maxilla is derived from the premaxilla, also called the incisive bone. In the mid-line, anteriorly, behind the alveolar ridge, is the incisive foramen, through which nerves and blood vessels pass. Posteriorly and laterally, in the palatine bone, is the greater palatine foramen, through which the largest vessels and nerves to the soft tissues of the hard palate pass. Further back, and still laterally, the *pterygoid hamulus* is located (Fig. 6.5), a bony process around which the tendon of the palatal tensor muscle makes a right-angle turn before spreading in the aponeurosis of the soft palate. The most posterior end of the hard palate is extended a little bit in the mid-line, and this process is called the *posterior nasal spine*. Although sometimes difficult to locate precisely on lateral X-ray films, particularly in children, where a dental germ may block the 'view', it is often used as a landmark for cephalometric analyses, e.g. in determining the palatal plane and in measuring the depth of the pharynx. There is a corresponding *anterior nasal spine* (Fig. 6.6), easily detected on lateral X-ray films, in the mid-line below the anterior osseus openings of the nasal cavities.

The bony structures of the hard palate are covered by the mucous membrane of the mouth, which is firmly attached to the periosteum by fibrous tissue. (Periosteum is a dense membrane of connective tissue which covers all bony tissue in the body.) Anteriorly, these soft tissues are raised into a number of small folds which extend from side to side, the transverse palatine folds. In cleft palate surgery, the mucous and fibrous tissue and the periosteum, loosened from the bone, constitute the mucoperiosteal flap, which is pushed backwards and sutured in the mid-line to its counterpart on the other side.

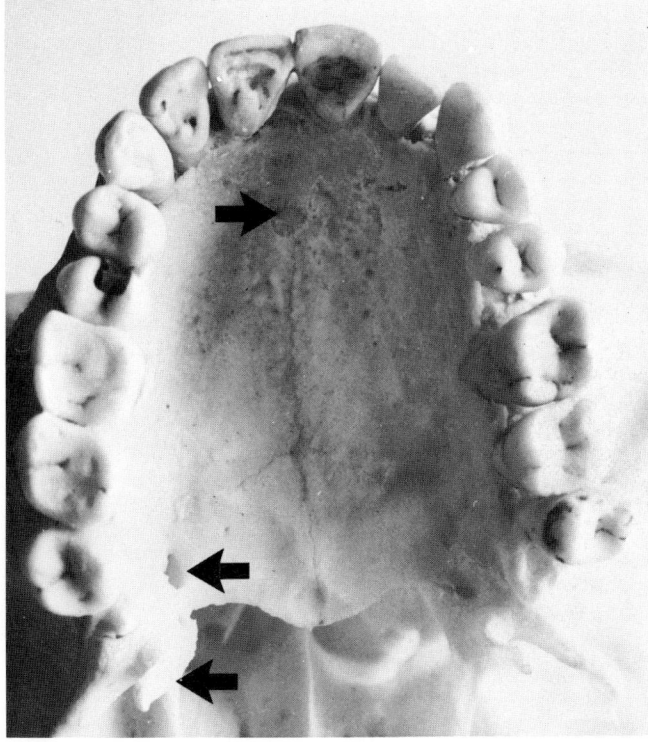

Fig. 6.5 The hard palate, alveolar ridge and teeth from below. The incisive foramen, the greater palatine foramen and the pterygoid hamulus are indicated by arrows

The hard palate separates the oral and nasal cavities. When there is a palatal cleft, this separation can be achieved by a prosthesis, until surgical palatal repair can be carried out. Sometimes there remains a fistula after surgery, an opening between the oral and nasal cavities, through which liquid food may pass into the nasal cavities. A fistula may affect speech by preventing the building up of adequate intra-oral air pressure necessary for articulation of the 'high pressure' consonants, notably the voiceless plosive and fricative sounds.

In the examination of patients with hypernasal speech without overt clefts, palpation of the posterior border of the hard palate is a routine procedure (the examiner extends his forefinger into the mouth of the patient and presses it

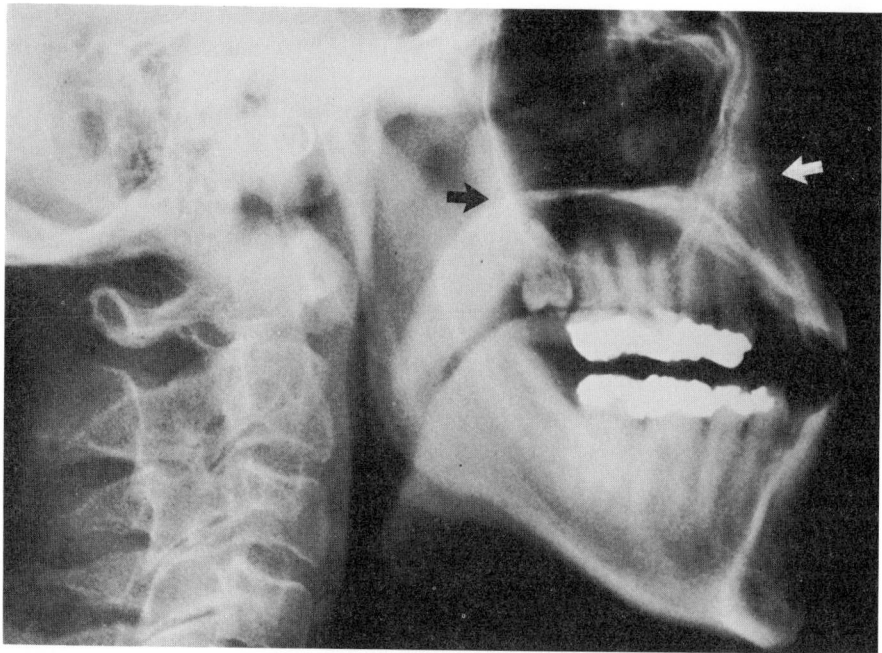

Fig. 6.6(a) From a cephalogram taken during rest. The soft palate is relaxed and allows air to pass through the velopharyngeal port. Arrows indicate the anterior (white) and posterior (black) nasal spines

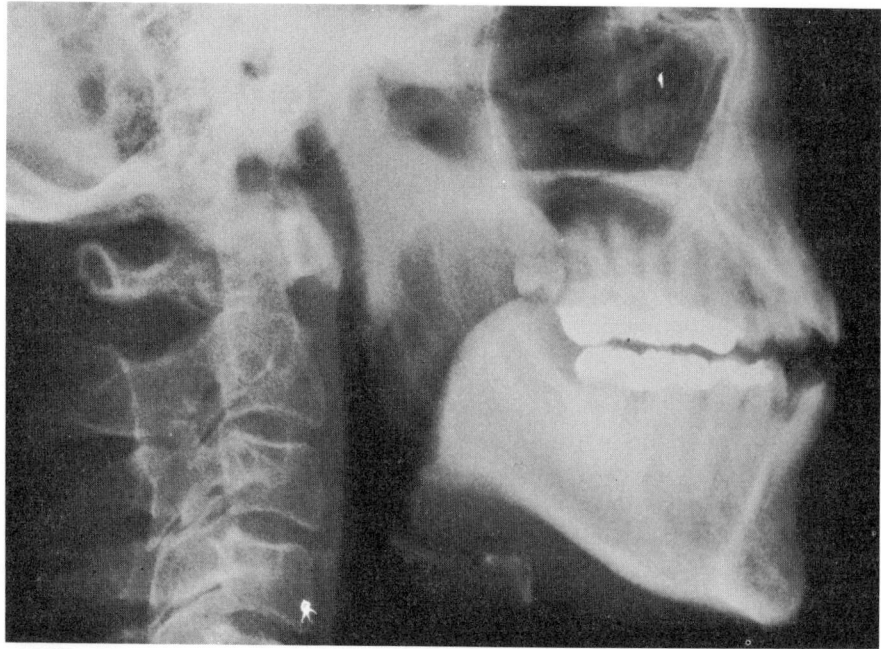

Fig. 6.6(b) From a cephalogram taken during the production of a sustained [s] sound. The soft palate is elevated and there is velopharyngeal closure

against the palate). If a notch is felt in the mid-line posteriorly—a triangular defect of the bone—the patient has a submucous cleft.

SOFT PALATE

The soft palate—or velum—is the posterior continuation of the hard palate. It is attached to the lateral walls of the pharynx and the palatal arches, which run from the soft palate downwards on both sides, in front of and behind the tonsils. The posterior margin is free, and the mid-line is extended to form the uvula (Fig. 6.7). At rest the soft palate hangs down, while during swallowing and speech it is elevated to contact the posterior pharyngeal wall, thus separating the nasal cavities and epipharynx from the middle and lower parts of the pharynx.

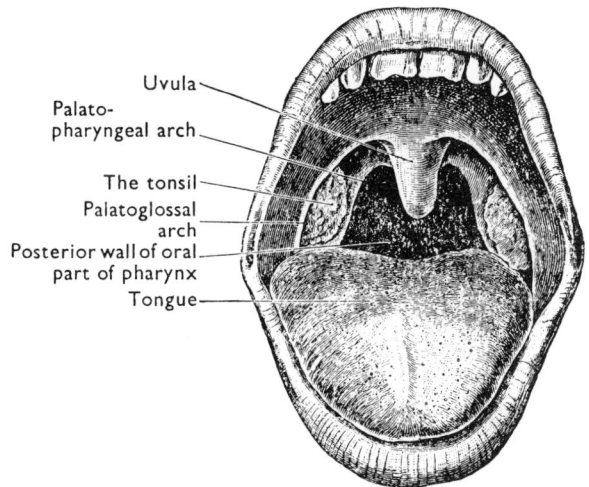

Fig. 6.7 The cavity of the mouth. (From Morley 1970: Cleft palate and speech, 7th edn)

The anterior part of the soft palate is relatively thick, with the posterior part thinning towards the free margin. The anterior two-thirds of the upper surface of the velum is covered by ciliated, cylindrical epithelium similar to that of the nose, the posterior third and the undersurface is covered by stratified squamous epithelium, as in the mouth and pharynx. Immediately beneath the mucous membrane of the upper surface is the muscular layer of the velum, consisting primarily of the levator and palatopharyngeus muscles (and in the mid-line the uvular muscles). These fibres are attached to the *aponeurosis* of the soft palate, a tendinous layer which may be looked upon as the extension of the hard palate and the continuation of the tendons of the tensor muscles. From below, fibres of the palatoglossus muscles insert into the aponeurosis. Between this musculo-tendinous layer and the mucous membrane of the oral surface, there is a com-paratively thick layer of fatty tissue and mucous glands, especially in the anterior part.

THE VELOPHARYNGEAL MUSCLES

Normally, the most anterior part of the soft palate has no muscle fibres, but the rest of the velum is to a large extent formed by muscles, and its movements are produced by these muscles. They are all paired. Their function (Fig. 6.8) can best be studied by means of electromyography and cineradiography (Fritzell 1969; Lubker 1975).

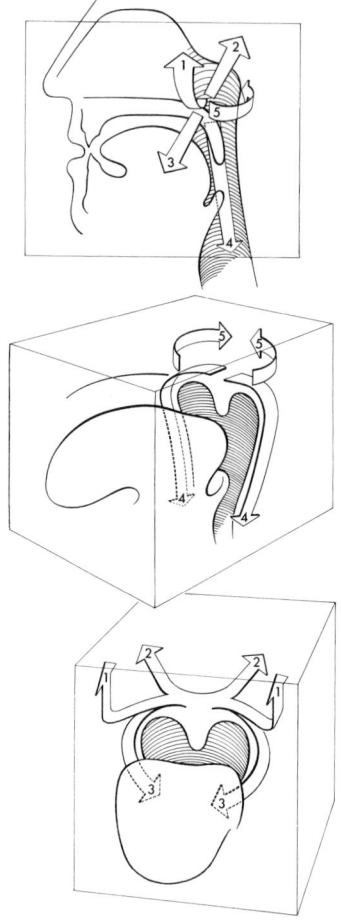

Fig. 6.8 Schematic presentation of the velopharyngeal muscles. The arrows indicate the approximate direction of their action and influence on the soft palate. 1, Tensor. 2, Levator. 3, Palatoglossus. 4, Palatopharyngeus. 5, Superior constrictor. (From Fritzell 1969)

The *levator veli palatini* is a slender muscle of even dimensions along its course from a small area in front of the carotid canal at the base of the skull to the velum. It is similar in shape to the muscles of the arm and leg, and it is capable of a considerable degree of shortening.

In the velum, the levator fibres spread somewhat and meet the levator fibres of the opposite side to form a sling, which pulls the velum upwards and backwards. The motor nerve supply of the levator muscle is from the palatopharyngeal plexus, which is composed of branches from the glossopharyngeus and vagus nerves and the sympathetic trunk. However, there is some evidence that the levator also receives motor fibres from the facial nerve (Ibuki et al 1978). The levator muscles are no doubt the most important ones in accomplishing velopharyngeal closure, as evidenced by electromyography (Fig. 6.9).

The *palatopharyngeus muscle* is the largest velopharyngeal muscle. It has its origin in the back and side walls of the pharynx and in the thyroid cartilage.

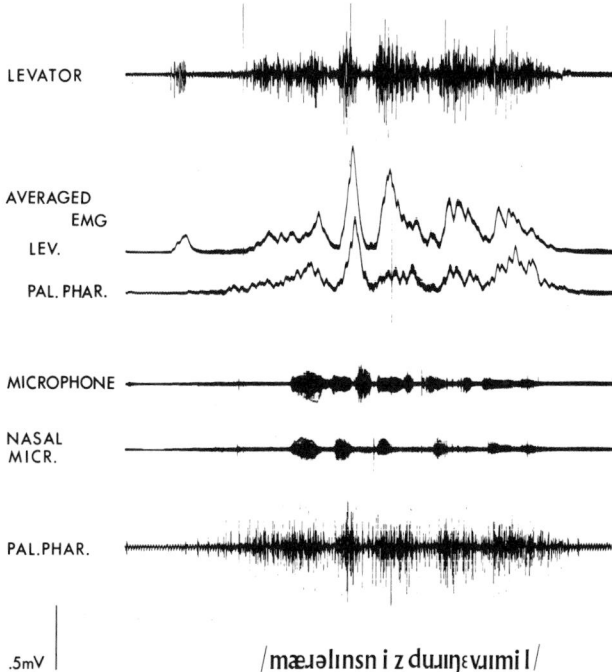

Fig. 6.9 An electromyographic recording of the sentence, 'Marilyn sneezed during every meal.' The levator muscle is active before the onset of phonation, but only to a moderate degree. Alternating periods of high and low activity follows, related to the production of oral and nasal speech sounds, respectively. The highest peak is for the [s] between the two nasal sounds. The palatopharyngeus activity is apparently synchronous with that of the levator; the only major difference seems to be that [iz] shows a peak in the averaged levator EMG, but no corresponding peak in the palatopharyngeus envelope. Duration 3.3 s. (From Fritzell 1969)

The vertically oriented anterior fibres of the muscle form the body of the posterior pillars of the fauces. When the palatopharyngeus muscles contract, the velum is pulled backwards and downwards, the lateral pharyngeal walls are brought medially, and the larynx and pharyngeal walls are elevated. The motor nerve supply is from the pharyngeal plexus. The palatopharyngeus muscles are moderately active in speech, often in synchrony with the levators (Fig. 6.9). When the levator and palatopharyngeus muscles contract simultaneously, the upward pull of the levator is more or less counteracted by the downward pull of the palatopharyngeus, and the resulting movement of the velum is directed backwards (Luschkǎ 1868; Podvineč 1952). The palatopharyngeus is more active in the production of the [ɑ] sound than for any other vowel, probably for the narrowing of the lateral pharyngeal walls typical for [ɑ] (Minifie et al 1970). During swallowing, the palatopharyngeus muscles contract much more vigorously than during any other activity.

The *salpingopharyngeus muscle* is inconsistently found in dissections. When present, it is formed by a single or a few muscle fascicles from the palatopharyngeus which pass in the salpingopharyngeal fold—behind the posterior pillars— and insert into the torus tubarius (Dickson & Dickson 1972). The salpingopharyngeus muscle has probably very little, if any, functional significance.

The *superior pharyngeal constrictor muscles* form the muscular coat of the upper pharynx. Its fibres are oriented largely in a horizontal direction. In most subjects some of these fibres are inserted into the soft palate. The motor nerve supply is from the pharyngeal plexus. When the superior constrictor contracts, the pharynx is narrowed and the velum is pulled backwards. In speech, the constrictor acts in synchrony with the levator, but, like the palatopharyngeus, it contracts much more forcefully during swallowing.

In some clefts patients, a transverse fold, a shelf-like forward bulging, of the posterior pharyngeal wall may be observed during speech. This is called Passavant's ridge. It is, no doubt, produced by contraction of constrictor fibres. It is usually regarded as a compensatory phenomenon, but its effectiveness as such has been questioned (Calnan 1957). When seen, it is most often located somewhat below the normal velopharyngeal closure level and does not meet the elevated velum.

The *tensor veli palatini* is a flat muscle of triangular shape, with its base and origin from the skull along the anterior wall of the auditory (Eustachian) tube, and its apex at the pterygoid hamulus. It descends almost vertically, and its tendon makes a right-angled turn around the hamulus, from where it spreads horizontally or slightly upwards to form the aponeurosis of the soft palate, to which the other palatal muscles are attached. The motor nerve supply is from the mandibular branch of the trigeminal nerve, which also supplies the muscles of mastication. The tensor is of vital importance for the opening of the auditory tube. When contracting, it also makes the soft palate tense and depresses its anterior part (Bloomer 1953). Electromyographic recordings from the tensor muscle have failed to demonstrate any systematic, consistent activity during speech, but as far as we know it is always active during swallowing (Fritzell 1979).

The *palatoglossus muscle* is small. It arises from transverse fibres within the tongue and ascends in the anterior pillar of the fauces to the palate. The motor nerve supply is from the pharyngeal plexus. When the palatoglossus muscles contract, the velum is lowered and drawn forward. In speech, palatoglossus is active in the production of sounds which require elevation of the back of the tongue, and often in the production of nasal sounds, although perhaps not in all subjects. This is a controversial issue. Bell-Berti (1976) could not corroborate the findings of Fritzell (1969) and Lubker & May (1973) of palatoglossus activity for nasal consonant production. A consistent palatoglossus activity has been demonstrated before the end of an utterance, an activity which probably accounts for the very quick opening of the velopharyngeal port observed when a metal mirror is held under the nostrils.

The *uvular muscle* has its origin from the palatal aponeurosis somewhat behind the posterior margin of the hard palate, close to the mid-line. It runs backwards and inserts into the connective tissue and mucosal basement membrane of the uvula (Azzam & Kuehn 1977). The function of the uvular muscle has not received much attention until recently. There is apparently reason to believe, however, that the uvular muscles by contracting produce a bulge on the upper side of the velum, which contributes to velopharyngeal closure (Pigott 1969).

VELOPHARYNGEAL CLOSURE—MECHANISM AND FUNCTION

During swallowing and speech, as well as during other activities like blowing and whistling, the oropharynx must be separated from the nasopharynx. This is done by velopharyngeal closure. Its main component is *elevation of the soft palate* to meet the posterior pharyngeal wall, slightly above the tubercle of the atlas—the uppermost cervical vertebra—as seen on X-ray films in a lateral projection (Fig. 6.6). *Inward movement of the side walls of the pharynx* also contributes to velopharyngeal closure, as demonstrated by various means of observation (see Chapter 13). Forward movement of the posterior pharyngeal wall is rarely observed in normal subjects.

The mechanism of velopharyngeal closure during speech is different from that during swallowing. According to Shprintzen et al (1974, 1975), during speech the side walls of the pharynx adduct, just at the level of the full length of the velum and the hard palate, but do not meet (Fig. 6.10). During swallowing, however, the side walls of the pharynx approximate over a long distance from the level of the palate and downwards (Fig. 6.11). This is in agreement with the electromyographic findings of much more intense constrictor and palatopharyngeus contractions during swallowing than during speech.

Observations of the velopharyngeal port from above or below by means of endoscopes or X-ray procedures have demonstrated variations in the closure mechanism during speech. Pigott (1969) used nasal pharyngoscopy and noted 'medial movement of the salpingopharyngeus in many subjects'. Skolnick et al (1973) used multiview videofluoroscopic techniques in lateral, base and frontal projections and found 'multiple patterns of sphincteric closure of the velopharyngeal portal' (Fig. 6.12). They found it useful to view the closure mechanism as consisting of two components, the velar and the pharyngeal. The contribution of each of these two is variable, particularly in non-normal subjects. Zwitman et al (1974) used an orally inserted endoscope and cineradiography in a submentovertical projection and described four variations in velopharyngeal closure in normals; the subjects differed in the degree of pharyngeal side wall activity.

In speech, the velopharyngeal closure mechanism is one of the articulators, since we use it to make the distinction between oral and nasal sounds. In English, there are three nasal speech sounds, m, n and ng. During their production, the velopharyngeal port is open, and the palate is kept in a somewhat raised position between full elevation and complete relaxation. All other speech sounds are classified as oral, and, in principle, they are produced with a closed velopharyngeal port.

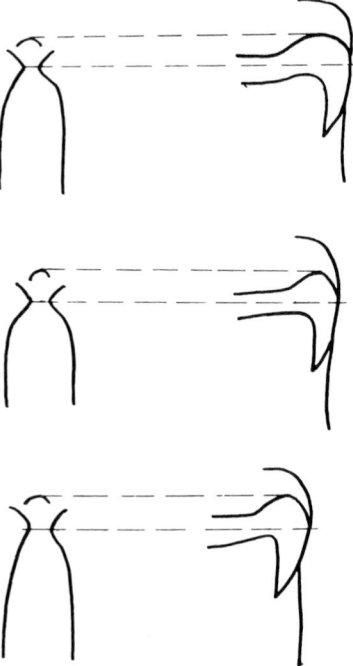

Fig. 6.10 Tracings of velopharyngeal closure from cinefluorographic video-recordings made in frontal and lateral projections simultaneously, during speech (top), whistling and blowing (bottom). It can be seen that the maximum medial excursion of the lateral walls of the pharynx occurs at the level where the velum contacts the posterior pharyngeal wall. (From Shprintzen et al 1975. Published by courtesy of The Cleft Palate Journal)

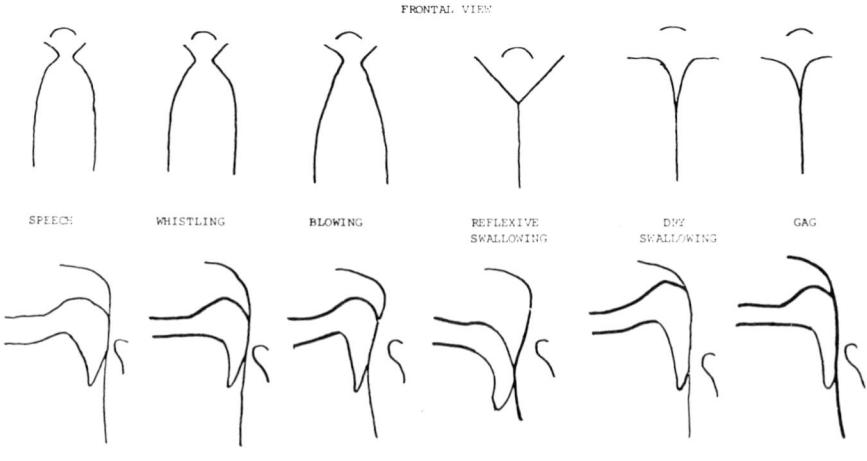

Fig. 6.11 Approximation of the lateral pharyngeal walls and velopharyngeal closure during speech, whistling, blowing, reflexive swallowing, dry swallowing and gagging. Tracings from cinefluorographic video-recordings in frontal and lateral projections. (From Shprintzen et al 1974. Published by courtesy of The Cleft Palate Journal)

The velopharyngeal closure has two important functions for the production of oral speech sounds. In the first place, it is necessary for normal non-nasal vowel quality. If the velopharyngeal port is open, nasal resonance is added, which distorts the quality. High vowels, like [i] and [u], are more distorted than low ones, [ɑ] and [æ]. This is due to the fact that the low vowels are produced with a wide open mouth, and the opening to the epipharynx and nasal cavities is comparatively small. The high vowels, however, are produced with a small opening of the mouth and the tongue raised close to the palate, and in this case the velopharyngeal insufficiency is relatively more important. Secondly, velopharyngeal closure is essential for the build-up of intra-oral air

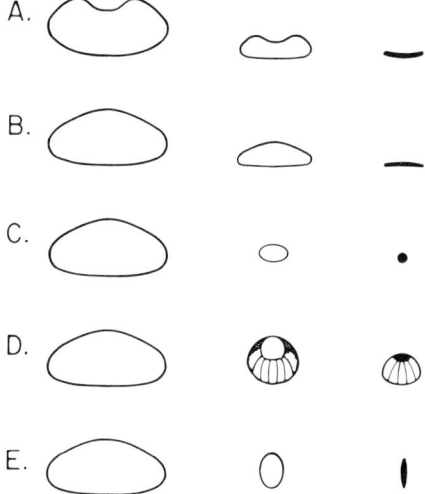

Fig. 6.12 Variations in the velopharyngeal closure mechanism as seen in a cinefluorographic base projection. Left column represents contour of velopharyngeal partial closure. A, Normal subject; note convex projection of uvula portion of velum into velopharyngeal portal at rest. B, Repaired cleft palate subject; note absence of uvula muscular bulge at rest; pattern of closure is coronal, similar to normal subject A. C, Repaired cleft palate with circular closure pattern. D, Repaired cleft palate with circular closure pattern and Passavant's ridge; ridge is represented by stippled and lined area in middle and extreme right columns. E, Repaired cleft palate with sagittal closure pattern. (From Skolnick et al 1973. Published by courtesy of The Cleft Palate Journal)

pressure to a level necessary for the distinct articulation of stop sounds and sibilants. If there is a leak through the velopharyngeal port, adequate pressure cannot be achieved, and the resultant consonant articulation will be weak, or an accompanying nasal snort will be heard.

We perceive the speech sounds as discrete units, but the movements that produce them are usually smooth and continuous, and articulatory events which mark the differences between sounds do not always occur simultaneously. For this reason, neighbouring sounds often influence each other, a phenomenon called co-articulation. Thus the velopharyngeal port may open during the production of sounds preceding a nasal consonant, e.g. before the tongue is raised to occlude the oral cavity. And correspondingly, the velopharyngeal port may remain open for a while during the following sounds, after the tongue has been lowered. This is most likely to occur when the nasal sound is preceded and followed by oral sounds which do not necessarily require high intra-oral air pressure and firm velopharyngeal closure. In this way, many so-called oral speech sounds are often produced with slightly open velopharyngeal port and therefore have a certain nasal quality. We usually do not perceive this, however. It is part of the normal amount of nasal resonance in speech.

Our traditional classification of sounds into oral and nasal ones is derived from observations of sounds produced in isolation, and this, of course, is a simplification. As indicated above, in connected speech adjacent sounds influence each other, and what is true for isolated sounds may not be true for the same sounds in connected speech. This is important to bear in mind during the clinical examination of patients with hypernasal speech. Predictions about velopharyngeal closure in spontaneous, running speech cannot be safely based on observations made during the production of sustained, isolated sounds.

Many studies have shown that the degree of velar elevation varies between oral sounds. Thus, during the production of closed vowels, like [i] and [u], the velum is higher than during open vowel productions like [ɑ] and [æ]. There is a corresponding variation in the degree of electromyographic activity of the levator muscles.

In cinefluorographic films it can be seen that the velum does not have a fixed position during velopharyngeal closure. If a sentence with only oral sounds is spoken and there is continuous velopharyngeal closure, small fluctuations in velar elevation may be observed. These movements may also be indirectly demonstrated by recordings of the nasal air flow. During exaggerated articulation in particular, a certain amount of nasal air flow may be recorded, which is obviously not coming from the lungs but presumably caused by pumping movements of the velum.

The adduction of the side walls also appears to vary between sounds, as demonstrated by Minifie et al (1970). This observation can also easily be substantiated by asking a subject to say [ɑ] and [æ] with the mouth wide open. Under such conditions one is likely to observe side wall adduction for [ɑ] but not for [æ].

In cleft palate, the muscles from the two sides do not meet. The levator and palatopharyngeus fibres insert into the posterior rim of the hard palate (Dickson 1972). There have been very few studies on this subject, however, and little has been published on submucous cleft palate anatomy. Recently, a clinical entity of occult submucous cleft palate was described (Kaplan 1975; Croft et al 1978), and one of its features is a supposedly hypoplastic or absent musculus uvulae. It might be hypothesized that there is a continuous scale of variation from the entirely normal palatal muscle anatomy to the apparent and grossly anomalous muscle anatomy of the complete cleft.

In children with cleft palate, as well as in children with other types of congenital palatopharyngeal incompetence, the development of speech and language may be influenced. Although the techniques for cleft palate repair have made very rapid progress during recent decades, there is still a certain number of children in whom the surgical habilitation is not completely successful. These children must learn to speak without being able to make velopharyngeal closure.

Their vowel quality tends to be hypernasal and their consonant articulation weak because they cannot raise their intra-oral air pressure sufficiently. Swallowing, however, usually presents no problems once the cleft has been repaired.

FINAL COMMENT

In cleft lip and palate, the structure and function of the upper airway and digestive system are grossly disturbed. The repair is very complicated and difficult, and it takes nearly two decades before the final results can be assessed. Today, in spite of these most serious problems, the habilitation of children with this malformation is amazingly successful, and in quite a few subjects near-normal anatomy and function is achieved. In others, however, the outcome is not what we would like it to be. There are still many questions to ask, problems to solve, and research to be done.

REFERENCES

Azzam N A, Kuehn D P 1977 The morphology of musculus uvulae. Cleft Palate Journal 14: 78–87

Bell-Berti F 1976 An electromyographic study of velopharyngeal function in speech. Journal of Speech and Hearing Disorders 19: 225–240

Bloomer H H 1953 Observations on palatopharyngeal movements in speech and deglutition. Journal of Speech and Hearing Disorders 18: 230

Calnan J S 1957 Modern views of Passavant's ridge. British Journal of Plastic Surgery 10: 89

Croft C B, Shprintzen R J, Daniller A, Lewin M L 1978 The occult submucous cleft palate and the musculus uvulae. Cleft Palate Journal 15: 150–154

Dickson D R 1972 Normal and cleft palate anatomy. Cleft Palate Journal 9: 280–290

Dickson D R, Dickson W M 1972 Velopharyngeal anatomy. Journal of Speech and Hearing Disorders 15: 372–381

Fritzell B 1969 The velopharyngeal muscles in speech. Acta Otolaryngologica, suppl, 250: 1–81

Fritzell B 1979 Electromyography in the study of velopharyngeal function—a review. Folia Phoniatrica

Ibuki K, Matsuya T, Nishio J, Hamamura Y, Miyazaki T 1978 The course of facial nerve innervation for the levator veli palatini muscle. Cleft Palate Journal 15: 209–214

Kaplan E N 1975 The occult submucous cleft palate. Cleft Palate Journal 12: 356–368

Leanderson R, Persson A, Öhman S 1971 Electromyographic studies of facial muscle activity in speech. Acta Otolaryngologica 72: 361–369

Lubker J F 1975 Normal velopharyngeal function in speech. Clinics in Plastic Surgery 2: 249–259

Lubker J F, May K 1973 Palatoglossus function in normal speech production. Papers from the Institute of Linguistics, University of Stockholm 17: 17–26

Luschkä H von 1868 Der Schlundkopf des Menschen. H Laupp, Tübigen

Minifie F D, Hixon T J, Kelsey C A, Woodhouse R J 1970 Lateral pharyngeal wall movement during speech production. Journal of Speech and Hearing Research 13: 584–594

Pigott R W 1969 The nasendoscopic appearance of the normal palatopharyngeal valve. Plastic and Reconstructive Surgery 43: 19–24

Podvineč S 1952 The physiology and pathology of the soft palate. Journal of Laryngology and Otology 66: 452

Shprintzen R J, Lencione R M, McCall G N, Skolnick M L 1974 A three-dimensional cinefluoroscopic analysis of velopharyngeal closure during speech and nonspeech activities in normals. Cleft Palate Journal 11: 412–428

Shprintzen R J, McCall J N, Skolnick M L, Lencione R M 1975 Selective movement of the lateral aspects of the pharyngeal walls during velopharyngeal closure for speech, blowing, and whistling in normals. Cleft Palate Journal 12: 51–58

Skolnick M L, McCall G N, Barnes M 1973 The sphincteric mechanism of velopharyngeal closure. Cleft Palate Journal 10: 286–305

Zwitman D H, Sonderman J C, Ward P H 1974 Variations in velopharyngeal closure assessed by endoscopy. Journal of Speech and Hearing Disorders 39: 366–372

7

Growth and development

POSTNATAL GROWTH OF THE JAWS

One of the most striking features of the cleft lip and palate malformation is its effect on the postnatal growth of the jaws. At the same time, one of the most intriguing features of the malformation is the variability of this effect. Normal variation exists in all aspects of growth, but in growth of the jaws in cleft lip and palate, variation may range within normal limits or may extend to the realms of pathological variation.

Aberrant growth in cleft lip and palate can only be assessed by the yardstick of normal growth and variation. In this chapter, therefore, it is proposed to outline normal growth of the jaws and the extent of normal variation, and then to describe and examine the reasons for the wide range of variation which can occur in the cleft malformation.

NORMAL GROWTH OF THE JAWS

The current concept of growth is that it is a response to a dual control. Given a normal nutritional and hormonal background most body structures have an inherent capacity to grow to a certain form and size, this capacity being largely genetically determined. On the other hand, structures will only reach their final form and size under the influence of normal function. It has been postulated that growth of the head, including the jaws, is also dependent on this dual genetic–functional control. Moss (1971) has suggested that the head is the seat of a number of functional matrices, each with its own supporting skeletal unit. These functional units include those of mastication and deglutition, respiration, hearing and balance, and speech, as well as the neural integration function of the brain. Each functional matrix and supporting skeletal unit has its own inherent potential for growth, but growth can be affected if either the growth mechanism itself or the function of the unit is deficient, usually as a result of some pathological condition or structural malformation.

The possible growth mechanisms of the skeletal units of the head are those of cartilaginous, sutural and periosteal and endosteal growth. All these mechanisms are important in various parts of the skull and jaws.

Cartilaginous growth is largely confined to the base of the skull and the nasal septum, these areas having originally developed from the cartilaginous basal plate. Secondary cartilage at the head of the mandibular condyle forms one of the mechanisms for mandibular growth.

Sutural growth can be considered as a continuation of the intramembranous ossification by which bones of the cranial vault and most of the facial bones develop. Growth at the sutures enlarges the periphery of the bones, and eventually joins together and sometimes fuses the originally separate elements of the various skeletal supporting units of the head.

Periosteal and endosteal growth, by adding and removing tissue from the surfaces of bones, enlarges and changes the shapes of the skeletal units during growth. In addition, together with other mechanisms of bone growth, it changes the relative positions of the skeletal units from their original positions at birth to their final relationships at maturity.

There has been some controversy over the exact role of these growth mechanisms. Some authorities have felt that they are primary features of growth, acting independently of other influences apart from nutritional and hormonal factors. The more recent concept is that they are secondary features, responsive to the growth and activity of the functional elements of the head. Thus it is considered that even if the mechanisms for bone growth are normal, the mandible will only reach its full potential size and form with normal growth and function of the muscular elements of mastication and deglutition, or the cranium will only reach its potential with normal growth of the brain.

According to this concept, therefore, growth can be adversely affected either by a direct pathological effect on the growth mechanisms themselves, such as trauma or infection, or as a secondary effect of a functional deficiency. There is ample evidence to support this concept from pathological conditions. For example, stripping the periosteum from a growing bone will directly affect one of its growth mechanisms and will result in a change in its final form. Inherited achondroplasia, which inhibits cartilaginous growth at the skull base, has a marked secondary effect on the position of the maxilla. Severe cerebral palsy, by reducing brain growth and function, not only results in reduced cranial growth but has secondary effects on the size of the jaws, probably through its influence on speech, mastication and other neuromuscular functions (Foster et al 1974).

In cleft lip and palate there are many possible factors which could affect growth, both by their primary effect on growth mechanisms and as a secondary result of their effect on function. In the initial defect, the sutural growth mechanism between the two sides of the maxilla is absent. In the operative procedure, periosteal stripping or postoperative scarring may occur. If there is a major defect, the function of the speech, chewing and swallowing mechanisms may be impaired. Add to this the possibility of an initial tissue deficiency or of more remote growth defects, perhaps at the base of the skull, and it becomes hardly surprising that growth is often adversely affected.

Before considering the effects on jaw growth of the cleft malformation, it is necessary to outline and exclude the effects of normal variation.

NORMAL VARIATION IN JAW SIZE AND FORM

Normal variation in jaw size, form and relationship is generally considered to be largely the result of genetic factors. Many studies of twins have been carried out which suggest that inheritance is the major factor involved. Setting aside the basic racial variations, the genetic mixtures which have occurred in most present-day populations can explain the range and extent of most normal variation which is to be seen (Fig. 7.1). The accepted ideals of jaw size and relationship occur in only a relatively small proportion of most mixed populations. Thus only a little over one-half of the population of the United Kingdom are thought to have upper and lower jaws which match in size and relationship. Over 40 per cent have a lower jaw relatively too small for the upper jaw, and about 5 per cent have an upper jaw too small to match the lower jaw. These discrepancies in jaw size range from slight to severe, though the total proportion of the normal population having severe discrepancies is probably fairly small. It is against this background of normal variation that growth variation in cleft lip and palate must be judged.

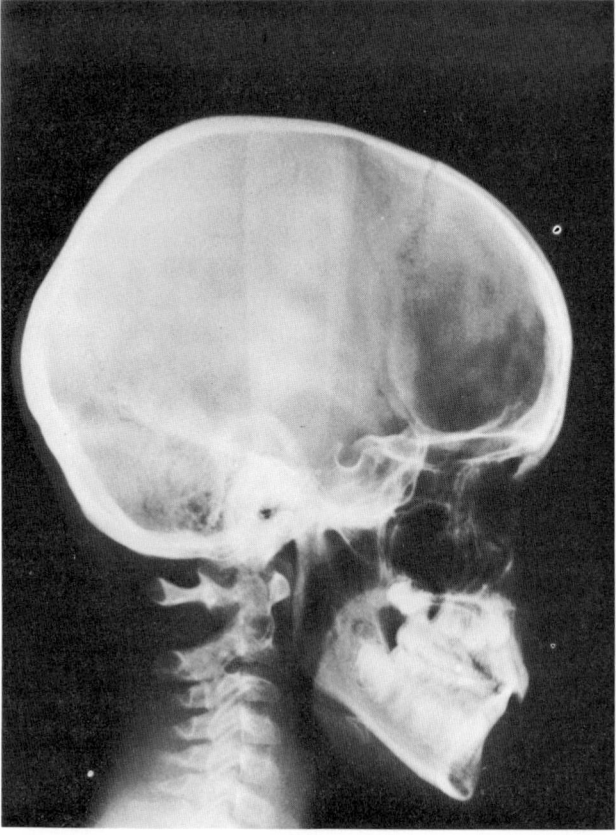

(a)

Fig. 7.1 Normal variation in jaw size and relationship. (a) Balanced size and relationship of maxilla and mandible. (b) Mandibular retrognathism and maxillary prognathism. (c) Mandibular prognathism relative to maxillary position

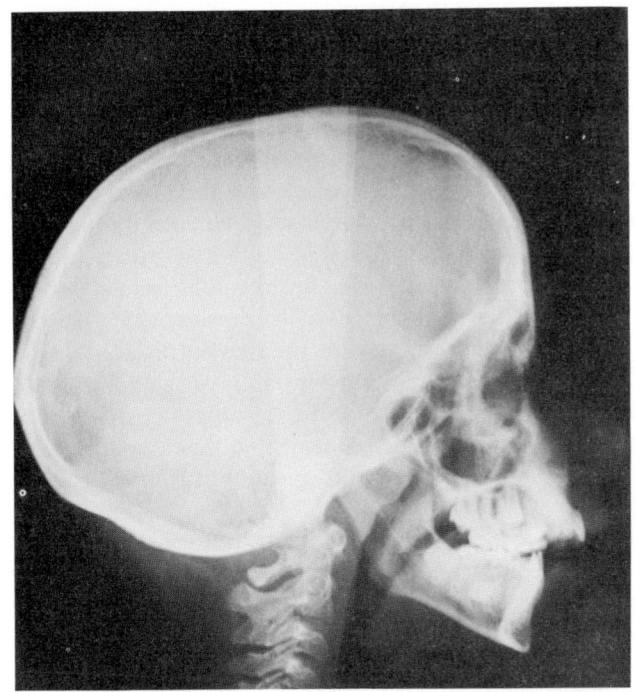

(b)

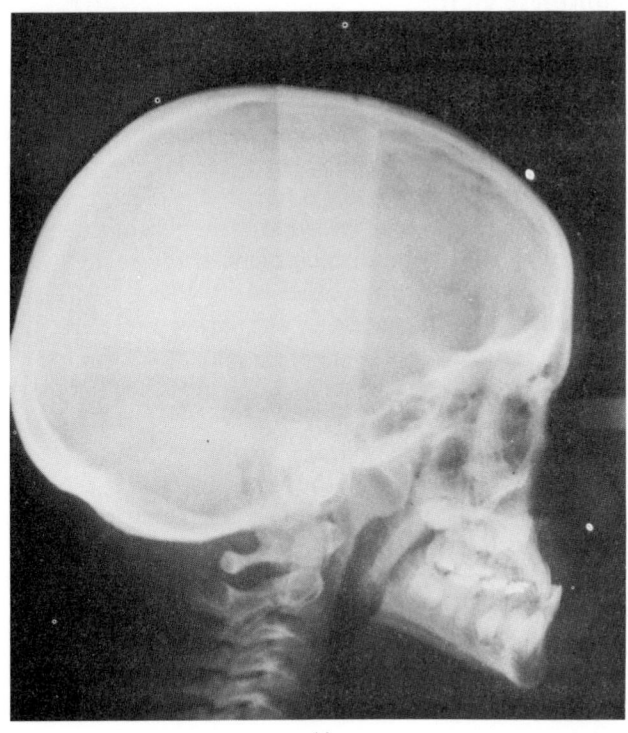

(c)

THE CLEFT PALATE AT BIRTH

At birth, and for the first few months of life, the infant with a cleft exhibits the basic defect, uninfluenced by any operative procedures. It is at this stage that variation is at its most striking, and perhaps this initial variation provides the key to the future variation in growth and development. However, there do not appear to have been any studies correlating the initial form and size of the facial and jaw structures with the dimensions attained at maturity. Those studies which have been made of the condition at birth have either outlined the extent of individual variation or have reported mean values for the various parameters of the head, and particularly of the jaws. Pruzansky (1953) has emphasized the remarkable range of variation found in the newborn, including differences in the separation of the segments, the positioning of the component parts of the jaws, the size of the palatal shelves and the completeness of the lip or palate cleft (see Figs 13.1 and 13.2). Added to this should be the differences in relationship between upper and lower jaw, and in the positions of the jaws relative to the cranial base.

In the light of these extensive individual differences it is difficult to outline general trends. However, studies involving measurement of the facial structures, by reporting mean values, have given information on some of the general trends and differences between cleft and normal infants. It is convenient to consider these within the various categories of cleft lip and palate.

Unilateral complete clefts

Several investigators have studied the form and dimensions of the jaws at birth in unilateral complete clefts (Aduss & Pruzansky 1968; Huddart et al 1969; Wada & Miyazaki 1975). The consensus of opinion is that the maxillary arch is wider than normal, with lateral displacement of the segments of the jaw. The anterior portion of the larger segment, which carries the premaxilla, tends to be protruded. Huddart et al (1969) have reported a mean deficiency of palatal tissue of 13.7 per cent and an excessive slope of the palatal shelves. These latter features, together with the lateral displacement of the segments, contribute to the width of the palatal cleft. On the other hand, Shaw (1978) has found little deficiency of maxillary alveolar tissue in a group of unilateral complete clefts at birth. There is not, however, complete agreement on the form of the upper arch. Ishiguro et al (1976) have reported that the mean arch breadth in complete unilateral cleft is narrower than normal. Individual variation and the choice of the sample could influence such findings.

With regard to other dimensions of the facial structures, Ishiguro et al (1976) have found that the height of the upper face is greater in unilateral complete clefts, but facial breadth is no greater than in normal infants. Mazaheri et al (1977) have reported that both the thickness and length of the soft palate and the height and depth of the nasopharynx are less in clefts than in non-cleft infants.

There has been little attention paid to mandibular dimensions at birth, though Ishiguro et al (1976) found that the mean breadth of the mandibular arch was less in clefts than in normal infants.

A feature which is not part of facial structures but which probably has a marked influence on the position of the facial bones is the degree of flexure of the cranial base. There is some evidence that excessive cranial base flexure is an important part of the cleft palate malformation, and Krogman et al (1975) have found excessive flexure of the cranial base in infants with unilateral complete clefts.

Bilateral complete clefts

Many of the findings reported on facial form in unilateral clefts apply to bilateral clefts. Thus Huddart (1970) and Robertson et al (1977) have reported wider maxillary arches and palatal tissue deficiency, with lateral displacement of the maxillary segments. Again, Ishiguro et al (1976) found narrower arch breadths in the cleft group. The pharyngeal and soft palate dimensions have been reported as less than normal (Mazaheri et al 1977) and the cranial base flexure as greater than normal (Krogman et al 1975). The most obvious differences are in the position of the premaxilla and the breadth of the face. Facial breadth would appear to be greater in bilateral clefts than in other types of cleft or in normal infants (Ishiguro et al 1976). The protrusion of the premaxilla is a fairly common feature, often accompanied by deviation of the nasal septum and rotation of the premaxilla (Fig. 7.2a). This is not, however, a universal feature in bilateral clefts. Occasionally the premaxillary position conforms to a correct relationship with the maxillary segment (Fig. 7.2b).

Cleft palate

There have been relatively few investigations into facial form at birth in isolated cleft palate. Ishiguro et al (1976) have found that facial breadth was no greater than normal, but facial height in clefts was greater than in normal infants. They also found that maxillary arch breadth was less than normal, but since their findings in this respect on unilateral and bilateral complete clefts were contrary to those of other authors there may have been ethnic or sampling differences in the populations studied. Nasopharyngeal and soft-palate dimensions were reported to be less than normal (Mazaheri et al 1977). Cranial base flexure was found to be greater in cleft palate than in normal controls, but less than in subjects with unilateral and bilateral complete clefts of lip and palate (Krogman et al 1975).

One of the difficulties of investigating isolated cleft palate is that there is greater variability in the degree of cleft. A unilateral or bilateral cleft of lip and palate can be designated as 'complete' in the sagittal dimension, though there is obvious potential for variation in other aspects. Isolated clefts of the palate on the other hand may vary in length as well as in width, involving only the soft palate or the soft and hard palate to varying degrees. Grouping these clefts into a single entity brings in a further source or error, unless the number studied is large enough to include the whole range of variation.

Cleft lip

There seems to have been no detailed study of facial and jaw dimensions at birth in those subjects with clefts confined to the lip. It could be assumed on

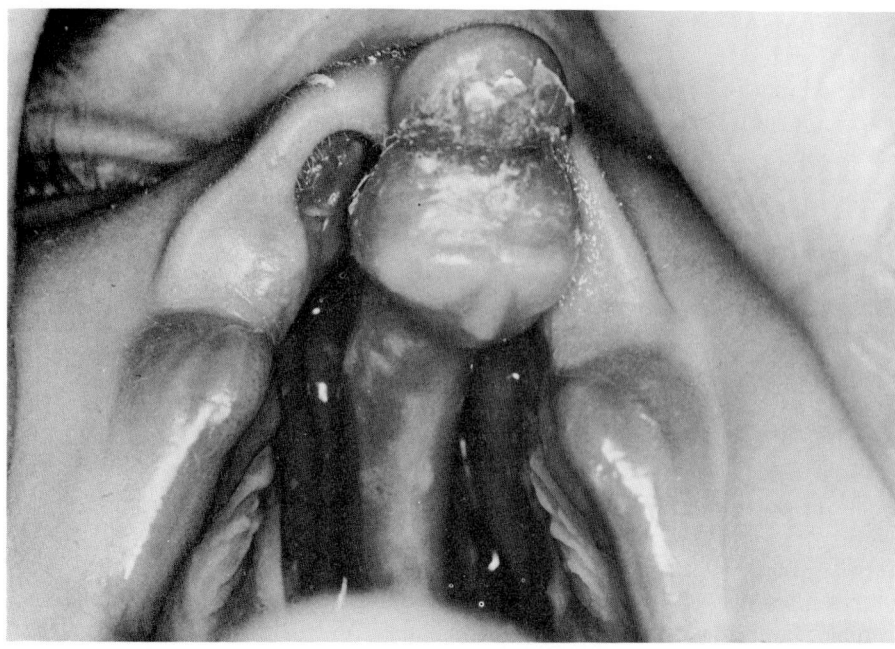

(a)

(b)

Fig. 7.2 Variation in premaxillary position in newborn infants with bilateral complete cleft of lip and palate. (a) Premaxilla protruded and nasal septum deviated. (b) No protrusion of the premaxilla

grounds of general clinical impression that clefts of the lip do not bring any major differences in other structures, or in facial growth. However, this assumption may not be valid, since lip clefts are essentially partial manifestations of the same pathological condition which produces more severe clefts in other cases, and there may be defects in other more remote structures which have hitherto gone unnoticed. Further study in this field is indicated.

GROWTH AFTER SURGICAL REPAIR

Surgical repair is a major incident in the life of the infant with cleft lip and palate. Before repair, growth has proceeded for a relatively short time, in an aberrant fashion because of the structural and functional anomalies resulting from the cleft. The objective of repair is to correct these anomalies, but in addition it brings potential for further anomalies in the form of trauma and continuing structural defects, and it seems to have a profound effect on growth, particularly of the maxilla.

In the immediate postoperative period, Aduss and Pruzansky (1968) have found a narrowing of the maxillary tuberosity width following lip repair and a further decrease in width following palate repair. This effect would be readily explained on a simple mechanical tension basis. The forces applied by a functioning repaired lip could readily move the maxillary segments closer together. Similarly the function of an intact soft palate would be sufficient to narrow the maxillary arch in the presence of a mid-palate bony defect, even though no physical tension existed in the repair process. Thus it is not surprising to see that the initial repair seems to reduce palatal width. On the other hand, this is not a universal finding. Mazaheri et al (1967) report that they have found no significant reduction in bituberosity width after initial lip or palate surgery. The width of the cleft was found to reduce after lip repair, presumably through reduction of anterior palate width and growth of the palatal shelves.

In the longer term the general finding is that maxillary growth is reduced after surgery. Osbourne (1966) and Hayashi et al (1976) have found a progressive reduction in maxillary prominence, with facial convexity becoming progressively less throughout the growth period. Measurements of mean values towards the end of the growth phase have shown the maxilla to be smaller, more retropositioned and more suprapositioned in relation to other facial structures than in normal individuals. Alveolar growth is also inhibited, in particular growth of the smaller segment in unilateral complete clefts. Again, there is some difference of opinion in the findings of various studies. While agreeing that there is a growth lag immediately after surgery, Mapes et al (1974) have found this lag to be transitory. They report that later growth rate may even exceed normal rates, and there is some catch-up growth both in the bony structures of the maxilla and in the soft palate.

With regard to other facial structures, the mandible has been reported to be shorter than normal at all ages up to maturity (Hayashi et al 1976) and normal in size at all ages (Osbourne 1966; Narula and Ross 1970; Krogman et al 1975). Again there may be ethnic differences in the populations studied, or sampling variation may account for the differences found. Similar comments apply to the findings on growth of facial height. Hayashi et al (1976) found the upper face height to be smaller and the lower face height larger than normal, the differences tending to increase with age. Ishiguro et al (1976) found the upper face height in cleft patients to be greater than normal, while Ross and Johnston (1967) found the upper face height in clefts to be no greater than normal. Other studies have given equally conflicting results.

In a study of 322 subjects with repaired clefts of all types, at ages ranging from 5 years to maturity, Foster (1967) found a high prevalence of maxillary retrusion, of medial displacement of the segments of the upper jaw and of lack of vertical growth of the jaw immediately posterior to the alveolar cleft. Relative

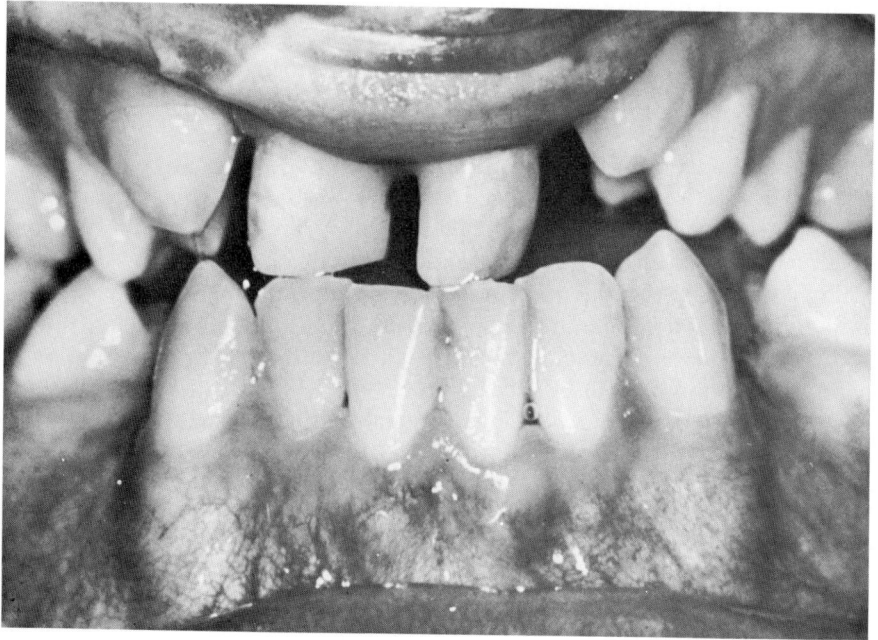

Fig. 7.3 Dentition of 12-year-old child with complete bilateral cleft lip and palate, showing relative maxillary retrusion, medial displacement of the maxillary segments and deficiency of vertical development immediately behind the alveolar clefts, which are the characteristic growth defects exhibited by many cleft subjects

retrusion of the maxilla affected 48 per cent of unilateral complete clefts, 37 per cent of bilateral complete clefts and 26 per cent of isolated palate clefts. The corresponding figure for the normal population is approximately 5 per cent. Some two-thirds of the subjects with complete clefts showed medial displacement of one or both segments of the maxilla, and the same proportion showed deficiencies of vertical growth of the maxillary alveolar segment adjacent to the cleft (Fig. 7.3).

The consensus of opinion seems to be that growth of the maxilla in repaired cleft lip and palate tends to be reduced in all planes of space. Thus the length, breadth and height of the jaw tends to be affected so that the maxilla is more retroposed and more supraposed and the face is more concave than normal.

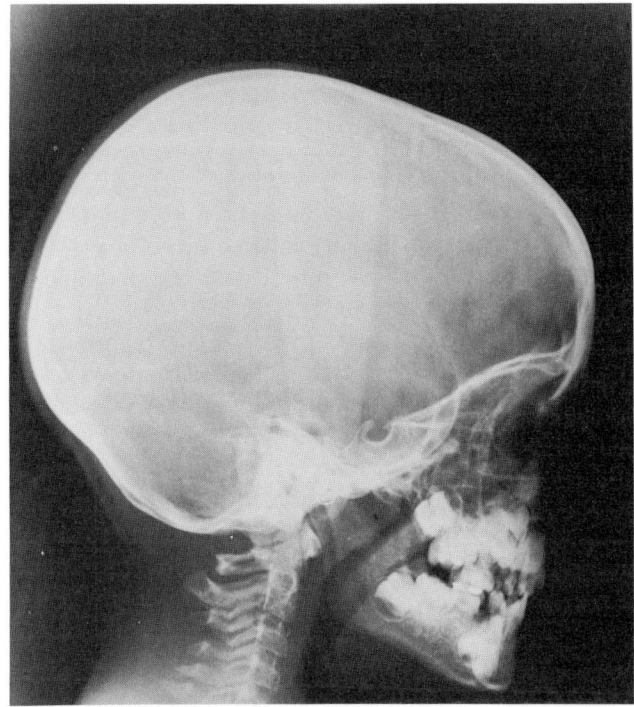

(a)

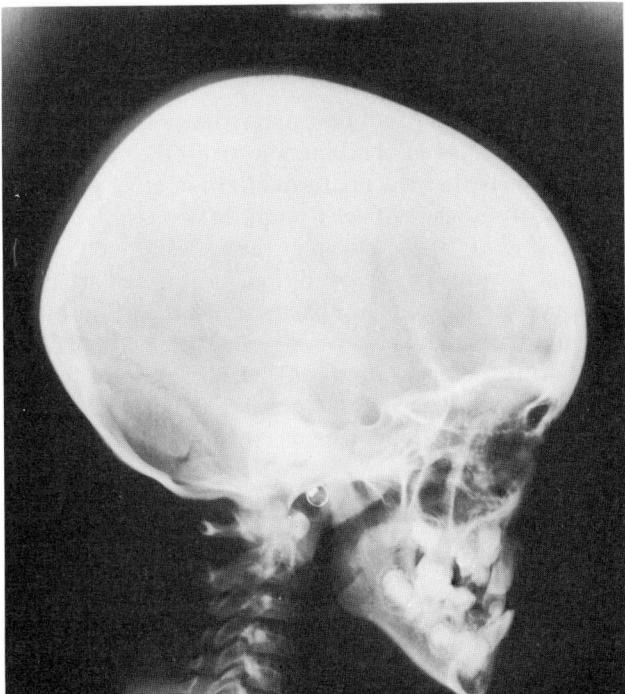

(b)

Fig. 7.4 Radiographs of
two 7-year-old children
with repaired complete
unilateral cleft lip and
palate. Variation in
maxillary growth is shown,
with little or no growth
deficiency in (a), but
relative maxillary
retrognathism in (b)

These effects are evident throughout the growth period and clinically sometimes seem to be progressive. They are also more marked in complete clefts, less evident in isolated palate clefts and often not evident when the cleft only involves the lip.

There is less agreement on the effects on growth of other structures, particularly the mandible, though many investigators have found that mandibular growth is reduced and the mandibular angle more obtuse. More remote from the facial structures, there is evidence that the cranial base exhibits a greater flexure, especially in complete clefts, and this may reflect the basic pathological process leading to the cleft malformation.

It must be emphasized that there is great variation in the effects on growth in cleft lip and palate. Some children show severe defects from an early age. In others an apparently minor growth defect becomes progressively worse. Still others, with a similar basic cleft type, may show no growth deficiency at all (Fig. 7.4).

The studies which have been quoted above and, which in some cases have seemed to be contradictory, have all reported mean values from populations. This tends to mask individual variation which makes a great deal of difference to the final form and dimensions of the face. In cleft lip and palate the potential source of such variation is manifold. It can include inheritance, the severity of the original defect and the effects of repair and repositioning procedures, as well as aspects of neuromuscular function so often overlooked.

SOURCES OF VARIATION IN GROWTH

Genetic differences

Cleft lip and palate is not a single entity with a single cause. It is likely that several different genetic mechanisms can produce a predisposition to the malformation, either as an isolated defect or in combination with other congenital deformities. Furthermore, it is likely that the malformation can arise purely as a developmental defect without an inherited background. It is possible, therefore, that differences in growth and in the final form of the face and jaws reflect differences in the causative mechanisms of the condition. Drillien et al (1966) have pointed out that their survey of cleft lip and palate subjects in Edinburgh showed differences between those subjects with a positive and those with a negative family history for clefts. While there was no significant difference in height and weight for age between the cleft subjects with a positive family history and their siblings, there were significant differences between cleft subjects with a negative family history and their siblings. In general, those cleft subjects with no family history of clefts tended to be worse affected with regard to birth weight, physical growth and intelligence than those with positive family history.

This suggests that the basic cause of the cleft may play a part in determining its overall effects, particularly in relation to the growth potential of the individual. There does not seem to have been any comparative study of facial growth differences between those clefts appearing in isolation and those appearing in combination with other congenital abnormalities, nor between those with and without a family history of cleft malformation. Although these divisions may not be absolute, such studies may throw more light on the reasons for variation in growth.

Sex differences

There is some evidence that growth of the jaws in cleft lip and palate varies between the sexes. In particular, there is evidence that females are more severely affected by the cleft malformation than males. In two separate studies Foster (1961, 1970) found that both the length of the maxilla and its position in relation to the cranial base were significantly more adversely affected in female than in male subjects with complete unilateral cleft lip and palate when compared with non-cleft controls matched for age and sex. Hayashi et al (1976) found that at all stages of growth, females with complete unilateral clefts showed more under-development of both maxilla and mandible than did males. Bimm et al (1960) found a consistent tendency towards reduction in mandibular growth in children with cleft lip and palate, with females being more severely affected than males.

Apart from these studies of growth, there is evidence from studies of the cleft malformation at birth which suggests that females tend to have more severe clefts than males. The work of Fogh-Andersen (1942), and Knox & Braithwaite (1963) has shown that, in isolated cleft palate, females exhibit a greater proportion of the more severe clefts involving both hard and soft palate and a smaller proportion of the less severe clefts involving only the soft palate than do males. Meskin et al (1968) found that, in all types of cleft, females exhibit a greater tendency to develop complete clefts and males to develop incomplete clefts. This finding is in accord with that of Drillien et al (1966), who found that, in general, cleft lip defects were more severe in females and that, in isolated cleft palate, females showed a severe degree of cleft more frequently than males. There was a highly significant excess of complete clefts of palate in females as compared with males.

Thus it would appear that females tend not only to develop more severe clefts but also to exhibit more severe growth restrictions. This could be due to genetic factors, with the genetic mechanisms producing the more severe defects exhibiting some sex limitation, or to environmental factors. Steigler & Berry (1958), for example, found that iron deficiency anaemia in pregnancy had affected 20 per cent of the mothers of females with clefts of the lip and palate, but only 10 per cent of the mothers of males.

There is, however, very little evidence as to the cause of these apparent differences between the sexes, and further study of this interesting phenomenon would be of value.*

The effects of operative repair

Taken at face value, surgical repair might be thought to be the most potent source of growth disturbance. It is usually performed at an early age, during one of the most rapid growth phases, and differences in techniques might reasonably be thought to result in differences in growth. Graber (1949, 1950) was one of the first to point out that growth differences might result from operative

---

* The slightly earlier fusion of the palate in the male may be relevant to this problem (see Chapter 3).

differences, and he advocated that palate repair should be delayed until the end of the fourth year of life, by which time five-sixths of the growth in width of the maxillary denture was completed. However, it should be pointed out that Graber's comparisons were between some very traumatic, multiple surgical procedures, which considerably inhibited growth, and which would be very unlikely procedures in the present day, and some more modern operative techniques which, as illustrated, had little effect on growth. Furthermore, the concept that five-sixths of the growth of the maxilla is completed by the age of 4 years is perhaps misleading. It has been shown (Foster et al 1972) that the maxillary dental arch in normal subjects increases in width by less than 5 per cent between the ages of $2\frac{1}{2}$ and $5\frac{1}{2}$ years. Further increases occur at the time of development of the permanent dentition, between 7 and 12 years. Other dimensions of the jaw increase throughout the growth period, and there is a considerable change in the relationship between the maxilla and the cranial base, with considerable increase in facial height, after the age of 4 years, and particularly during the pubertal growth spurt. The effects of surgery on growth, therefore, need to be looked at on a broader perspective than simply the dimensions of the maxillary arch, and it seems likely that the timing of surgical repair during the first few years of childhood is relatively unimportant.

It does, however, also seem likely that very traumatic surgery and more refined surgery will have different effects on growth, as illustrated by Graber, Mapes et al (1974), in a study of maxillary growth after surgical repair, clearly indicated surgery as a growth inhibitor, but found that if the surgery was sufficiently atraumatic the maxilla could recuperate by accelerating its rate of growth in the year following surgery.

The effects of different surgical procedures
If the older, more grossly traumatic methods of repair are excluded, it would be interesting to see whether modern surgical techniques differ in their effects on growth. The major problem in studying this aspect of cleft lip and palate is that it is unlikely that the surgical technique will constitute the only difference. If the results of different cleft palate centres are compared, there may be ethnic and nutritional differences in the populations, differences in timing of the operation, differences in nursing management and differences in surgical skills as well as the basic difference in the method of repair. For these and other reasons there is a dearth of good comparative studies which could isolate the various repair procedures in use at the present time. In one such study, Onizuka & Isshiki (1975) compared the effects of four different methods of lip and palate repair on the form and dimensions of the maxillary arch. They concluded that there was little difference in the results of the four methods, and any of the methods studied could be expected to result in maldevelopment of the maxilla. This does not, of course, mean that there is no method in current use which generally has less adverse effect on growth than other methods, but if such a method exists its effects have not been clearly demonstrated.

Growth in unrepaired clefts of lip and palate
As previously mentioned, most authorities feel that surgical repair has some potential for limitation of growth. There have been claims that the results of

careful operative procedures do not show any defects in growth (Bill et al 1956; Ross 1970), but any large group of repaired cleft palate subjects will usually exhibit some growth defects. Whether this is due to periosteal stripping, scar contraction, interference with blood supply, alterations in muscular function or to any other factor has not been established. The role of the basic tissue deficiency has also not been established. There is, however, one way in which the overall effects of surgery could be determined, and that is by means of a good comparative study between adults who have and who have not undergone surgical repair of the cleft. To date, work on these lines has been limited, for good reasons. In most developed countries almost all children born with clefts undergo surgical repair. Only in relatively underdeveloped countries are there substantial numbers of individuals who reach maturity with no repair of the cleft, and many of these are in fairly isolated communities. Even if they were more readily accessible there would still be the problem of ethnic differences between the repaired and unrepaired individuals, and there might also be differences in the causative background to the malformation, such as different genetic or environmental influences, which have been previously mentioned. These factors mean that comparisons between repaired and unrepaired clefts are not only difficult to make but also of less value than might be supposed. Nevertheless there have been a number of reports of facial and jaw dimensions in unoperated clefts, from which some general tentative conclusions may be drawn.

Two main findings emerge from studies of unoperated adults. The first is that major growth defects, which markedly affect the size and the position of the maxilla, do not seem to occur. Mestre et al (1960), Ortiz-Monasterio et al (1966) and Bishara et al (1976) have all studied adults with unoperated clefts of various types, and have found no significant differences in the overall size of the jaws and in the position of the maxilla when compared with normal adults. In a separate study, comparing operated and unoperated subjects with isolated clefts of the palate, Bishara (1973) found that all the cleft subjects had more retroposed maxilla and mandible than a normal adult group, but there were no significant differences in any parameters between operated and unoperated clefts. Apart from this, findings have generally been that in the absence of surgical repair, major growth defects are avoided.

The second general finding is that there is evidence of localized growth defects in unoperated subjects, particularly in the immediate region of the cleft of the alveolar arch. Several investigations have pointed to this finding, among them a study by Atherton (1967) of a number of skulls of various ages with unoperated clefts. Atherton reported that the general development of the facial bones was good, except in the region of the cleft, where there were various relatively minor growth deficiencies and deviations in the direction of growth. Pitanguy & Franco (1967) found a regional mesodermal deficiency in 84 subjects with unoperated clefts, although there was better general harmony of growth than in operated cases. Crabb & Foster (1977) have outlined the localized growth defects in a number of unoperated subjects. Defects occurred particularly in lateral and vertical growth at the region of the alveolar cleft (Fig. 7.5).

Thus, although comparisons are difficult and the numbers are limited, from

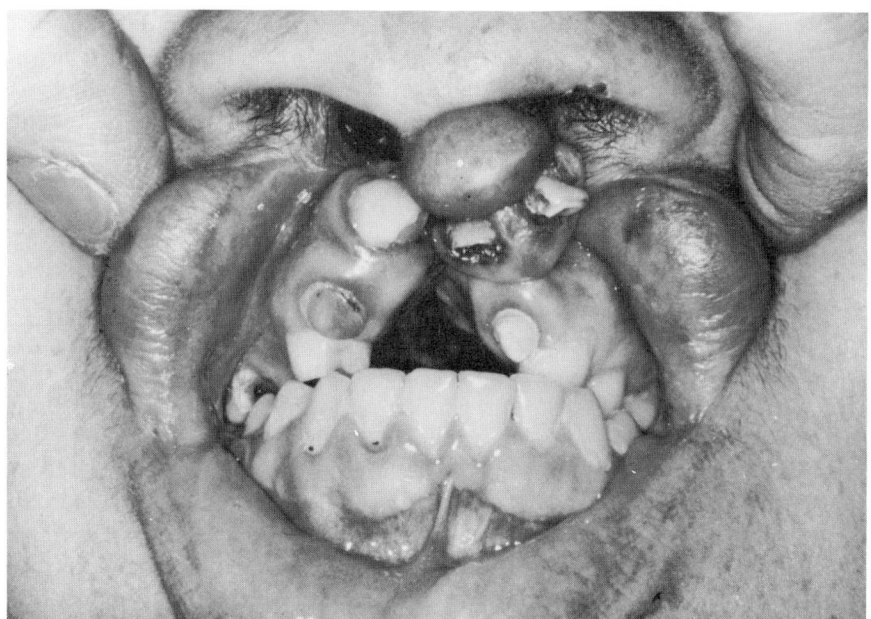

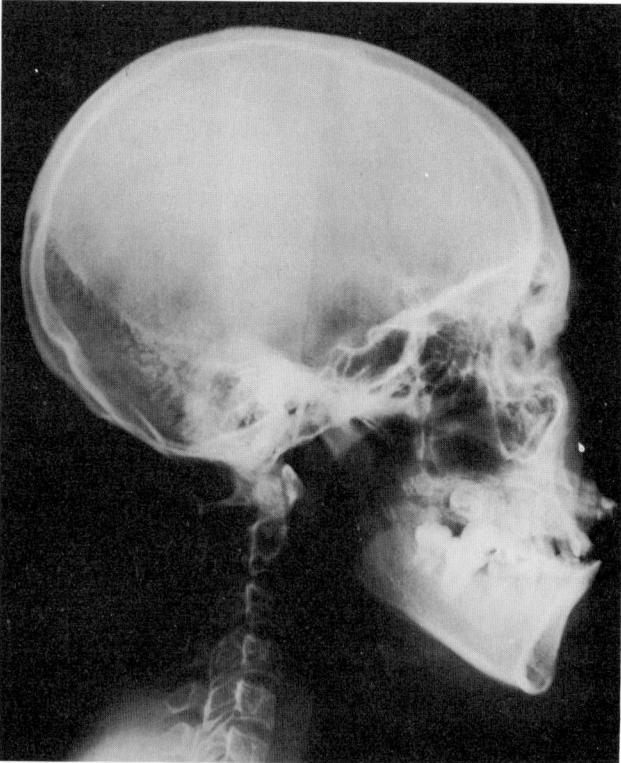

Fig. 7.5 Twenty-one-year-old adult with unoperated complete bilateral cleft lip and palate. Growth deficiencies are localized, with vertical and lateral growth in the vicinity of the alveolar clefts being affected, and the original protrusion of the premaxilla persisting

the evidence available it seems that the basic tissue deficiency provides the main variable in unoperated clefts, and this is usually not sufficient to produce major growth defects.

Tissue deficiency

A deficiency of mesodermal tissue, rather than a mere failure of fusion of embryonic elements, is generally felt to be the pathogenic background to most clefts (Stark 1968). The degree of tissue deficiency must constitute one of the variables which affect growth, and in some cases may be the overriding factor. Clefts at birth show a wide range of tissue deficiency in the visible elements of the upper jaw, and attempts have been made to quantify the basic deficiency of the palatal shelves. In addition there are variations in the size of the segments of the alveolar arches and in the width of the alveolar cleft and there may well be variation in structures as yet not investigated, such as the other facial bones, cranial base elements and the muscular elements of the head. Foster & Lavelle (1971) found that the teeth in cleft subjects were significantly smaller than in normal controls. In a study of skulls with unoperated clefts, Atherton (1967) found that the reduction in size of the elements of the maxilla was present at all ages, and did not seem to be progressively greater with age. This suggests that the size reduction was the result of tissue deficiency rather than growth deficiency. If this is the case, even the most meticulous operative repair, if it does not add tissue in some way, would be unlikely to overcome the basic problem, and it is likely that later results in terms of growth, speech and other oral function depend to a large extent on the amount of tissue originally present.

AREAS FOR FURTHER STUDY

While much has been discovered regarding growth in cleft lip and palate, there are many areas where it would seem that further investigation would be rewarding.

There is a need for long-term investigations comparing the original condition at birth with the final achievements at maturity, particularly with regard to growth and speech. Such studies would throw light on the range of tissue deficiency in the original defect, not only in the immediate vicinity of the jaw but also in other parameters of head and body growth, and would give an indication as to what extent we are dealing with basic defects.

Growth studies to date have tended to lay emphasis on hard tissues. Hard tissue, however, is the end result of inheritance, function and nutrition. Future studies might place more emphasis on muscular function and its relationship to growth.

With regard to inheritance, more detailed study of variation related to different genetic backgrounds to clefts is indicated. In particular a study of jaw and facial dimensions and speech function in subjects with a positive and a negative family history of clefts, and in subjects where the cleft has occurred in conjunction with other congenital deformities, might throw light on the causative nature of the cleft as a source of variation. Similarly the differences between the sexes which have been already noted warrant further investigation.

Finally, since operative repair appears to be a major factor in growth restriction, a careful study of the results of different methods of repair might be valuable. Such a study would eliminate other differences, including ethnic variation, general management, nutrition, timing of operation and skills, possibly by one surgical team carrying out different types of repair on a randomly selected basis.

Investigations such as these would need to be broad in nature, encompassing a full range of basic variations, and would obviously be long-term. However, careful prospective studies are necessary if we are to move aside some of the residual barriers to knowledge of growth variation in cleft lip and palate.

SUMMARY

Growth of the jaws in cleft lip and palate exhibits variation well beyond the range of normal. While in some cases deficiencies of growth may not exist, in others defects, particularly of maxillary growth, are very marked. There is a consensus of opinion that, at maturity, the maxilla is more retroposed, the facial profile more concave and the height of the upper face more reduced in a larger proportion of cleft individuals than in the normal population. There is also evidence that the cranial base flexure is greater and the mandible more retroposed in cleft lip and palate than in normal subjects.

However, the study of growth in cleft subjects has usually been the study of growth in repaired clefts, since by and large subjects available for study have had repair operations carried out. There do not seem to have been any true growth studies on unrepaired clefts, though there is some evidence regarding facial parameters in mature unrepaired clefts. The sources of variation in growth could therefore conveniently be divided into two main groups, these being basic sources on the one hand and the repair procedure on the other.

At birth, cleft palate subjects already exhibit a wide range of variation quite apart from differences in the cleft type. In particular this variation includes differences in the degree of tissue deficiency, and differences in the relative positioning of the component parts of the jaws. There may well be other differences more remote from the facial structures which have not yet been investigated. Tissue deficiency may have a profound effect on future growth, and on growth-related activities such as speech performance. There is evidence to suggest that variation in the degree of tissue deficiency may have its source in the causative mechanisms of the cleft. In particular, differences in the genetic background to the cleft and in the intrauterine environment may result in differences in growth, as well as in other factors such as intelligence. There is strong evidence that sex differences exist both in the extent of the original defect and in the growth of the jaws to maturity.

The repair procedure has clearly been shown to be a potential source of disturbance of growth. Whether this is due to the trauma of periosteal stripping, effects on blood supply, scar tissue contraction or any other cause has not been determined. Physical change in the position of the components of the jaw could readily be seen to occur as a result of changes in muscle function following lip repair or palate repair, but in addition there is evidence of progressive reduction of growth after repair which could not be explained simply by changes in muscle function. On the other hand, many repaired clefts grow to within normal limits, and there is almost certainly a difference in effect between the careful, skilled operative procedure and the more traumatic or repetitive procedure now happily becoming a thing of the past. There is evidence that, although a relatively atraumatic operation can cause an immediate reduction of growth, the effect may be transitory, and an acceleration of growth may occur in the later postoperative period. It seems, however, that even the most careful procedure is unlikely to produce normal growth in the presence of severe tissue deficiency, unless some way can be found to make up that deficiency.

The limited studies which have been made on unoperated clefts in adults have suggested that there are no major growth defects in the absence of operative repair. There are localized defects, particularly of lateral and vertical growth in the region of the cleft, which must be accounted for by basic tissue deficiency and functional aberrations. However, the limited nature of the studies and the differences in the populations make it impossible to draw firm conclusions.

Further study is needed to throw more light on the variations in growth. In particular, the reasons for the differences in basic tissue deficiency and the effects of those differences need more investigation. There is also a need to look further than the immediate vicinity of the maxilla in assessing the discrepancies, growth and treatment of children with cleft lip and palate.

REFERENCES

Aduss H, Pruzansky S 1968 Width of cleft at the level of the tuberosities in complete unilateral cleft lip and palate. Plastic and Reconstructive Surgery 41: 113–123

Atherton J D 1967 Morphology of facial bones in skulls with unoperated cleft palate. Cleft Palate Journal 4: 18–30

Bill A H, Moore A W, Coe H E (1956) The time of choice for repair of cleft palate in relation to the type of surgical repair and its effect on bony growth of the face. Plastic and Reconstructive Surgery 18: 469–473

Bimm J A, Eisner D A, Ibanez C D 1960 Cleft palate: morphology of the human mandible. American Journal of Orthodontics 46: 791 (Abstract)

Bishara S E 1973 Cephalometric evaluation of facial growth in operated and non-operated individuals with isolated clefts of the palate. Cleft Palate Journal 10: 239–246

Bishara S E, Kraus C J, Olin W H, Weston D, Ness J E, Felling C 1976 Facial and dental relationships of individuals with unoperated clefts of the lip and/or palate. Cleft Palate Journal 13: 238–252

Crabb J J, Foster T D 1977 Growth defects in unrepaired unilateral cleft lip and palate. Oral Surgery, Oral Medicine, Oral Pathology 44: 329–335

Drillien C H, Ingram T T S, Wilkinson E M 1966 The causes and natural history of cleft lip and palate. Livingstone, Edinburgh

Fogh-Andersen P 1942 Inheritance of harelip and cleft palate. Busck, Copenhagen

Foster T D 1961 Some aspects of jaw growth in cleft palate. European Orthodontic Society Transactions, p 384–395

Foster T D 1967 Malocclusions in 322 patients with cleft lip and palate who have not had presurgical dental orthopaedic treatment. European Orthodontic Society Transactions, p 445–454

Foster T D 1970 Sex differences in maxillary growth of cleft subjects. Cleft Palate Journal 7: 347–352

Foster T D, Lavelle C L B 1971 The size of the dentition in complete cleft lip and palate. Cleft Palate Journal 8: 177–184

Foster T D, Grundy M C, Lavelle C L B 1972 Changes in occlusion in the primary dentition between $2\frac{1}{2}$ and $5\frac{1}{2}$ years of age. European Orthodontic Society Transactions, p 75–84

Foster T D, Griffiths M I, Gordon P H 1974 The effects of cerebral palsy on the size and form of the skull. American Journal of Orthodontics 66: 40–49

Graber T M 1949 Craniofacial morphology in cleft palate and cleft lip deformity. Surgery, Gynaecology and Obstetrics 88: 359–369

Graber T M 1950 Changing philosophies in cleft palate management. Journal of Paediatrics 37: 400–415

Hayashi I, Saduka M, Takimoto K, Miyazaki T 1976 Craniofacial growth in complete unilateral cleft lip and palate: A roentgeno-cephalometric study. Cleft Palate Journal 13: 215–237

Huddart A G 1970 Maxillary arch dimensions in bilateral cleft lip and palate subjects. Cleft Palate Journal 7: 139–155

Huddart A G, MacCauley F J, Davies M E H 1969 Maxillary arch dimensions in normal and unilateral cleft palate subjects. Cleft Palate Journal 6: 471–487

Ishiguro K, Krogman W M, Mazaheri M, Harding R L 1976 A longitudinal study of morphological craniofacial patterns via P.A. X-ray head films in cleft patients from birth to 6 years of age. Cleft Palate Journal 13: 104–126

Knox G, Braithwaite F 1963 Cleft lip and palate in Northumberland and Durham. Archives of Disease in Childhood 38: 66–70

Krogman W M, Mazaheri M, Harding R L, Ishiguro K, Bariana G, Meier J, Canter H, Ross P 1975 A longitudinal study of the craniofacial growth pattern in children with clefts as compared to normal, birth to 6 years. Cleft Palate Journal 12: 59–84

Mapes A H, Mazaheri M, Harding R L, Meier J A, Canter H E 1974 A longitudinal analysis of the maxillary growth increments of cleft lip and palate patients. Cleft Palate Journal 11: 450–462

Mazaheri M, Harding R L, Nanda S 1967 The effect of surgery on maxillary growth and cleft width. Plastic and Reconstructive Surgery 40: 22–30

Mazaheri M, Krogman W M, Harding R L, Millard R T, Mehta S 1977 Longitudinal analysis of growth of the soft palate and nasopharynx from 6 months to 6 years. Cleft Palate Journal 14: 52–62

Meskin L H S, Pruzansky S, Gullen W H 1968 An epidemiologic investigation of factors related to the extent of facial clefts. 1 Sex of patient. Cleft Palate Journal 5: 23–29

Mestre J C, deJesus J, Subtelny J D 1960 Unoperated oral clefts at maturation. Angle Orthodontist 30: 78–85

Moss M L 1971 Functional cranial analysis and the functional matrix. In: Patterns of Orofacial Growth and Development. American Speech and Hearing Association reports no. 6, Washington DC

Narula J K, Ross R B 1970 Facial growth in children with complete bilateral cleft lip and palate. Cleft Palate Journal 7: 239–248

Onizuka T, Isshiki Y 1975 Development of the palatal arch in relation to unilateral cleft lip and palate surgery: A comparison of the effects of different surgical approaches. Cleft Palate Journal 12: 444–451

Ortiz-Monasterio F, Rebeil A S, Barrera G, Hoffman H R, Vinageras E 1966 A study of untreated adult cleft palate patients. Plastic and Reconstructive Surgery 38: 36–41

Osbourne H 1966 A serial cephalometric analysis of facial growth in adolescent cleft palate subjects. Angle Orthodontist 36: 211–223

Pitanguy M D, Franco T 1967 Non-operated facial fissure in adults. Plastic and Reconstructive Surgery 39: 569–577

Pruzansky S 1953 Description, classification and analysis of unoperated clefts of the lip and palate. American Journal of Orthodontics 39: 590–611

Robertson N R E, Shaw W C, Volp C 1977 The changes produced by presurgical treatment of bilateral cleft lip and palate. Plastic and Reconstructive Surgery 59: 86–93

Ross R B 1970 The clinical implications of facial growth in cleft lip and palate. Cleft Palate Journal 7: 37–47

Ross R B, Johnston M C 1967 The effect of early orthodontic treatment on facial growth in cleft lip and palate. Cleft Palate Journal 4: 157–164

Shaw W C 1978 Early orthopaedic treatment of unilateral cleft lip and palate. British Journal of Orthodontics 5: 119–132

Stark R B 1968 Mesodermal deficiency as a pathogenic factor in facial anomalies. In: Longacre J J Craniofacial anomalies. Lippincott, Philadelphia

Steigler E J, Berry M F 1958 A new look at the etiology of cleft palate. Plastic and Reconstructive Surgery 21: 52–73

Wada T, Miyazaki T 1975 Growth and changes in maxillary arch form in complete unilateral cleft lip and palate children. Cleft Palate Journal 12: 115–130

8

Speech and language disability

The term 'cleft palate speech' at one time provided a shorthand term which readily evoked a syndrome of speech disability characterized by hypernasal resonance with pharyngeal and glottal realization of many sounds. Faced with such markedly abnormal and even unintelligible utterance it was to be expected that the main focus of attention should have been concentrated on attempts to improve structural and physiological conditions which contributed to this state. Understandably other aspects of speech and language tended to receive scant attention.

In present-day practice only a small proportion of children with cleft palate find their way to speech therapy and, of those who do, a large percentage require remediation for a range of disability which extends beyond that traditionally associated with cleft palate. New techniques of surgery whereby it has become possible to produce effective closure of the velopharyngeal sphincter at an early age are largely responsible for the change in the pattern of the caseload.

As well as including a description of those disorders arising directly from malfunction of the velopharyngeal sphincter, this chapter will consider some of the more recently observed patterns of disability. Any description would, however, be incomplete if it were confined to a discussion of speech and language problems as isolated entities. As cleft palate is almost invariably a congenital condition, the resultant disorder of communication must be considered in the context of the normal processes and sequences of emerging language and must also take into account the backcloth of environmental influence.

SPEECH AND LANGUAGE DEVELOPMENT

There have been few linguistically orientated studies of language development in cleft palate children. Many of the studies reported in the 1950s and 1960s were restricted to items such as mean length of utterance and vocabulary recognition. Similarly, investigations of articulatory behaviour tended to address themselves to the physiological rather than to the phonological aspects of production. Furthermore, many of these studies relied upon a criterion of 'intelligibility', a term usually ill-defined and one which appeared to have considerable dependence on a subjective evaluation.

The search for definitive evidence of delay or deviance directly attributable to the structural condition is influenced by many issues which confuse a straightforward appraisal, so that a direct correspondence cannot be assumed. To begin with, the cleft palate population is a heterogeneous one. Quite apart from the diversity of structural anomalies, in other respects too those with cleft palate are subject to the same variations of intelligence, social and environmental influences as is any growing child. These are all factors which are known to influence the course of language development. Indeed, there are some syndromes of which cleft palate is only one feature, e.g. Klippel-Feil and Treacher-Collins, and in such cases any language disorder may well causally be more directly related to an intellectual deficit rather than to the cleft palate condition.

Another important point is the way in which mother–child interaction may be affected by the condition. Emotional reactions to children born with malformations have been described by Bentovim (1972). In a chapter describing the influence of obstetric circumstances on later development, Stratton (1978) discusses at length a transactional model of mother–child relationship. This relates to the mother's attitude specifically to the preterm infant, but the points made have potentially equal application to the child born with cleft palate. The basis of the thesis is: 'Recognition of the continuing interplay of influences throughout development, such that the child elicits responses from his environment according to his characteristics at the time; the environmental influence will produce a response from the child which may in turn modify his environment and so on.' If by reason of his cleft palate and particularly so if he also has a cleft lip the child evokes a different reaction in the mother, this in turn may produce different behaviour from him. Other points to bear in mind are the different mode of feeding and the currently prevalent practice of consigning babies born with handicapping conditions to special care units during early life. These circumstances may impose constraints upon the growth of close social realationships and also possibly subsequently upon cognitive and linguistic development. Furthermore, because of the handicap, the expectation of the mother with regard to her child's level of language attainment may be different. It has been shown that mothers tend to continue to regard children with congenital handicap as being different long after they have in fact moved towards normality.

Thus speech and language is vulnerable to the influences of attitude and environment and in particular it seems possible that the development of pragmatic aspects of language may be restricted by these conditions.

Evans & Renfrew (1974), in a paper discussing the timing of surgery, cite evidence of the adverse effect on behaviour of children admitted to hospital after the age of 7 months and link this with reported findings that children undergoing cleft palate surgery past the age of 12 months appeared to suffer regression in language development whereas those treated at 6 months developed along normal lines. The implication is that separation at the later age is likely to produce considerable emotional trauma with attendant interruption of language development. A further inference from this study relates to the quality of verbal interaction experienced by the later-treated children both in hospital and at home. Certainly the age between 12 and 18 months is a critical time of linguistic development, and it could be argued that traumatic events, particularly those which involve oral structures, might well in some cases have a bearing on subsequent disability. There is a great need for well-organized evaluative studies which can elucidate more precisely the nature of any delay in speech development.

Among the many variables which need to be considered there is one constant factor common to all children with cleft palate. This is that they all learn to speak in the presence of articulatory organs which differ structurally and possibly physiologically from the norm. However successful the surgical intervention, early oral sensation derived from sucking and feeding will be different. Also, the high incidence of hearing impairment directly associated with the condition even when of a mild degree or of a fluctuating nature leads to the belief that impairment of auditory perception may adversely influence developing speech. Another factor which may influence speech development is the presence of dental and occlusal abnormalities. This is particularly likely where there is also involvement of the alveolus. It is therefore against a setting of these conditions, some inferential as in the case of psychosocial factors, and some, such as structural deviation, established, that speech and language disability has to be discussed.

Phonological development

Certainly there is evidence that phonological as against articulatory disability exists. Ingram (1976) reports on deletion of final consonants, unstressed syllables, and of the reduction of clusters (also reported in many other investigations). These are all maturational features which when they persist give rise to typical patterns of delay. Some studies report inability in making binary contrasts but such difficulties could be articulatory as in the case of, for example, nasal v. oral contrast where failure may be a function of structure and movement. Similarly a stop v. continuant opposition may prove difficult to realize if there is inadequate control of the air stream. Crystal (1980) has noted that where there is deviant realization of voiced/voiceless consonants, each member of the pair may maintain a phonological contrast, using features such as place and manner. Thus as an example he cites [s]–[z] where [s] is realized as a pharyngeal fricative and [z] as a glottal stop.

Syntax

There is also little evidence at syntactic level since most studies predate current methods of analysis. Whitcomb et al (1976) investigated production of language of eight cleft palate children and compared this with that of eight children without language impairment. The developmental sentence scoring protocol was used. Findings indicated depressed scores for the cleft palate group especially in relation to both length and complexity of sentence production.

Faircloth & Faircloth (1972) contended that physiological abnormality may adversely influence syntactic integrity. This conclusion was based on a two-minute sample of spontaneous speech obtained from ten children aged 6 to 11 years with cleft palate. Analysis of the samples indicated an inverse relationship between articulatory precision and syntactic adequacy. That is to say, those children who concentrated on achieving the best possible articulatory patterns often did so at the expense of syntactic complexity, while those who used more elaborate sentence forms sacrificed articulatory accuracy in order to do so. The authors' explanation for this was that in the cleft palate group the physiological set of the oral structures betokens excessive tension which extends to respiration, phonation and resonance. Limitation of inspiration and thus of expiration imposes a restriction on the number of syllables per breath. In an unconscious effort to achieve intelligibility the child may therefore confine himself to syntactically simpler utterances. It is also tempting to conjecture upon the influence of strongly articulatory biased therapy programmes in reinforcing this condition. Again the definition of syntactic complexity is not very clear.

It is likely that such physiological constraints will also produce abnormal prosody, particularly in relation to stress and pause.

The study is an interesting one in that it samples contextual speech, demonstrates the likely effect upon extrasegmental features and also serves as a cautionary warning of the danger of placing undue emphasis on articulatory performance at the expense of expressive language.

Pannbacker (1975), investigating the language skills of a group of adults with repaired clefts of the palate, found that they used shorter responses than normal speakers but that there were no significant differences in syntactic structures nor in vocabulary. Edwards (1974) studied aspects of speech and language in a group of twenty children with repaired cleft palate whose intelligence, hearing and resonance was in the normal range. On the Reynell scales expressive language showed a mean score of -1 SD but within the group there was a wide range of score from -3 SD to $+2$ SD. Interestingly there was a somewhat similar spread of scores in the comprehension scales and a high correlation between the two measures ($P=0.001$). The Reynell expressive language scale yields little information about the type of syntactic structures the child employs, but gives overall useful data on his ability to use language.

Subsequent analysis using LARSP procedure of three recorded samples of lower scores indicated a pattern of delay rather than of deviant production. This was evidenced by a preponderance of less complicated, two- and three-element stages, e.g. 'Him bad. It big book. Mum see me. Ride bike,' thus substantiating other studies cited. But apart from a small range of specific articulatory defects not related to resonance these children did not have to contend with the problems encountered by those in the Faircloth study. The argument that syntactic complexity is sacrificed in the cause of syllabic integrity would not therefore apply here.

At the present time there is no very effective method by which this concept of 'Language in use' can be evaluated. Yet its importance is surely unchallenged since the need to convey meaning is one of the prime functions of communication, and the other levels which we analyse are means towards achieving this end.

ARTICULATORY DEFECTS

Reference has been made to the persisting pattern of maturationally earlier phonology found in children with cleft palate. In one respect, however, there is a marked deviation from the developmental hierarchy. This is manifest in the tendency towards backward displacement of production of some anterior sounds. A partial explanation can be found in the compensatory movement of pharyngeal imbalance (coupling deficiency). This posterior displacement of the body of the tongue has been reported (Westlake 1967; Morley 1970), as has evidence demonstrating diminished use of the tongue tip. Lawrence and Philips (1975) demonstrated, by means of telefluoroscopic recording, deviant lingual contact in a group of cleft palate subjects. Their findings indicated a significant relationship between defects of resonance and deviant lingual contact. That is to say, those subjects with inadequate velopharyngeal closure and with hypernasal resonance, resorted more frequently to posterior displacement of the tongue. The relationship of tongue position to defects of resonance and phonation will be discussed in more detail later in this chapter.

Edwards (1974), in a study of language skills in children aged 4 to 6 with repaired cleft palates (groups II and III, Kernahan & Stark), delineated a group with a characteristic pattern of articulatory disorder. From an initial number of 38, 20 were selected for further study. On the Edinburgh Articulation Test they had a mean score of 77 (between 1 and 2 SD below the norm). A qualitative analysis revealed no features of immaturity and all the deviant realizations fell into the atypical category.

The subjects demonstrated some, or all, of the following realizations:

$$[t] \rightarrow [ʕ]$$
$$[d] \rightarrow [ʝ]$$
$$[S] \rightarrow [ʕ][ɬ]$$
$$[tʃ] \rightarrow [tɬ]$$
$$[dʒ] \rightarrow [d̥ɬ]$$

Placement for all these phonemes involved the tongue tip remaining behind the lower incisor teeth and the front and body of the tongue being raised towards the palate. The voice/voiceless contrast was appropriate but in the realization of plosives there was an error of manner (friction v. stop) and of place.

Lateral realization of [s] has been reported in other studies, particularly in the presence of dental malocclusion, notably Angle Class III and certainly 75 per cent of the group had this occlusal pattern. Palatal realization of alveolar stops does not, however, appear to be related to this. Obviously the question of diminished sensation in the alveolar region resulting from the presence of scar tissue is another factor to be considered. This same pattern of articulation had, however, been observed in two cases not included in the study, where the cleft did not extend to the alveolus. Hochberg & Kabcenall (1967), in their study of oral discrimination in subjects with cleft palate, found no significant difference in scores either with or without a prosthesis. This reinforces the evidence from other studies (Dixon 1962; Hardcastle 1976) that the tongue tip is the area of most prolific sensory endowment.

Morley (1970) also drew attention to this characteristic and discussed possible reasons. Evidence that abnormal patterns of tongue carriage are prenatally determined is conflicting and thus inconclusive. A consensus of views appears to favour the possibility that this posterior displacement derives from early sensorimotor patterning related to abnormal sucking and feeding. The baby with an unoperated cleft is required to adopt compensatory tongue movements in order to effect the negative pressure within the oral cavity which is necessary for the channelling of food. These negative functions impose kinaesthetic 'blueprints' which are established at an early age and which may at a later stage influence the range of babbling patterns. Attention has been drawn by investigators to the paucity of front sounds in the babbling repertoire of infants with cleft palate. Olsen (1965), in a study of babbling, compared the distribution of consonants in normal and cleft palate infants aged between 5 and 12 months. The repertoire of the normally developing infant was much wider by comparison and in particular with reference to inclusion of anteriorly produced consonants.

Cleft palate infants: ʔ h fi m w n
Normal infants: ʔ h k b t d n m z

It would be interesting to know whether the early use of feeding plates has any influence on subsequent patterns of babbling. At the present time the writer is unaware of any published studies, though anecdotal evidence appears to indicate that children who are fitted with feeding appliances soon after birth are less likely to have articulatory problems later on. This evidence is, however, too imprecise for any definite conclusions to be drawn, and a properly controlled study taking into account the multiplicity of variables impinging upon language development is needed.

The role of tactile and proprioceptive feedback in relation to speech development has until recently been a relatively neglected area of study, the focus of attention having been largely auditorily biased. The general view is that auditory feedback has primacy of place in relation to development of speech and language and that tactile and proprioceptive feedback is responsible for the maintenance of speech (for conflicting view see Liberman et al 1967). Hardcastle (1976), discussing sensory feedback in speech production, described the role of tactile feedback as one which provides information *after* the event while the proprioceptive system gives an ongoing account *during* the event. Additionally, facilitation of the monitoring process through a *predictive* function is suggested. This priming aspect of speech control has been described comprehensively by Lashley (1951) in a classic paper on seriation. Because of the rapidity of movement involved in ongoing articulation, it is likely that some type of individual schema (neural correlate of movement) is laid down against which rapid comparison and necessary modification can take place. Such a schema would be the product of synthesis of all principal sensory systems, auditory, visual and proprioceptive.

There have been many investigations into the part played by proprioception (in this context the term is taken to be synonymous with kinaesthesis) in the monitoring of speech and deviations in articulatory patterns comparable to those seen in patients with cleft palate have been observed. Many studies have been based on the artificial interruption of tactile and proprioceptive feedback by oral anaesthesia (Bosma 1967, 1970). Gammon et al (1971) attempted to evaluate the relative importance of auditory and proprioceptive feedback in speech by an experiment in which they differentially masked the auditory and tactile proprioceptive channels. In both conditions there were marked misarticulations. Interruption of auditory feedback produced changes in prosodic features and in vowel production, while oral anaesthesia resulted in changes in articulation of consonants, notably in a trend towards backward displacement of sounds normally produced anteriorly. These characteristics are sometimes heard in the speech of those with acquired deafness, who presumably rely heavily on proprioceptive monitoring.

Table 2.3 (p. 25) illustrates either a growing trend or a growing awareness of a trend towards the pattern of articulation described in the study by Edwards (1974). Anterior realizations of [s] which might represent immaturities remain more or less constant (1.6 per cent, 2.5 per cent). There is a marked increase in the incidence of medial realization (3.3 per cent, 52 per cent) and a decrease in posterior (i.e. glottal and pharyngeal) realizations (78 per cent, 17 per cent).

Such compelling evidence of changes in pattern gives rise to questions as to possible reasons. Undoubtedly one answer may be found in the major advance in surgical techniques. Whereas historically the main focus of attention was on the structural aspects of surgery—that is, the closure of the palate, with physiological efficiency as a secondary factor—the dynamics of the velopharyngeal sphincter are now a matter of prime concern to most teams operating on cleft palates. The improved understanding of the interrelationship of different factors in the vocal tract which contribute to acceptable speech has been brought about in part by new methods of study. No longer is it sufficient to rely upon an open mouth, a tongue depressor and production of 'Ah' to determine future course of action. The advent and use of lateral cine- and videoradiography, then of nasal endoscopy and of multiview video fluoroscopy have provided workers with much valuable additional information. A fuller account of the methods of assessment which have brought about this change are discussed elsewhere in this book (Chapter 15).

Another type of assessment of oral sensation is that relating to stereognosis. This is the ability to differentiate between different shapes and textures, in this case orally. Surprisingly few studies have been carried out on subjects with cleft palate, and this may in part be due to the fact that most of the North American literature has concentrated on problems of resonance and articulation as they are related to velopharyngeal dysfunction. Edwards (1974) included a test of oral form recognition in her cleft palate study. This was based on the forms used by Hochberg and Kabcenall which differed either in shape or texture. Instead of visual to oral matching, however, which is dependent on cross-model coding, discrimination was based upon recognition on a 'same/different' basis. The cleft palate subjects showed significantly poorer ability in this task when compared with a matched group of normal speakers. However, these results are somewhat inconclusive. Because the group was young (age 4 to 6 years) the number of trials was limited to ensure that the response did not become random through fatigue and boredom. It appears that this is a skill which improves with age and some investigators would for this reason exclude children under the age of 6. A pilot study carried out on 20 normal 4- to 6-year-olds, however, indicated that they were able to manage this task adequately.

Impaired ability in carrying out rapid alternating movement of the articulatory organs is a characteristic feature of dyspraxic-type disorders. Fletcher (1978), in his study of Alabama children with cleft palate, assessed diadochokinesis. This was based on the rate of production of five syllables [pʌ][fʌ][lʌ][tʌ][kʌ], and of four different syllable combinations [pʌtə][pʌkə][tʌkə]. Of the sample ($n=70$) 18.6 per cent failed to produce the syllables in rapid repetition. There was a hierarchy of difficulty, with the trisyllable pʌtʌkə being failed most frequently. All failures related to production of lingual plosive sounds. When times for production were compared with those of a control group the cleft palate subjects were consistently slower. Discussing the study, Fletcher noted that in no case was the production of the bilabial syllable pə affected, thus ruling out the question of velopharyngeal insufficiency. Production was at a normal rate when no lingual activity was involved. The suggestion is made that these results appear to reflect some degree of reduction in tongue function, an observation already made with reference to the Hochberg and Kabcenall study, when subjects' performance in oral recognition did not appear to be affected by the presence of a prothesis.

Dentition and occlusion

Studies of the possible effect on speech of defects of dentition in the non-cleft palate population indicate that most people are capable of achieving acoustically acceptable speech through compensatory strategies. A cleft of the palate involving the alveolus may, however, contribute to articulatory defects. The presence of palatal, or supernumerary teeth or of markedly rotated upper dentition may restrict tongue movement. Such conditions are likely to be temporary and are usually remedied by orthodontic treatment.

Commonly there is a disparate relationship between the maxillary arches and mandibular arches. Failure of maxillary growth, collapse of the maxillary arches or hyperplasia of the mandible will produce a Class III Angle occlusal pattern and is often associated with a lateral open bite. The most vulnerable consonants are then [ʃ][ʒ][ʧ] and [ʤ] together with /s/ clusters. Foster & Greene (1960) demonstrated a significant relationship between /s/ realized laterally and collapsed maxillary arch in a group of cleft palate children. This pattern of misarticulation reflects the rank order of frequency of defect in speech disorders in the cleft palate population. It involves sounds which require a considerable degree of fine neuromuscular co-ordination and also high intra-oral pressure. Thus these patients are 'at risk' from several sources.

Where there is hypoplasia of the mandible, as for example in the Pierre Robin syndrome, there may well be restriction of tongue movement. If the arch disproportion is marked, difficulty may be experienced in bilabial closure and /p//b//m/ will be realized more readily by labiodental approximation. Because of the abnormal occlusion, difficulty may also occur with alveolar stops /t//d/ and these will be realized either as dental or palatal stops [t̪, d̪] [ʈ, ɖ] or even [c, ɟ].

It is very rarely that a repaired cleft of the lip has any direct effect on speech production. Factors which might impair ability to round and stretch the lips would be scarring and limitation of tissue, but in the younger population these conditions are seldom encountered.

HEARING IMPAIRMENT

More detailed discussion of this takes place elsewhere in this book (Chapter

9) and here it is referred to passim as a possible aetiological factor in articulatory defect. It cannot be stressed too strongly that all children with cleft palate and associated speech disability should have a full audiological investigation as a routine measure. It has been the practice in many cases to offer a screening test on a once-off basis, and where evidence of hearing loss above 20 dB has not been found no further action has been recommended. Such a procedure is not adequate. Mainly because of Eustachian tube anomalies, hearing loss in cleft palate children is most commonly of the conductive type and is subject to fluctuation particularly where there is evidence of upper respiratory infection. A slight overall loss or, even more so, a variable or intermittent loss, is likely to have a deleterious effect upon developing speech, since the child will have no stable model against which adequate comparison for discriminatory purposes can be made. Walton (1973), reporting on audiometric screening procedures, cited the findings on threshold audiometric data for 93 school-age children with clefts of the palate. Of these, 61 per cent would have passed conventional screening tests; yet, of these, approximately 50 per cent were found to have conductive hearing loss and otoscopic abnormalities. Heed should also be given to the possible co-existence of sensorineural impairment.

DISORDERS OF RESONANCE

The most common manifestation of deviant resonance is perceived hypernasality. Less commonly hyponasal resonance may be a feature of disorder associated with cleft palate. This appears in many cases to be related to the outcome of secondary surgical procedures, as, for example, when pharyngeal flaps occlude the nasopharynx, though it may also arise from structural anomalies of the nasal septum. An anterior occlusion of this type gives rise to cul-de-sac resonance (mixed hyper- and hyponasality).

Velopharyngeal function has been one of the central themes of North American research for many years and this has yielded interesting data. Fritzell's (1969) comprehensive study of the velopharyngeal muscles in speech has also provided valuable normative data. As a result, it is now widely accepted that an efficient velopharyngeal valve depends on many other factors as well as the ability of the soft palate to elevate, move back and make contact with the posterior pharyngeal wall. Advances in instrumentation have served to emphasize the three-dimensional nature of velopharyngeal function. Thus closure is seen as a result of sphincteric action in which posterior *and* lateral walls of the pharynx play an active part in synchrony with the soft palate. The sphincteric nature of the activity cannot be gauged by techniques of oral examination, since much of the activity takes place above the level of the mouth in the epipharynx. Furthermore, an evaluation based on lateral cine- or videoradiography alone provides information only about anteroposterior relationships and tells nothing of the nature of the mesial shelving movement of the lateral pharyngeal walls.

For speech therapists, these techniques of evaluation have far-reaching implication in remedial work. This is not to say that evidence of ears and eyes should be unheeded. Perception can indicate *what* the abnormal factors are, but not *why* they may be abnormal. A telling example is the case of a child in whom

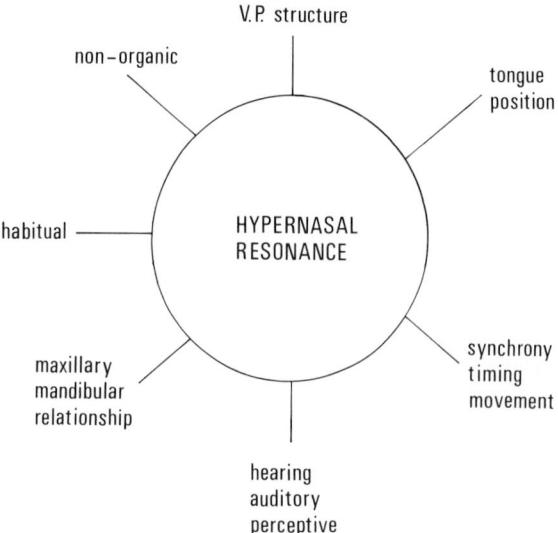

Fig. 8.1 Hypernasal resonance

nasality was perceived but where lateral cineradiography showed what appeared to be adequate closure. Continued speech therapy had produced disappointingly little improvement and increasing frustration and diminishing motivation. Nasendoscopy demonstrated that closure was incomplete, that there was little movement of the lateral pharyngeal walls with resultant guttering. In such a case, surgical procedure was the only means whereby amelioration could be expected.

Saxman (1972) differentiates between hypernasality which is the direct result of velopharyngeal insufficiency and that which is indirectly related to it. This seems to be an important distinction since it may account in some measure for a small percentage of cases who fail to improve following apparently successful surgery.

Hypernasality, which is related directly to faulty velopharyngeal function, is associated with markedly reduced intra-oral pressure and is frequently accompanied by audible nasal emission of air. It is consistent throughout speech production and is not subject to great fluctuation. Such conditions are the result of velopharyngeal incompetence, and this can be assessed qualitatively by techniques to which reference has been made. For these conditions surgery is indicated.

Hypernasality arising as an indirect result of velopharyngeal malfunction can be related to a number of factors. These include: defects of oronasal coupling; deviate placement of tongue; timing of velopharyngeal closure.

Defects of nasal coupling
In normal speakers there is a balance between oral and nasal resonance which is connected with the relative dimensions of the oro and nasal pharynx. Where this balance is not maintained, resulting speech will be perceived as either more or less 'nasal' in quality. There is a range in degree of acceptable quality. This

type of nasality differs from that arising from velopharyngeal insufficiency and is probably acoustically determined by a particular configuration and relationship of muscle tension in the pharyngeal walls which is conducive to the reinforcement of higher frequency harmonics (Counihan 1971). Studies have demonstrated a high incidence of increased dimensions of the nasopharynx in cleft palate subjects even following repair. This may, however, lessen with maturation.

Deviate placement of tongue

The relationship between articulation and nasality has already been commented upon. Moore and Sommers (1975) studied correspondence between various phonetic contexts and perceived nasality. Their findings suggested that an interaction between tongue height and lateral wall movement may be related to increased nasality. Tongue positioning in cleft palate is to some extent influenced by the need to adopt compensatory posture to produce efficient valving. The typical at rest position therefore is one where the tongue tip lies behind the lower incisors while the back is retracted and raised towards the soft palate. These two conditions, viz. the abnormal tongue positioning together with associated tension, affect the position of the larynx.

Timing of velopharyngeal closure

The temporal sequence of movements is a critical factor in the co-ordination of velopharyngeal movement. Seriation of neuromuscular activity is vital to effective organization of behaviour and in particular to the effective production of speech. Lashley's (1951) paper, in which this theory was propounded, postulated a selector and a programming function which ensures the correct sequence and timing of neural commands. An impairment or failure of this mechanism may explain the pattern of disorder characteristic of one type of articulatory dyspraxia. It is interesting to note the clinical example of a 4-year-old child with a dyspraxic-type disorder involving palatal function for speech who sounded exactly like a child with cleft palate, the principal differences being the variability of the condition and the evidence of normal vegetative function. Electromyographic studies (Fritzell 1969) may, if taken together with nasopharyngoscopy, be a fruitful source of more precise information on this important aspect in future research.

Other factors not directly related to velopharyngeal function, although coexisting, are hearing loss and maxillary/mandibular relationships and presence of anterior fistulae. Appropriate velopharyngeal closure is to some extent monitored by auditory feedback. A characteristic of speech in those with impaired hearing ability is hypernasal resonance, and there was evidence of this in a videotape demonstrating nasal endoscopy (Piggott & Makepeace 1974) when palatopharyngeal malfunction was demonstrated in the case of a deaf subject without cleft of the palate. The fluctuating type of hearing loss suffered by a significant number of children with cleft palate must make absolute discrimination between nasal and non-nasal contrasts somewhat difficult, even more so when taken in conjunction with an already less than perfect mechanism for effecting this.

Stengelhofen (personal communication) states that the size of the anterior fistula does not appear to relate to the degree of hypernasality. Improvement in speech is noted in some cases following closure by obturator, but other factors relating, for example, to tongue movement need to be taken into account. The fitting of an obturator is recommended as a diagnostic procedure.

Hypernasality arising from other conditions

Many therapists have experience of seeing patients who present with severe hypernasal resonance and yet whose soft palate musculature appears to be intact and functioning normally. In these cases other possibilities need to be considered. The first is to consider where there may be a submucous cleft; the second is through multiview fluoroscopy to determine that there is no anomaly of the musculus uvulae. To some extent such an anomaly may be regarded as a variation of the sub-mucous cleft condition. This muscle has for long been considered as playing a somewhat insignificant and passive role contributing to velopharyngeal closure. In support of this view, it was said that, in olden days, the uvula was removed with the tonsils as a possible seat of infection with no deleterious effects on speech. Recent studies ascribe to this muscle a far more active function: a series of cases reported by Shprintzen (1979) have demonstrated that even apparently minor deviations in its structure can result in disorders of resonance, which might otherwise be labelled as of 'non-organic origin'. Thirdly, there is a need to establish that there is no hearing impairment.

There are also many neuropathological conditions which affect resonance; indeed, this symptom is one of the early indications of myasthenia gravis and therefore the possibility of some type of neuropathology may need to be considered, as may the results of traumatic interruption of the nerve supply to the palate. Adenoidectomy may result in increased nasality, although normally this is a transient state. It is only when differential diagnoses such as these have been convincingly eliminated, however, that the clinician is justified in seeking a non-organic explanation for this condition. A detailed consideration of these aspects lies outside the scope of this book.

Phonation

The presence of dysphonia can easily be overlooked when there are overriding defects of resonance and articulation. Indeed, it is often difficult to differentiate between those problems arising from laryngeal dysfunction and those which have their origin in velopharyngeal incompetence. To attempt to so do is, however, important because of the somewhat different focus of attention for remediation. Frequently the two conditions co-occur, the dysphonia being the outcome of compensatory efforts to overcome the hypernasality.

The presence of an aspirate type of disorder should be considered. Here the voice is weak and breathy. It may be a habitual reaction adopted to minimize nasality, and ironically its encouragement may even be part of the speech therapy procedure as a strategy adopted by the clinician to eliminate glottal realizations. As perceived nasality increases with intensity, the encouragement of a soft breathy voice may also give the illusion of diminished nasality.

Dysphonia may be the result of different reactions to the velopharyngeal insufficiency. Because there is a reduction in overall vocal intensity efforts to compensate for this may involve either increase in subglottic pressure or changes in synchrony of movement of laryngeal muscles. Alternatively it has been suggested that raised tongue posture produces elevation of the larynx through the action of the hyoid. This is seen as a means of valving to overcome nasal escape of air. Whatever forces operate, there is additional strain on the vocal cords sufficient to produce pathological changes in some cases. McWilliams et al (1969), in a study of children with cleft palate, found that out of 32 with accompanying hoarseness 27 had vocal nodules. A follow-up study five years later showed that 70 per cent of the cases still had some abnormality of vocal cords. Maturation must be taken into account when assessing phonation of young children. The voice is developing and is influenced by changing structure and function of the vocal tract. A longitudinal study reported in 1977 (Mazaheri et al 1977) discussed the earliest age at which secondary surgery should be carried out. It concluded that since improvement in all aspects of speech, including voice quality, is aided by maturation, secondary procedures such as pharyngoplasty are not recommended before the age of 6 years.

This chapter has looked at some of the speech and language difficulties which occur in the condition of cleft palate and in particular it has described these in the context of recent research in the fields of neurophysiology, linguistics and of social psychology.

REFERENCES

Bentovim A 1972 Handicapped preschool children and their families. British Medical Journal 3: 579–581, 634–637

Bosma J F (ed) 1967 First symposium on oral sensation and perception. Thomas, Springfield, Illinois

Bosma J F (ed) 1970 Third symposium on oral sensation and perception. Thomas, Springfield, Illinois

Counihan D T 1971 In:Grabb W C, Rosenstein S W, Bzoch K R (eds) Cleft lip and palate. Little Brown, Boston

Crystal D 1980 Clinical linguistics and phonetics. Springer, Berlin

Dixon D A 1962 Sensory nerve terminations in the oral mucosa. Archives of Oral Biology 7: 38–48

Edwards M 1974 Perceptual processes underlying speech. Unpublished MPhil thesis, University of Aston in Birmingham

Evans D, Renfrew C E 1974 The timing of primary cleft palate repair. Scandinavian Journal of Plastic and Reconstructive Surgery 8: 153–155

Faircloth S R, Faircloth M A 1972 Delayed language and linguistic variations. In: Grabb W C, Rosenstein S W, Bzoch K R (eds) Cleft lip and palate. Little Brown, Boston

Fletcher S G 1978 Diagnosing speech disorders from cleft palate. Grune & Stratton, London

Foster T D and Greene M C L 1960 Lateral speech defects and dental irregularities in cleft palate. British Journal of Plastic Surgery XII 4: 367–377

Fritzell B 1969 The velopharyngeal muscles in speech. Acta Otolaryngologica Suppl 250

Gammon S A, Smith P J, Daniloff R G, Kim C W 1971 Articulation and stress juncture production under oral anaesthetization and masking. Journal of Speech and Hearing Research 14: 271–282

Hardcastle W J 1976 Physiology of speech production. Academic Press, New York and London

Hochberg I, Kabcenall J 1967 Oral stereognosis in normal and cleft palate individuals. Cleft Palate Journal 4: 47–57

Ingram D 1976 Current issues in child phonology in normal and deficient child language. Morehead D, Morehead A (eds). University Park Press 3: 27

Lashley K S 1951 The problem of serial order in behaviour. In: Jeffress L A (ed) Cerebral mechanisms in behaviour. Wiley, New York

Lawrence C A, Philips B J 1975 A telefluoroscopic study of lingual contacts made by persons with palatal defects. Cleft Palate Journal 12: 85–94

Liberman A M, Cooper F S, Shankweiler D P, Studdert-Kennedy M 1967 Perception of the speech code. Psychological Review 74: 431–461

Mazaheri M, Krogman W M, Harding R L, Riski J L 1977 Pattern of Velopharyngeal growth in cleft palate patients with or without pharyngeal flaps. Proceedings of third international congress on cleft palate and related craniofacial anomalies, Toronto

McWilliams B J, Bluestone C D, Musgrave R H 1969 Diagnostic implications of vocal cord nodules in children with cleft palate. Laryngoscope 79

Moore W H, Sommers R K 1975 Phonetic contexts: Their effects on perceived intelligibility in cleft palate speakers. Folia Phoniatrica 27: 410–422

Morley M E 1970 Cleft palate and speech. Churchill Livingstone, Edinburgh, 7th edn

Olsen D A 1965 PhD dissertation, North Western University. Quoted in Westlake 1967

Pannbacker M 1975 Oral language skills of cleft palate speakers. Cleft Palate Journal 12: 95–106

Pigott R W, Makepeace A P W 1974 Videotape nasal endoscopy. Frenchay Hospital, Bristol

Saxman J H 1972 A call for new directions in cleft palate research. Cleft Palate Journal 9: 274–279

Shprintzen R J 1979 Velopharyngeal insufficiency in the absence of overt or submucous cleft palate. Palatoglossal malfunction. R E Ellis, F C Flack (eds) College of Speech Therapists, London

Stratton P M 1978 Criteria for assessing the influence of obstetric circumstances on later development. In: Benefits and hazards of the new obstetrics clinics in dev. medicine 64. Heinemann

Walton W K 1973 Audiometrically 'normal' conductive hearing losses among the cleft palate. Cleft Palate Journal 10: 99–103

Whitcomb L, Ochsner G, Wayte R A 1976 Comparison of expressive skills of cleft palate and non cleft palate children. Journal Oklahoma speech and hearing association 3: 25–28

9

Associated conditions

INTRODUCTION

The impact of clefts of the lip and palate on the child and his/her family has been extensively studied and documented. Evidence of the fact that cleft palate constitutes more than a facial anomaly has changed greatly over time from that of survival to the involvement of a countless number of pervasive associated conditions. The growth and application of the interdisciplinary approach in the management of the individual with cleft palate has provided a corresponding growth of knowledge and perception of the variety of problems inherent in the condition. Advances in the technology of habilitation have produced a tremendous output of research and clinical studies describing the incidence, classification, symptoms and management of conditions associated with clefting. In essence, the area of conditions associated with clefts of the lip and palate is vast and the subject matter is further confused by differences in research and clinical methodology. The purpose of this chapter will be to provide a summary overview of associated conditions of cleft lip and cleft palate reported in the recent literature and will cover the most commonly associated problems including: (1) hearing loss, (2) submucous cleft palate, (3) bifid uvula, and (4) syndromes associated with clefting.

HEARING LOSS

In any discussion of the types and kinds of associated conditions inherent in clefts of the lip and palate the most universal is bilateral conductive hearing loss and middle ear disease. Historically reports of the incidence of hearing loss in the cleft palate population have ranged from 0 per cent (Goetzinger et al 1960) to 90 per cent as reported by Sataloff & Fraser (1952). The presence of middle ear disease with attendant hearing loss in children is well documented and summarized by Nober (1968) and Bluestone (1971). Most of these studies reporting on the incidence of hearing loss were done with children over 3 years of age. In a pioneer and widely quoted study, Skolnik (1958) was among one of the first to report on the incidence of hearing loss in children according to age. He found 6 per cent conductive loss in infants under 1 year of age, 27 per cent in the 1- to 4-year age group and 67 per cent in the group from 5 to 13 years. Of the total group of 401 children he found only five with sensorineural loss. For a number of years the problem of hearing loss in children, stemming in part from Skolnik's study, was considered to be a condition of early and middle childhood. It was not until 1967 that Stool & Randall reported their finding of middle ear disease in infants with cleft palate under 1 year of age. They examined the tympanic membranes and middle ears bilaterally of 25 infants ranging in age from 9 days to 12 months using a binocular operating microscope with magnification. They found mucoid material (middle ear fluid) in 94 per cent (47 of 50 ears), and 10 biopsy specimens revealed the presence of granulation tissue suggesting that the process may have taken place *in utero*. At about the same time Paradise & Bluestone (1969) began their series of studies with infants. They examined 69 infants with cleft palate 24 months of age or younger using a standard diagnostic otoscope. Of this group 16 were 1 month of age or less and 20 were 2 to 3 months old. They found that only six of the 138 middle ears were normal and within a short time these became diseased. In another study, Paradise et al (1969) examined 50 infants with cleft palate and found evidence of bilateral otitis media in 47 of the 50 children. Within two months, four of the initially normal ears had become diseased. On the basis of these findings, the authors concluded that few, if any, infants with cleft palate can long remain free of significant middle ear disease. Furthermore, they indicated that it seems reasonable to assume that otitis media develops quite early in most, if not all, infants with cleft palate and that it probably develops within the first month of life.

The discovery that middle ear effusion is almost invariably present in the infant with cleft palate suggests that the disease process begins very early in life. Middle ear effusion is defined as sterile fluid in the middle ear, whereas there is no evidence of mucous or other fluid in the normal newborn. Middle ear effusion has many names, including serous otitis media, secretory otitis media, glue ear, mucoid ear, middle ear catarrh, tubotympanitis, allergic otitis media and others (Greydanus et al 1977). The presence of middle ear disease found in all ages of children with cleft palate under 24 months of age suggests that spontaneous resolution rarely occurs. Glassock (1971) has indicated that prolonged middle ear effusion may cause permanent damage to the middle ear mechanism and may result in sensorineural as well as conductive loss. Many causes of middle ear effusion have been proposed and the most commonly ascribed to the population of individuals with cleft palate is dysfunction of the muscles controlling the Eustachian tube. Inability to move foreign particles from the nasopharynx and difficulty in equilibrating pressure changes have also been demonstrated by X-ray and air-flow studies. Soudijn & Huffstadt (1975) report a somewhat different cause in a group of children they examined ranging in age from $2\frac{1}{2}$ to 19 months. These authors suggest that in infants with cleft palate the Eustachian tube has never opened and therefore air has never entered the tympanic cavity. They state that the fluid in the middle ear was present before the child was born and because of the malfunction of the Eustachian tube the fluid cannot be discharged into the nasopharynx.

In an attempt to evaluate the status of the nasopharynx, Eustachian tube and middle ear mastoid areas of infants with cleft palate, a number of investigators have conducted roentgenographic investigations using radio-opaque contrast material and fluoroscopy. Bluestone's (1971) roentgenographic findings support the hypothesis, proposed by Holborow (1962), that the Eustachian tube dysfunction of infants with cleft palate consists of inability of the nasopharyngeal end of the tube to open actively. If the Eustachian tube fails to open, the middle ear cannot be adequately aerated, and fluid usually accumulates in it. Bluestone concluded that the nasopharyngeal orifice of the Eustachian tube in infants with cleft palate appears to act as a 'flutter valve'. Fluid and air are able to clear passively but the orifice must open actively to allow flow of the liquid. Since opening results from contraction of the tensor palati muscle, its failure to function effectively must be integrally involved in the Eustachian tube obstruction of infants with cleft palate.

In 1972, Bluestone et al conducted a roentgenographic study of the Eustachian tube in infants and children with cleft palate ranging in age from 7 days to 8 years. Their population consisted of children with unrepaired cleft palates, children with normal palates who had received a myringotomy with fluid aspiration and tympanostomy tube insertion because of chronic or recurrent secretory otitis media, and children who served as controls with normal palates and middle ears and no history of middle ear disease. In the control group the Eustachian orifice was observed to open with every swallow. By contrast, in the children with unrepaired cleft palates, the nasopharyngeal orifice of the Eustachian tube failed to open on swallowing. In the group of children with normal palates who had previously had middle ear disease and whose middle ears were intubated and aerated, obstruction of the Eustachian tube occurred in slightly fewer than half the cases. Although abnormal Eustachian tube function occurred in association with middle ear disease in infants and children with both cleft and normal palates the type of abnormality appeared different in the two groups. Those children with cleft palate invariably demonstrated obstruction at the nasopharyngeal end of the Eustachian tube, but the obstruction was of a one-way 'functional' type. In those children with normal palates, if they had obstruction at all, they tended to have roentgenographic findings compatible with two-way 'mechanical' obstruction.

Another cause of middle ear effusion studied by Bluestone et al (1975) dealt with Eustachian tube ventilatory function in relation to cleft palate. They examined infants with unrepaired clefts of the palate, children with repaired palatal clefts, and children and adults with normal palates who had sustained traumatic perforation of the tympanic membranes but who otherwise had negative otologic histories. They found that the Eustachian tubes of the children with unrepaired clefts appeared more pliant than in those with repaired palates, and that theirs in turn appeared more pliant than those of the persons with normal palates. The authors indicate that their findings suggest abnormal auditory tube distensibility. The apparent superiority in tube function observed in the children with repaired palates might therefore be related to an increase in overall tubal stiffness, alteration in muscle vectors, or both.

Although the literature indicates a high incidence of otitis media during the first two years of life in infants with cleft palate, palatal repair appears to result in significant improvements in middle ear status in most children. Several studies have indicated that this may be one of the benefits of early corrective surgery (Bluestone et al 1972; Bluestone et al 1975; Gerwat 1975; Yules 1975).

Although Eustachian tube function improves with surgical correction of the palate the question of the role of craniofacial growth in the alleviation of middle ear disease has not yet been fully answered. Several studies have indicated that in many children Eustachian tube function improves with age regardless of soft palate closure. Maue-Dickson (1977) reports that recent studies have shown that by 5 years of age, middle ear fluid is no more common in cleft palate or hearing impaired groups than it is in normal groups. Cole & Cole (1974) reported normal Eustachian tubes in cleft palate patients and that poor Eustachian tube function is not characteristic of cleft palate in the young adult age group. Möller (1975) reports that of a total of 113 children evaluated over time the otologic picture had changed from birth when 100 per cent had otopathologic findings to 50 per cent in the 6-year age group, and that serous otitis media decreased from 19 per cent in the 6-year-old group to 6 per cent in the 15-year-old group. To date, present knowledge concerning the reasons for the decrease of middle ear effusions remains unclear. Despite the fact that some studies cite the benefits of corrective surgery, none of these studies rules out the possibility that cranio-facial growth may be an important consideration and that spontaneous improvement may occur even without corrective surgery (Maue-Dickson 1977).

The treatment of middle ear effusions in individuals with cleft palate presents an area marked with some controversy. Two of the most common treatment methods include decongestants and myringotomy and tympanostomy (Paradise et al 1969; Bluestone 1971; Paradise & Bluestone 1974; Yules 1975; Crysdale 1976). The theory behind the use of decongestants, either local or systemic, is that they will establish Eustachian tube drainage. The use of decongestants has, however, produced generally poor results in the cleft palate population (Yules 1975). The consensus opinion of most otologists is that tonsillectomy and/or adenoidectomy, often employed for serous effusions in the non-cleft population, is contraindicated for individuals with cleft palate. The single and most common procedure currently used is myringotomy and/or middle ear ventilating tubes. A great many variations concerning the shape, type of material and point of insertion have been made since the concept of ventilating tubes was published by Armstrong in 1954. One of the problems with the tubes is that they are not easily retained and repeated insertions are necessary, usually for a period of years. Some studies have reported significant complications associated with the use of ventilating tubes. Paradise & Bluestone (1974) found that purulent otorrhea occurred in 68 per cent of infants with cleft palate after tube insertion. Crysdale (1976) found otorrhea in four of 57 of his patients with cleft palate. He also noted that more serious complications such as persistent perforations, tympanoclerosis and cholesteatoma also occurred but were less frequent. In an appraisal of the use of ventilating tubes, Crysdale states that the usual mild hearing loss associated with middle ear effusion prior to palatal surgery does not by itself justify ventilation tube surgery.

SUBMUCOUS CLEFT PALATE

The term submucous cleft palate (SMCP) was first coined by Kelly in 1910. In 1954 Calnan described what have come to be known as the three classic features of overt SMCP, namely (1) bifid uvula, (2) palatal muscle diastasis and (3) bony notch of the hard palate. The overt physical signs of an underlying anatomic abnormality include insertion of the levator and other palate muscles onto the hard palate instead of forming a sling across the mid-line. As a result of the muscle malposition, velar function may be abnormal and velopharyngeal incompetence may result (Kaplan 1975). The often unnoticed SMCP has been studied by plastic surgeons yet the true incidence, natural history and patho-physiology of the condition is not well known (Beeden 1972; Stewart et al 1971; Weatherley-White et al 1972).

Submucous cleft palate in itself tends to be relatively asymptomatic with re-spect to abnormal speech and nasal regurgitation (Bergstrom & Hemenway 1971). The diagnosis of SMCP is not usually straightforward because muscle divarication may not be extensive, the length of the palate may be adequate in spite of the lack of muscle, and there may be sufficient pharyngeal wall mobility to close off the nasopharynx. These factors may account for the small incidence of speech problems particularly if the individual has not had an adenoidectomy and/or tonsillectomy. Furthermore, although a bifid uvula is present in almost all cases of SMCP, clinical examination, even under anaes-thetic, may be misleading (Beeden 1972). In order to determine the incidence of SMCP Stewart et al (1971) were among the first to study a random population for this defect. Of a total of 10 836 school children examined the authors found nine children with previously undiagnosed SMCP, an incidence of 1 : 1200. Six of the nine children were asymptomatic; one had a speech defect with articulation errors but not hypernasality, and one had recurrent otitis media. Subsequently, the authors studied 50 persons with SMCP, 42 of whom had been detected as a coincidental finding during evaluation for unrelated prob-lems. Each of the 50 persons received the following evaluations: paediatric his-tory and physical examination; pedigree and examination of family members; audiogram; otolaryngologic examination; speech evaluation; dental examina-tion; and examination by a plastic surgeon. Table 9.1 presents Stewart et al's (1971) list of characteristics of individuals with SMCP, the incidence and type of complications.

Inspection of the findings in Table 9.1 indicate that the incidence of complica-tions appears to be lower in those individuals in whom the SMCP is an isolated defect and that only 45 per cent of those persons with an isolated SMCP were symptomatic. Additionally, ear problems, hearing loss and speech defects were also considerably lower in the isolated SMCP.

Weatherley-White et al (1972) reported the findings of their study of patients with SMCP 5 years of age and over. To qualify as a diagnosed SMCP the indivi-duals had to exhibit a bifid uvula, a bony notch in the hard palate and a muscle diastasis. Submucous cleft palate, as an isolated anomaly, was found in 35 per cent of the patients. Sixty-five per cent had other abnormalities including neuro-sensory hearing loss, chronic serous otitis media, congenital heart disease, cleft lip, microtia, talipes deformity, syndactylism and mental retardation. Rarer defects included one case each of associated Klippel-Feil and Treacher-Collins syndromes. Although the true incidence of SMCP has been thought to be rela-tively small the studies by Stewart et al (1971) and Weatherley-White et al

(1972), all conducted at the University of Colorado Medical Center, report an incidence of 1 : 1200, which is comparable to the incidence of true cleft palate. This group of researchers attribute the probable lack of recognition of the incidence of SMCP to the cryptic nature of the condition in which a large percentage of the patients have normal speech and often minimal muscle defect. Although 50 per cent of the SMCP patients studied by Weatherley-White et al had speech abnormalities of some type, these were often due to other defects such as mental and motor retardation and hearing loss from serous otitis media, rather than true velopharyngeal incompetence. On the basis of their findings Weatherley-White et al (1972) state that any treatment plan prior to the development of speech is contraindicated. Surgery should not be considered until the child is 4 to 6 years of age, at which time a valid speech evaluation can be obtained

Table 9.1 Types of associated conditions found in 50 submucous cleft palate individuals (modified from Stewart et al 1971, p 65)

SUBMUCOUS CLEFT PALATE

Male	29	(58%)	Caucasian	29
Female	21	(42%)	Spanish surname	20
			Oriental	1
			Negro	0

Isolated defect	29	(58%)	
Other abnormalities	21	(42%)	
Treacher Collins		Cleft lip	
Klippel-Feil		Choanal atresia	
Fanconi syndrome		Moebius syndrome	
Congenital rubella		Ring 18 chromosome	
Albinism		Mental retardation	

Complications

	Isolated defect	Other abnormalities	Total
Ear problems	34%	62%	44%
Hearing loss	24%	54%	33%
Speech defects	28%	75%	38%
Total	45%	85%	55%

and significant velopharyngeal incompetence appears to be the cause of the speech defect.

In 1971 Bergstrom & Hemenway reported on one of the first studies of the incidence of ear disease in patients with SMCP. Of a group of patients ranging in age from 2 months to 50 years they found an incidence of 39.6 per cent of recurrent and chronic diseases ranging from otitis media to cholesteatoma. Thirty-four per cent had conductive hearing loss and 25 per cent had either pure sensorineural or mixed hearing losses. Of the total group of patients with SMCP, 44.8 per cent were completely asymptomatic and about half of the patients with significant middle ear disease did not have speech disorders. On the basis of their study and findings Bergstrom & Hemenway (1971) indicate that many of the SMCP persons in their group shared many of the otologic problems of persons with overt cleft palate and that most of the ear disease seemed clearly related to poor function of the Eustachian tube.

Another type of SMCP reported in the literature is the 'occult' submucous cleft. Recent studies have indicated that muscle malposition can occur in the absence of the classical triad of overt signs and this condition is designated occult submucous cleft palate. In a comprehensive study of 240 cases of velopharyngeal incompetence without cleft lip or cleft palate Kaplan (1975) identified 23 cases of occult submucous cleft. These individuals had the same type of anatomic abnormality that leads to velar dysfunction, that is the insertion of the palate muscles onto the hard palate rather than onto the mid-line soft palate raphe. Kaplan concludes that isolated cleft of the secondary palate, submucous cleft palate, and occult submucous cleft are variations in the expression of the same embryologic disorder, and that there is a continuous spectrum of severity of muscle malformation and actual clefting.

BIFID UVULA

The bifid, or cleft uvula, is usually defined as a partial or total bifurcation of the uvula. Unlike the situation in submucous cleft palate the incidence and natural history of the bifid uvula is well known. The seemingly minor anatomical variant of an isolated bifid uvula may be indicative of a more serious physiological abnormality. Taylor (1972) considered the bifid uvula to be a sentinel manifesting a disturbance of the normal embryological development of the palate and related structures. As such, he considered it to be a microform of the fusion defects consisting of cleft lip, cleft palate, or both. Beeden (1972) indicated that the bifid uvula sometimes represents the most obvious sign of the presence of a submucous cleft in the soft palate. Shapiro et al (1971) indicated that the incompletely fused uvula might be considered to be between malformation and normal development in the palatal fusion process. Meskin et al (1965) considered the bifid uvula to be transmitted as an autosomal dominant trait, whereas Cervenka & Shapiro (1970) indicated that their findings were consistent with polygenic inheritance. Shapiro et al (1971) supported the contention that bifid uvula is a microform of facial clefts and that their findings were most consistent with a quasicontinuous polygenic basis for these conditions.

The occurrence of bifid uvula has attracted increased attention in recent years because of the assumption that it is (a) a microform of cleft palate, (b) the significantly greater incidence of otological diseases in persons with the anomaly than in controls and (c) because the incidence varies widely in different racial populations (Lindemann et al 1977). In a study of more than 10 000 school children Stewart et al (1971) found 108 bifid uvulas, of which 100 were isolated and eight were associated with SMCP, an incidence of about 1:100. This figure closely approximates the incidence reported by Meskin et al (1964). Shapiro et al (1971) found an incidence of 9.95 per cent of Japanese, 6.8 per cent of Chinese, 0.2 per cent of Afro-Americans, 10.5 per cent of American Indians of Chippewa ancestry and 18.8 per cent in Navajo Indians. Lindemann et al (1977) found an incidence of 1.3 per cent in the Danish population, and the prevalence was of the same order of magnitude in both children and adults. Because of the apparent parallel between the frequency of bifid uvula in different racial groups, Chosack & Eidelman (1978) undertook a study of the incidence and mode of inheritance of bifid uvula in a group of 70 000 children in Israel between the ages of 6 and 18 years. The population was made up of people of Ashkenazi, non-Ashkenazi and Israeli origin. They found an incidence of 0.44 per cent, which is considerably lower than the incidence reported for most other racial and ethnic groups. Within the total group, they found that the non-Ashkenazi group had a significantly higher incidence than the Israeli and Ashkenazi groups. When the factor of mode of inheritance was analysed the results of this study indicated that the prevalence of bifid uvula in parents and siblings was 7.7 per cent and 7.5 per cent respectively. These findings lead the authors to support the hypothesis of a polygenic mode of inheritance for bifid uvula in their population.

SYNDROMES ASSOCIATED WITH CLEFTING

The literature dealing with cleft lip and cleft palate has described the impact of other anomalies on the population of individuals with clefts with a frequency varying from 10 to 50 per cent. Fogh-Anderson (1942) indicated that cleft lip and cleft palate are most likely associated with other severe malformations in 10 per cent or more of the cases, while the normal frequency of these malformations hardly exceeds 1 per cent. He identified the anomalies as clubfoot, polydactyly, syndactyly, inguinal hernia and congenital heart disease. Lis (1965) estimated an incidence of 50 per cent congenital anomalies for children with clefts. He categorized these anomalies to include: (1) defects in tissues or organs of branchial origin, (2) chromosomal abnormalities, (3) defects of the central nervous system which may include sensory, motor, intellectual, and/or perceptual neurological disturbance and (4) defects of the heart and genitourinary systems. In an overview of associated anomalies Wells (1971) listed the additional conditions of microcephalus, defects of the external ears, microstomia, spina bifida, ectopia cordis, micrognathia with Pierre Robin syndrome, hypospadias, and defects of the musculoskeletal system. The subject of other physical conditions associated with cleft palate is endless and is further confused by the differences in definition of an anomalous condition.

To date, many anomalies reported in association with cleft lip and cleft palate are not recognized as constituting syndromes of known genesis (Cohen 1978). At the present time it is difficult to know how frequently cleft palate has to occur in a syndrome to be considered a feature of that syndrome. According to Cohen (1978) if a given abnormality occurs with greater frequency in the syndrome population than it does as an isolated abnormality in the general population, it should be considered part of a syndrome. A review of the literature during the past 10 years indicates a tremendous increase in the incidence of clefting associated with syndromes. In 1971 Gorlin et al reviewed 72 syndromes in which clefting occurred, and in 1976 Gorlin et al described approximately 117 syndromes with orofacial clefts (excluding lateral and oblique facial and mandibular clefts). In 1978 Cohen delineated 154 syndromes in which clefting of various types occur. In a comprehensive documentation Cohen has compiled tables of syndromes associated with clefting which describe type of syndrome, striking feature of each syndrome, relative frequency of cleft lip and palate in

Table 9.2 Summary of syndromes with cleft lip and cleft palate (modified from Cohen 1978, p 307)

(a)

Category	Number
Syndromes with cleft lip–palate	28
Syndromes with cleft palate	77
Syndromes with Robin complex	18
Chromosomal syndromes with clefts	29
Median cleft lip	7
Associations with clefting	17

(b) Syndrome breakdown by aetiology

Aetiology	Number
Monogenic	79
Autosomal dominant	(35)
Autosomal recessive	(39)
X-linked	(5)
Experimentally induced	6
Chromosomal	29
Unknown genesis	40
Total number of syndromes	154

each syndrome, aetiology of each syndrome and the bibliographical reference for each condition. A summary of the 154 syndromes which include cleft lip and palate is presented in Table 9.2.

SUMMARY

Among all of the orofacial and sensory conditions associated with cleft palate the presence of conductive hearing loss is the most common, often the most debilitating, and in many instances the most difficult to control. To date, it is estimated that about 50 per cent of adults with cleft palate who were treated for middle ear disease in early and middle childhood have a conductive hearing loss. With the discovery in 1967 by Stool & Randall that middle ear effusion is present in infants with cleft palate within the first few months of life great strides have been made in early intervention. The current emphasis in both clinical research and management is in early detection and intervention of middle ear effusion in the infant. One of the goals is to minimize subsequent recurrent and chronic middle ear disease. Of equal importance is the prevention, where possible, of intermittent hearing loss during the crucial period of speech and language acquisition during the first three or four years of life. The methods and procedures of early intervention vary widely and are dependent upon the philosophy and orientation of the otologist. There have been significant advances made in the understanding and use of myringotomy and ventilating tubes. Some controversy remains concerning the age at which surgery should take place, the types and shapes of the ventilating tubes and the point of insertion. Another factor that has become clear in recent years is that submucous cleft palate is much more frequent than was formerly known. The incidence of conductive hearing loss in individuals with submucous cleft has been reported to approximate the incidence of hearing loss in the overt cleft palate population. Similarly, the effects of bifid uvula are becoming better understood with respect to hearing loss, and some reports indicate the incidence of hearing loss in individuals with bifid uvula closely parallels that of cleft palate. Another significant advance has been the tremendous growth of documentation concerning clefting and associated syndromes. These findings and the availability of newer diagnostic tools and methods enhances early diagnosis of associated conditions and the subsequent implementation of early intervention. With increasing advances in clinical research it can be anticipated that the application of these findings will provide the child born with cleft palate the opportunity for a much better total habilitation than was formerly possible.

REFERENCES

Armstrong B 1954 A new treatment for chronic secretory otitis media. Archives of Otolaryngology 59: 653–657

Beeden A G 1972 The bifid uvula. Journal of Laryngology and Otology 86: 815–819

Bergstrom L, Hemenway W 1971 Otologic problems in submucous cleft palate. Southern Medical Journal 64: 1172–1177

Bluestone C 1971 Eustachian tube obstruction in the infant with cleft palate. Annals of Otology, Rhinology and Laryngology 80: 1–28

Bluestone C, Wittel R, Paradise J 1972 Roentgenographic evaluation of Eustachian tube function in infants with cleft and normal palates. Cleft Palate Journal 9: 93–100

Bluestone C, Cantekin E, Berry Q, Paradise J 1975 Eustachian tube ventilatory function in relation to cleft palate. Annals of Otolaryngology 84: 333–338

Bluestone C, Cantekin E, Berry Q 1975 Certain effects of adenoidectomy on Eustachian tube ventilatory function. Laryngoscope 85: 113–127

Calnan J S 1954 Submucous cleft palate. British Journal of Plastic Surgery 6: 264–282

Cervenka J, Shapiro B 1970 Cleft uvula in Chippewa Indians: prevalence and genetics. Human Biology 42: 47–52

Chosack A, Eidelman E 1978 Cleft uvula: prevalence and genetics. Cleft Palate Journal 15: 63–67

Cohen M M 1978 Syndromes with cleft lip and cleft palate. Cleft Palate Journal 15: 306–328

Cole R, Cole J 1974 Eustachian tube function in cleft lip and palate patients. Archives of Otology 99: 337–341

Crysdale W 1976 Rational management of middle ear effusions in the cleft palate patient. Journal of Otolaryngology 5: 463–467

Fogh-Andersen P 1942 Inheritance of harelip and cleft palate. Busck, Copenhagen

Gerwat J 1975 The structure and function of the nasopharyngeal lymphoid tissue with special reference to the aetiology of secretory otitis. Journal of Laryngology and Otology 89: 169–174

Glassock M 1971 Pediatric otology. Journal of the Tennessee Medical Association 64: 19–28

Goetzinger C, Embry J, Brooks R, Proud G 1960 Auditory assessment of cleft palate adults. Acta Otolaryngologica 55: 551–557

Gorlin R, Cervenka J, Pruzansky S 1971 Facial clefting and its syndromes. Birth Defects 7: 3–49

Gorlin R, Pindborg J, Cohen M 1976 Syndromes of the head and neck. McGraw-Hill, New York, vol 2

Greydanus D E, O'Donnell E J, McDonald T J 1977 Middle ear effusions. Mayo Clinic Proceedings 52: 497–503

Holborow C 1962 Deafness associated with cleft palate. Journal of Laryngology and Otolaryngology 76: 762–773

Kaplan E N 1975 The occult submucous cleft palate. Cleft Palate Journal 12: 356–368

Kelly A B 1910 Congenital insufficiency of the palate. Journal of Laryngology and Otolaryngology 25: 281, 324

Lindemann G, Riis B, Sewerin I 1977 Prevalence of cleft uvula among 2732 Danes. Cleft Palate Journal 14: 226–229

Lis E 1965 Other concomitant conditions: other physical conditions. In: Irwin J (ed) The proceedings of the conference: Communicative problems in cleft palate. ASHA Reports 1: 91–102

Maue-Dickson W 1977 Cleft lip and palate research: an updated state of the art. Section II
    Anatomy and physiology. Cleft Palate Journal 14: 270–287

Meskin L, Gorlin R, Isaacson R 1964 Abnormal morphology of the soft palate: I The prevalence
    of cleft uvula. Cleft Palate Journal 1: 342–346

Meskin L, Gorlin R, Isaacson R 1965 Abnormal morphology of the soft palate: II The genetics
    of cleft uvula. Cleft Palate Journal 2: 40–45

Möller P 1975 Long-term otologic features of cleft palate patients. Archives of Otolaryngology
    101, 605–607

Nober E H 1968 Hearing problems associated with cleft palate. In: Lencione R (ed) Cleft Palate
    Habilitation. Syracuse University Press, Syracuse, p 37–50

Paradise J, Bluestone C (1969) Diagnosis and management of ear disease in cleft palate infants.
    American Academy of Ophthalmology and Otolaryngology 73: 709–713

Paradise J, Bluestone C, Felder H 1969 The universality of otitis media in 50 infants with cleft
    palate. Pediatrics 44: 35–41

Paradise J, Bluestone C 1974 Early treatment of the universal otitis media of infants with cleft
    palate. Pediatrics 53: 48–54

Sataloff J, Fraser M 1952 Hearing loss in children with cleft palates. Archives of Otolaryngology
    55: 61–64

Shapiro B, Meskin L, Cervenka J, Pruzansky S 1971 Cleft uvula: a microform of facial clefts and
    its genetic basis. Birth Defects 7: 80–82

Skolnik E 1958 Otologic evaluation in cleft palate patients. Laryngoscope 68: 1908–1949

Soudijn E, Huffstadt A 1975 Cleft palate and middle ear effusions in babies. Cleft Palate Journal
    12: 229–233

Stewart J, Ott J, Lagace R 1971 Submucous cleft palate. Birth Defects 7: 64–66

Stool S, Randall P 1967 Unexpected ear disease in infants with cleft palate. Cleft Palate Journal
    4: 99–103

Taylor G 1972 The bifid uvula. Laryngoscope 82: 734–737

Weatherley-White R, Sakura C, Brenner L, Stewart J, Ott J 1972 Submucous cleft palate. Plastic
    and Reconstructive Surgery 49: 297–304

Wells C G 1971 Cleft palate and its associated speech disorders. McGraw-Hill, New York

Yules R 1975 Current concepts of treatment of ear disease in cleft palate children and adults.
    Cleft Palate Journal 12: 315–322

10

Psychosocial aspects of cleft lip and palate

INTRODUCTION

The effects of the kinds of physical, sensory and perceptual problems caused by clefts of the lip and palate have changed over time as methods of habilation have improved. Despite the advances in the technology of rehabilitation, society still attaches a stigma to an obvious physical anomaly. In a culture that attaches high values to physical attractiveness, especially facial attractiveness, the handicap of cleft lip and palate should be expected to have serious consequences on the psychological and social development of the individual. If in addition to the cosmetic problem the individual also has a speech and hearing handicap the magnitude of the psychosocial problems may be compounded (Goodstein 1968; Clifford 1973; Spriestersbach 1973). The presence of a facial anomaly affects not only the individual but also his family, peers, acquaintances and society itself. In essence, the psychological and social effects on the individual with a cleft lip and palate are shaped not only by his/her own perceptions about the condition and the meanings attached to them, but also by the feelings, attitudes and reactions of all the people in his environment (Clifford 1973). The literature on physical handicaps reflects an almost universal agreement that the psychological and social problems of the handicapped are of major importance in habilitation. In some instances, it is estimated that the psychosocial problems may more often adversely influence the final habilitative picture than does the primary disability. Given these assumptions, the child born with a cleft lip and palate seems almost preordained to sustain a number of debilitating psychosocial problems. Personality theory, particularly psychoanalytic theory, suggests that there should be definite personality and social adjustment differences between children and adults with and without clefts. To date, most of the studies reported in the literature dealing with the psychosocial aspects of the cleft problem do not bear out these assumptions. This may be due to problems of research design that include small sample populations, questionable control groups, methodological differences and the lack of refined measurement tools. At present it is difficult to compare the results of one study to another and this often restricts the usefulness of the findings (McWilliams 1970; Wirls 1971; Spriestersbach et al 1973). The following section presents a review of the literature dealing with the psychosocial aspects of the cleft problem relating to (1) parental attitudes, (2) intelligence, and (3) the psychosocial adjustment of cleft palate children and adults.

PARENTAL ATTITUDES

The literature dealing with the effects upon parents of the birth of a physically handicapped child are in general agreement that it usually causes a number of complex and serious problems in parent–child relationships. Most of the reports of parental reactions to the birth of a child with a cleft of the lip and palate indicate that it unquestionably causes shock and anxiety feelings. It is to be expected that the parents' reactions may be translated into a variety of attitudes and subsequent behaviours towards their handicapped child. These reactions can range from rejection or overprotection, to an almost total preoccupation with the child's appearance and physical management, and ultimately in maintaining realistic expectations for the child's accomplishments (Wirls 1971). The influence of parental attitudes and particularly the bonding between mothers and their infants is now widely acknowledged and has been documented by recent research in mother–child interaction. If mutually satisfying mother–child interactions do not begin early this may lead to problems in the child's social and intellectual development. The birth of a child with a cleft places the parents under the stress of being unable to carry out the usual social rituals associated with the birth of a new baby. In addition they do not know or cannot acquire alternative patterns of behaviour during the neonatal period. All of these assumptions would tend to indicate that the child born with a cleft is at high risk for developing psychosocial problems stemming from parental and other environmental influences. While some studies tend to verify this point of view an almost equal number report essentially normal parent–child interactions and parenting behaviours.

Parental reaction to the birth of a child with a cleft is a uniquely individual response. What the reaction will be is dependent in great measure upon the people who are the parents, how much of a threat a congenital anomaly in their child is to their egos, and their use of psychological defence mechanisms (McWilliams 1970). A number of studies have been conducted to determine whether there are any common variables in parental reactions and attitudes. In one of the earliest reports of a retrospective study Weachter (1959) identified ten areas of parental concern. These included (1) the child's appearance, (2) request for immediate surgery, (3) speech development, (4) feeding, (5) reaction of the spouse, (6) reaction of the siblings, (7) reaction of family and friends, (8) intellectual development, (9) financial problems, and (10) recurrence of the defect in other unborn children. Although the order of priority may have changed somewhat over the past twenty years, current clinical experience indicates that most parents usually express the same kinds of reactions. Tisza & Gumpertz (1962) reported that the mothers of infants with clefts of the lip and palate reacted with strong feelings of disappointment, helpless resentment and hurt at having given birth to a congenitally deformed child. They also indicated that the mother needs time to work through a period of mourning for the normal child she expected before she is able to accept her handicapped child and deal with the problems of habilitation.

In contrast to these findings Goodstein (1960a, b) found an almost total lack of differences between parents of children with clefts and physically normal children. Of significance was the finding that the parents of older cleft palate children were more poorly adjusted than were the parents of younger cleft children. Goodstein interpreted these findings as indicating that the effects on parental adjustment are not immediately evidenced but that these effects develop over time. Parental reaction shortly after the birth of a child with a cleft may tend to be optimistic because of the knowledge of remedial surgery and other therapies. If intervention strategies are not completely successful by the time the child reaches school age and there are resulting problems the parents may then again become increasingly concerned with the cleft problem. Spriestersbach's (1973) comprehensive study of the psychosocial aspects of the cleft problem tended to substantiate some of Goodstein's findings.

In another study designed to explore parental attitudes, Clifford (1969b) studied 60 pairs of parents whose children with cleft palate were under 2 years of age. He found that parents rated a cleft lip and palate as a more severe problem than either a cleft lip or a cleft palate. The parents in this group rated the more severe problem of a cleft lip and palate as having a greater emotional impact on their lives. The findings also indicated that mothers are more affected by the handicap than the fathers, but neither mothers nor fathers viewed the condition of cleft lip and palate as playing a major role in marital adjustment. The results of a study by Clifford & Crocker in 1971 indicated that contrary to what might have been expected the mothers of infants born with a cleft did not express profoundly debilitating emotional reactions. Comparatively speaking they mentioned that they were shocked upon being told about the facial defect but that it did not cause or precipitate a crisis within the family. In this study, the resolution of the crisis of having a child born with a defect appeared to have a cohesive rather than divisive effect on family relationships. Additionally the fact that the parents were told that remedial surgery was available provided them with their greatest comfort. These parents reacted as if the worst was over, and the existence of remedial measures served, in great part, to help dissipate their anxiety. A noteworthy finding in this study was that the mothers of cleft palate infants reported a high degree of marital satisfaction, and in this respect their reactions were similar to those of the control group of mothers. The authors conclude from their findings that giving birth to a cleft child produces an initial, highly intense period of shock which is of relatively short duration. The period of shock is rapidly dissipated because of the knowledge of remedial measures and, for this group, because of the positive support these women received from their marriages.

In a recent study, Richman (1978b) compared the responses of parents' and teachers' perceptions of the behaviour of cleft palate children between the ages of 7 and 12 years. The results indicated that teachers view cleft palate children, both male and female, as significantly more inhibited in the classroom than the parents report them to be at home. The parents were in agreement and differed from the teachers in that they did not view their cleft palate children as excessively inhibited. The author concluded that there were two important implications regarding the parents' rating of their cleft palate children's behaviour. One was the fact that the parents did not significantly disagree in their ratings, suggesting that parenthood of a child with a congenital anomaly does not necessarily create a disparity in parental perceptions of their child. Secondly, it is important to note that parents' behaviour ratings are consistent with other reports of teacher ratings of normal schoolchildren. This may indicate that while parents view their cleft children as behaviourally normal, external social influences may elicit different behaviours or a different perception of behaviours by others.

INTELLIGENCE

Among all of the components of the psychosocial problems inherent in cleft lip and palate perhaps the one variable that has been studied the most extensively has been the aspect of intelligence. Although the literature lacks consensus, the findings usually indicate that intellectual capacity in the cleft palate population is distributed throughout the total range of abilities with a trend towards studies reporting some degree of intellectual impairment (Goodstein 1968; Ruess 1968). In most of the studies dealing with the relationship of intelligence to the cleft condition the mean intelligence quotient (IQ) scores tend to be somewhat lower than that of the non-cleft population, although the lower mean scores usually fall within the limits of average intelligence (McWilliams 1970). As Spriesters-bach et al (1973) pointed out, although cleft palate children tend to achieve slightly lower scores on intelligence tests, no logical explanation for these find-ings has been provided. Before considering the published reports it is important to note that in many studies, and particularly in the earlier studies, there was very little methodological uniformity with reference to sample population age, type and severity of the clefting condition, use of control groups and the kind of intelligence tests employed.

Billig (1951) was among the first to report on the degree of intellectual impairment in cleft palate children based upon scores derived from standardized intelligence tests. She found that children between the ages of 2 months and 17 years had a mean IQ score of 94, or six points lower than the expected mean of 100. Means and Irwin (1954) found that the derived scores of cleft children were depressed, with the norm tending towards the lower end of the average range. Munson & May (1955) found that 63 per cent of their cleft palate popula-tion were within or above the normal range as compared with an expected 75 per cent of the general population. Similarly, Illingworth & Birch (1956) found that only 60 per cent of their cleft palate group fell within the average or above average range compared to expected norms. In 1961 Lewis compared the intelli-gence of cleft palate children with that of their siblings using the Standford–Binet intelligence scale. She found a significant difference between the two groups with a 10-point differential in favour of the sibling group. Lewis also found that cleft palate children with other anomalies had significantly lower IQ scores than cleft palate children without other anomalies. In a comprehensive study of 466 children with cleft lip and palate Estes & Morris (1970) found that the WISC full-scale IQ and Binet IQ scores were, on average, about five points lower than for normal children.

In contrast, Rattner et al (1958) and Cervenka & Drabkova (1965), in studies using very small sample populations, found that cleft palate children demon-strated normal intelligence and average IQs within the expected range. Studies by Morris (1962), Ruess (1965) and Smith & McWilliams (1969) also reported normal intelligence for children with cleft palate. However, significant differences were found by these investigators when they compared the IQ scores of the cleft palate and non-cleft groups. In all instances the higher IQ scores favoured the non-cleft groups.

With the development of more refined methods of evaluation, a number of investigators began looking at specific dimensions concerning the relationship of clefting and intelligence. In 1961, Goodstein, in one of the more controlled studies of intellectual capacity, administered the WISC to a group of children with cleft lip and palate, and to a comparable control group of children without known physical defects. The mean full-scale WISC was 94 for the cleft palate children and 104 for the control group. The cleft group had lower IQs than the control group on all three scales of the WISC. Of significance was the finding that the intellectual impairment of the cleft group was more substantial in the area of verbal skills than in the area of manipulative skills. In another well-controlled study of cleft palate children and their siblings, Ruess (1965) also found significantly lower verbal scores in the cleft palate group. A comparison of the scores on the performance tests, reading and writing skills, figure drawing and school progress indicated that there was essentially no difference between the two groups. The Goodstein (1961) and Ruess (1965) studies were among the first to document the finding that the lower scores in intellectual capacity found in children with clefts might be correlated to deficits in verbal functioning. In 1972, McWilliams & Musgrave's study tended to substantiate this variable. They evaluated cleft palate children based on the level of their speech adequacy. Children with completely normal speech had Binet IQ scores of around 109, and for those with normal voice quality and consonant articulation errors the mean Binet IQ score was 108. The mean WISC IQs for two groups were 104 and 105 respectively. However, for the cleft children who had hypernasal speech the Binet IQ mean was 97, a statistically significant difference. The scores for the hypernasal group of cleft children on the WISC did not reach significance, but the trend was in the direction of lower IQs as compared with the cleft children with normal speech and voice quality.

What began to emerge from the early pioneer studies by Goodstein (1961), Lewis (1961), Morris (1962), Ruess (1965), Smith & McWilliams (1966) and Phillips & Harrison (1969) was the concept that there were differences between verbal and performance abilities of cleft palate children as measured by intelligence scales. Similarly Estes & Morris (1970) found in their study that cleft palate children obtained higher WISC performance scale IQ scores than WISC verbal scale IQs. The authors indicate that these results tend to substantiate the finding of an apparent deficit in cleft palate children's skills as they relate to verbal activities. As Estes & Morris point out, there may be several possible explanations for these findings. The deficit may be developmental or the result of lack of language stimulation in the home. Nation (1970) found that vocabulary comprehension, as measured by the Peabody picture vocabulary test, was reduced in young normal hearing cleft palate children between the ages of 34 and 63 months, when compared to their non-cleft siblings and groups of selected normal children. Another possible cause of the verbal deficit in cleft palate children may stem from problems in both expressive language development and hearing disorders. These conditions may interfere with the development of intellectual skills which are assessed by intelligence tests. Morris (1962) reported significant correlations between articulation scores and verbal, performance, and full-scale WISC scores. Some investigators report that the effects of hearing loss have been shown to cause differences in IQ scores. Means & Irwin (1954) reported that a significantly greater per cent of cleft palate children without a hearing loss had IQs above 100 than did those children with a hearing loss.

In 1972 Lamb et al undertook a study of cleft palate children and their siblings to study the variables of intelligence, hearing loss and visual-perceptual-motor abilities. Each pair of children were administered the Peabody picture vocabulary test (PPVT), the Wechsler intelligence scale for children (WISC), Cohen's verbal comprehension factor (VC) and Cohen's perceptual organization factor (PO). A comparison of the results of the four tests indicated that there were significant differences between the two groups of children in verbal intelligence as measured by the PPVT and WISC verbal tests as well as in verbal comprehension as measured by the VC. The difference in the test scores was in favour of the sibling group. There were no differences between the two groups in performance IQ scores or in perceptual organization. When the test results of the normal hearing cleft palate children were compared to the poor hearing cleft children, these investigators found a significant difference between the two groups in verbal ability as measured by the PPVT, and a definite trend towards differences in performance as indicated by the scores for the WISC performance IQ and the PO factor.

Another area which has been investigated has been the relationship of the type and severity of the cleft condition to intelligence. In 1961, Goodstein reported that children with cleft palate only (CPO) were significantly more impaired intellectually than were children with cleft lip and palate (CLP) on scores derived on the WISC. Similarly, Drillien et al (1966) reported slightly lower IQs for children with CPO. In 1970, Estes & Morris compared the IQ scores of children with cleft lip only (CLO), CLP and CPO. They found that the relationship between type of cleft and psychological scores indicated that the scores for the CLP were higher than for the CPO group. In general, test means for the CLO group were higher than for the CPO group but were similar to the means for the CLP group. In this study, however, none of the differences between cleft types was significant.

In contrast, Lamb et al (1973) did not find any differences between types of clefting and intelligence in their sample population. The authors evaluated children between the ages of 5 and 16 years using the WISC and PPVT scales. The authors found no significant difference in intellectual function between the CLP and CPO cleft type groups. In an evaluation of the data with reference to sex and type of clefting condition their findings suggest that the more severe intellectual impairment may occur in the cleft palate individual of the sex with the less frequent incidence, that is the female CLP and the male CPO. Their results suggest that it may be the female CLP and male CPO groups who are the language deficient subgroups, and that the language skills of the male CLP and female CPO groups are approximately normal.

Most of the earlier studies dealing with the relationship of intelligence and type of cleft were based upon the results of cross-sectional investigations of children. In 1975, Musgrave et al reported on a longitudinal study conducted with two groups of cleft palate only (CPO) children over a 10-year period. Their study included a number of variables of which one was intelligence. The first examination was carried out in the preschool age years using the Stanford–Binet intelligence scale, form L–M. The mean IQ scores for the two groups of CPO infants were 95.6 and 97 respectively. At the preschool age level both groups demonstrated the commonly reported tendency to place somewhat below the expected average. On the second examination, conducted approximately 10 years later, the mean Binet IQ scores for the two groups were 106.7 and 111.2 respectively. Of interest in the results of this study was the finding that both groups showed an increase in IQ from the time of the first examination to the second examination, and that the scores on the second examination placed them somewhat higher than the expected mean for the general population.

In 1977, Starr et al were among the first to conduct both a longitudinal and cross-sectional study of cleft palate infants under the age of 2 years using the Bayley scales of infant development. The sample population consisted of infants with cleft palate only (CPO), cleft lip and palate (CLP), and cleft lip only (CLO). The results of the test scores indicated that there were no significant differences among the three cleft type groups on mental development as compared with the Bayley norms at 6, 12, 18 and 24 months. These findings were similar to those of Plotkin et al (1970), who reported that the developmental functioning of infants with cleft lip and palate, as measured by the Cattell infant intelligence scale, were normal for age levels. Starr et al (1977) indicated that, for their sample, the CPO group had higher scores than the CLO and CLP groups, with the CPO group contributing disproportionately to the higher scores for all the cleft types.

The current recognition of the benefits that may be derived by early intervention places a corresponding need on the development of methods of identification before the age of 3 years in all developmentally delayed children including children with clefts. Fox et al (1978) undertook a study to determine whether developmental delay could be documented in young cleft palate infants between the ages of 2 and 33 months, when compared to matched controls. Among the factors evaluated in this study was the effect of the severity of the cleft condition on linguistic and non-linguistic development. The sample cleft palate population consisted of infants with cleft palate only (CPO), and cleft lip and palate (CLP) and a control group of non-cleft infants. The two groups of children were administered the Denver developmental scale by Frankenburg and Dodds, 1969; the receptive expressive emergent language scale (REEL) by Bzoch and League, 1971; and the experimental version of the birth-3 scale by Bangs and Garrett, 1973. To test the effects of the severity of clefting on developmental scores, values were assigned to four different types of cleft conditions. A cleft of the soft palate only was rated the least extensive cleft condition, followed in order of severity by cleft of the hard and soft palate, cleft of the hard and soft palate with a unilateral cleft of the lip, and cleft of the hard and soft palate, with bilateral cleft lip, being rated the most severe type.

The results of this investigation indicated that the performance of the cleft palate infants paralleled, but fell below, the control group on all 11 behaviours as measured by the three tests. The cleft palate group scored from one to three months below the controls on all three of the developmental measures. Analysis of the two groups showed a significant difference between the cleft and control groups indicating that the performance scores represented populations from two distinct groups. The most powerful subtest in predicting the groupings of the children into cleft or non-cleft categories was the expressive language subtest of the REEL. When the effects of the severity of the cleft were analysed, these investigators found that, contrary to reports of lower IQ scores for CPO children, the results of this study supported the findings of McWilliams & Musgrave (1972) that children with the most extensive or severe type of cleft were at significantly higher risk for developmental problems. On the basis of their findings, Fox et al (1978) indicated that their sample population of cleft palate infants differed from the controls on both linguistic and non-linguistic measures. They suggested that the deficits usually documented in older cleft palate children can be identified during the first three years of life and may provide more adequate guides for early intervention strategies.

Most of the studies reviewed indicate that if children with clefts exhibit any intellectual impairment their scores usually fall within the lower limits of the average range. A recent study by Richman (1978a) shows that the cleft child's cosmetic appearance may, however, markedly influence teachers' appraisal of their cognitive abilities. There has been considerable research in the past few years relating children's physical attractiveness to adults', typically teachers', perceptions of intellectual ability. These findings generally support the contention that teachers view physically attractive children as possessing higher intellectual ability than physically unattractive children. In order to explore these findings, Richman evaluated teachers' reports of cleft palate children between the ages of 9 and 14 years. Each teacher was asked to rate the children on an intellectual ability scale. The results indicated that cleft children with noticeable facial disfigurement and above average intelligence were underestimated on the teachers' rating of ability. The children with noticeable facial disfigurement and below average intellectual ability were overestimated. The ratings of children with severe facial disfigurement and average or above average intelligence provided the expected finding. This would be in keeping with the culturally conditioned stereotype relating physical unattractiveness to decreased intellectual ability. Perhaps the unexpected finding, according to the author, was that the teachers overestimated the ability of children whose IQ scores indicated they were below average. Regardless of the reasons for these ratings, it is apparent from the results of this study that children with clefts, who also have cosmetic problems, are viewed differently in terms of their intellectual abilities by their teachers than are their non-cleft peers.

PSYCHOSOCIAL ADJUSTMENT OF CLEFT PALATE CHILDREN AND ADULTS

Psychosocial adjustment of cleft palate children

Children born with cleft lip and palate often experience a number of unique conditions in their life adjustments beginning at the moment of birth. Among these special conditions may be the reaction of their parents and family, problems in feeding during infancy, the traumas of repeated hospitalizations and surgery within the first three years of life and ultimately the reaction of their peers and teachers in school. In addition, the child with a cleft lip and palate may also have other types of physical handicaps which may include marked facial disfigurement, defective and/or delayed speech and language development, varying degrees of hearing loss and other physical anomalies. According to personality theories the effect of these atypical conditions early in life are usually considered to be predictive of a variety of psychosocial problems. Any one of these conditions, or a combination of these conditions, can be expected to produce a negative effect upon the child's personality development and social adjustment. It would seem, therefore, that children with clefts should exhibit a number of psychological characteristics that would differentiate them from children without clefts. Despite the logic underlying these assumptions the majority of the findings of clinical research and observations do not overwhelmingly confirm this point of view.

There is some evidence from studies using behavioural observations, clinical impressions and projective techniques that children with cleft exhibit a number of unique characteristics not shared by non-cleft children. Among the several studies that have reported that children with clefts are psychologically different from non-physically handicapped children was the one conducted by Goodstein in 1961. In his study on intellectual competence, Goodstein administered the Vineland social maturity scale (VSMS) to the mothers of the children with cleft palate and to mothers in a control group of physically normal children. He found a small but significant difference between the cleft palate and the control group. For the children below 5 years of age the cleft group had a mean social quotient (SQ) of 97 compared to an SQ of 109 for the control group, between the ages of 5 and 16 years the cleft group had an SQ of 100 compared to an SQ of 104 for the controls. The results of this cross-sectional study would tend to imply that cleft palate children begin their social adjustment more slowly, but that by the time they reach adolescence they have achieved almost the same level of social integration as their non-cleft peers. This inference needs to be viewed with some caution because of the unreliability of the VSMS. Estes & Morris (1970) found in a comparison of the results of scores on the WISC, Binet and VSMS, that of the three tests, results with the VSMS were in least agreement with the other two. They suggest that the role of the parent as interviewee probably contributed greatly to that variance.

Other studies suggest psychological differences. Tisza et al (1958) found in psychiatric observations of preschool cleft palate children that they demonstrated higher levels of muscular rigidity, bodily tensions, and distortions of psychomotor tasks as compared to physically normal children. Gluck et al (1965) found that cleft children were more frequently shy and enuretic, and had more physical anomalies and chronic illnesses than non-cleft children. Smith & McWilliams (1966), in a comparison of cleft and non-cleft children, found that the cleft group was less creative on both verbal and non-verbal tasks. In 1969, Tisza et al found that the dramatic play of cleft children between the ages of 5 and 8 years showed fantasies of unusual intensity involving oral aggression, and conflict between active-aggressive and passive wishes. In a study comparing concepts of self-image between children with asthma and clefts, Clifford (1969a) found that the children with clefts perceived themselves to be less well accepted at birth by their parents.

In studies dealing with the concept of personality differences in children with clefts, Spriestersbach (1973) found that cleft palate children were less confident, less aggressive, and less independent than their non-cleft peers. Richman's (1976) investigation supported the contention that cleft palate children display greater inhibition of impulses than non-cleft children, but the author indicated that this does not necessarily imply that these children are emotionally malad-justed. The child with a cleft palate may have learned to avoid situations which give rise to negative responses by others. Conversely, the results of a number of sytematic studies using structured personality tests and projective techniques have not convincingly demonstrated that children with clefts are markedly psy-chologically different than their non-cleft peers. As early as 1956, Sidney & Matthews compared the social adjustment of a group of cleft palate children with two control groups. The tests included the California test of personality, the thematic apperception test and a teachers rating scale. In general, the mean scores for the three groups were similar with no significant differences between the cleft group and the first control group. The authors concluded that their findings failed to provide any clinically significant evidence that children with clefts are different in social adjustment from non-cleft children. In a more de-tailed study of personality adjustment, Watson (1964) compared boys with clefts with a group of boys with chronic physical handicaps and physically normal boys. He found no significant differences among the mean scores for the three groups on the Rogers personal adjustment inventory. Similar results were obtained by Palmer & Adams (1962), Corah & Corah (1963), Ruess (1965) and Clifford (1967). As Wirls & Plotkin (1971) indicated, the overall negative results, in and of themselves, should not be interpreted to mean that there are no personality differences between cleft palate children, their non-cleft peers and their siblings. As has been suggested by McWilliams (1970) and Spriestersbach (1973), it may be that projective tests are not sufficiently sensitive instruments to assess personality differences in cleft palate populations. To date, the results of most of the studies dealing with the psychosocial status of cleft palate children are not conclusive. By and large, most of the studies indicate that while some differences exist between cleft groups and matched/ sibling groups there is no scientifically verifiable evidence that there are major or significant personality and adjustment differences in children with cleft palate.

Psychosocial adjustment of adults

The literature dealing with the psychosocial, vocational and educational integration and status of the cleft palate adult is somewhat limited. A trend in recent years has been the use of follow-up, self-administered questionnaires and check lists, and personal and phone interviews. There are advantages in gathering longitudinal information in this fashion in that it provides an overall view of the activities and social adjustment of large numbers of children who have reached adulthood. Conversely, with the passage of time, problems encountered during the school years and in adolescence may be forgotten or denied. As a consequence, the true effects of the influence of the cleft condition on subsequent life style and accomplishments may be obscured. Notwithstanding these procedural shortcomings, a number of studies during the past 10 years have provided some insight and trends concerning the psychosocial adjustment of cleft palate adults.

In a study to evaluate whether the presence of a cleft had influenced their social relationships, Van Demark & Van Demark (1970) interviewed 39 cleft palate teenagers. Of this group, 24 reported that the cleft had made no difference and 12 said that the cleft was a handicap in varying degrees of severity in their social activities. Despite this somewhat positive overall appraisal of the effects of having a cleft, 21 said they had never belonged to a social organization and four reported no social activity of any kind. Based on these responses, it would appear that this group of teenagers were observers rather than active participants in social interactions. Compared to non-cleft teenagers this group also appeared to be less active in dating. For example, 15 of the total group reported that they had never dated, or only once or twice a year, and 22 indicated that they had difficulty in dating, or felt they had been refused because of their cleft condition.

In 1972, Clifford et al evaluated 98 adults who had been operated upon by one surgeon 22 to 27 years prior to the follow-up study. The interviews and questionnaire explored each person's accomplishments, satisfaction with appearance and treatments, their perceptions of the influence of having a cleft and ratings of self-satisfaction and body satisfaction. Of this group of adults, their expressed satisfaction with their accomplishments in terms of employment was high. Seventy-seven were married and none was divorced. When the various items on the self-satisfaction scale were ranked according to mean satisfaction levels, the body items associated with clefts were, however, relatively low. The item with the lowest satisfaction level was teeth, closely followed by speech. Despite the low ratings for body image, this group perceived their clefts as having relatively little influence on their lives.

In a study to evaluate social adjustment from a behavioural point of view, McWilliams & Paradise (1973) interviewed cleft palate adults ranging in age from 18 to 38 years. They were interested in finding out how cleft palate adults compared educationally and occupationally with their parents and nearest-age siblings, and maritally with their siblings. The results indicated that both the cleft group and their siblings achieved a significantly higher level of education than did either their fathers or mothers. There were no significant differences, however, between the educational levels of the cleft palate group and their siblings. Differences in school drop-out rate indicated that more cleft palate adolescents dropped out of high school than did their siblings. However, at the college level there were no significant differences between the two groups. The results of marital status indicated that a significantly larger number of the cleft palate adults remained single compared to their nearest-age siblings.

Perhaps the most comprehensive studies dealing with the sociological aspects of cleft palate adults are those by Peter & Chinsky (1974a, b) and Peter et al (1975a, b). They evaluated the results of a self-administered questionnaire to 195 cleft palate adults, 190 of their siblings, and 209 randomly drawn control subjects between the ages of 24 and 54 years. In assessing marital status Peter & Chinsky (1974a) found that the cleft group marry at a significantly lower rate when compared with their siblings and the control group. Of the total cleft group, 26 per cent had never married as compared to 8.9 per cent of the siblings and 8.6 per cent of the controls. Overall, the cleft group was found to have been older at the time of first marriage, to have had fewer children per marriage, and to have had more childless marriages, indicating a substantive difference when compared to the sibling and control groups.

In an assessment of educational attainment for the three groups, Peter & Chinsky (1974b) found that there were no significant differences in the mean age for school attendance. The drop-out rate for the cleft group, in the elementary and high school years, was 2 per cent higher than for their siblings and 4 per cent lower than for the random controls. The rate of college attendance was slightly higher for both siblings and controls than for the cleft group, but for the clefts who attended college the percentage who graduated was the same as for the sibling and control groups. Overall, the results of this study tend to demonstrate that cleft palate individuals, as a group, achieve educational levels very similar to those of their siblings and random controls. In contrast with these findings, Birch & Lindsay (1971) found that most of the cleft palate adults in their study reported being teased about their facial deformities and speech defects during their school years. This group also indicated that they had experienced problems in social adjustment during the adolescent years, particularly in heterosexual relationships, which were later magnified in adulthood.

In a study of the vocational and social accomplishments of cleft adults, their siblings and a random control group Peter et al (1975a) found that the cleft group did not vary significantly in terms of income from that of the control group. However, the siblings scored significantly higher than the cleft group. In a comparison of the three groups, the clefts had the lowest median income, and their aspiration level was lowest in terms of the amount of desired increase in income. In another assessment of the same three groups, Peter et al (1975b) measured the degree of limitation which the cleft adult might experience in their integration with social groups. On the basis of their findings the authors reported that the interdependence of the cleft group with the extended family bordered on dependence. The cleft group was the least mobile of the three groups in terms of geographic mobility from their childhood residence. The cleft adults participated less frequently than their siblings and the control group in voluntary associations such as social clubs, fraternal orders and service groups. The cleft group tended to have fewer friends and their friendships were less cohesive.

Although the cleft adults in this study cannot be characterized as grossly different from the other two groups, the authors concluded that they are a definable population in that they demonstrate some degrees of limitation in their social interactions, and these limitations are presumed to stem from having a cleft.

SUMMARY

The literature dealing with the psychological and social aspects of cleft palate reveals a vast body of information covering a wide array of variables related to the psychosocial status of children and adults, and their families. Despite the assumptions that the effects of having a cleft lip and palate should markedly influence psychosocial relationships, most studies have not convincingly demonstrated that children and adults are psychologically different from their non-cleft peers. Of all the areas of investigation pertaining to personality development, intelligence, school achievement, and social and economic accomplishments only in the area of intelligence have differences been consistently reported. Most studies indicate that there is a tendency for cleft palate children to achieve slightly lower scores on intelligence tests than their non-cleft peers. However, intelligence scores usually fall within the limits of average intelligence. Although the parents of children born with a cleft usually report initial periods of shock and anxiety, most of the studies indicate that parents make rapid accommodation to the condition and tend to view their cleft children as behaviourally normal.

While most of the studies of cleft palate children have not supported the hypotheses which suggest major personality and maladjustment problems, many have alluded to differences which exist between cleft and non-cleft children. Some investigators have indicated that the failure to estimate these differences may be due to faulty research design and the lack of refined measurement tools. Similarly, most studies of the cleft palate adult show that while differences occur between the cleft groups, matched controls and their siblings, most of these differences do not approach significance.

A review of the literature dealing with the psychosocial aspects of the cleft condition indicates that the majority of the studies have been cross-sectional and included disparate groups of cleft individuals spanning a wide range of ages and types of clefts. Ongoing and future research in this area will need to develop well-designed longitudinal studies in order to provide more scientifically documented information about the behavioural, social and psychological status of cleft palate individuals.

REFERENCES

Billig A (1951) A psychological appraisal of cleft palate patients. Proceedings of the Pennsylvania Academy of Sciences p 29–31

Birch J, Lindsay W 1971 An evaluation of adults with repaired bilateral cleft lips and palates. Plastic Reconstructive Surgery 48: 457–465

Cervenka J, Drabkova H 1965 The intelligence quotient in cleft lip and palate. Acta Chirugica: A E Plasticae 7: 58–61

Clifford E 1967 Connotative meaning of concepts related to cleft lip and palate. Cleft Palate Journal 4: 165

Clifford E 1969a The impact of symptom: a preliminary comparison of cleft lip–palate and asthmatic children. Cleft Palate Journal 6: 221–227

Clifford E 1969b Parental ratings of cleft palate infants. Cleft Palate Journal 6: 235–244

Clifford E 1973 Psychosocial aspects of orofacial anomalies: speculations in search of data. In: Orofacial anomalies: Clinical and research implications. ASHA Reports no 8, p 2–29. American Speech and Hearing Association, Washington DC

Clifford E, Crocker E 1971 Maternal responses: the birth of a normal child as compared to the birth of a child with a cleft. Cleft Palate Journal 8: 298–306

Clifford E, Crocker E, Pope B 1972 Psychological findings in the adulthood of 98 cleft palate children. Journal of Plastic and Reconstructive Surgery 50: 234–237

Corah N, Corah P 1963 A study of body image in children with cleft palate and cleft lip. Journal of Genetic Psychology 103: 133–173

Drillien C, Ingram T T S, Wilkinson E 1966 The causes and natural history of cleft lip and palate. Livingstone, Edinburgh

Estes R, Morris H 1970 Relationship among intelligence, speech proficiency, and hearing sensitivity in children with cleft palates. Cleft Palate Journal 7: 763–773

Fox D, Lynch J, Brookshire B 1978 Selected developmental factors of cleft children between 2 and 33 months of age. Cleft Palate Journal 15: 239–245

Gluck M, Wylie H, McWilliams B J, Conkwright E 1965 Comparison of clinical characteristics of children with cleft palates and children in a child guidance clinic. Perceptual Motor Skills 21: 806

Goodstein L 1960a MMPI differences between parents of children with cleft palates and parents of physically normal children. Journal of Speech and Hearing Research 3: 31–38

Goodstein L 1960b Personality test differences in parents of children with cleft palates. Journal of Speech and Hearing Research 3: 39–43

Goodstein L 1961 Intellectual impairment in children with cleft palates. Journal of Speech and Hearing Research 4: 287–294

Goodstein L 1968 Psychosocial aspects of cleft palate. In: Spriestersbach D, Sherman D (eds) Cleft palate and communication. Academic Press, New York, ch 6

Illingworth R, Birch L 1956 The intelligence of children with cleft palate. Archives of Diseases of Children 31: 300–302

Lamb M, Wilson F, Leeper H 1972 A comparison of selected cleft palate children and their siblings on the variables of intelligence, hearing loss and visual-perceptual-motor abilities. Cleft Palate Journal 9: 218–228

Lamb M, Wilson F, Leeper H 1973 The intellectual function of cleft palate children compared on the basis of cleft type and sex. Cleft Palate Journal 10: 367–377

Lewis R 1961 A survey of the intelligence of cleft palate children in Ontario. Cleft Palate Bulletin 11: 83–85

McWilliams B J 1970 Psychological development and modification. In: Speech and the dentofacial complex: The state of the art. ASHA Reports no 5, 165–187

McWilliams B J, Musgrave R 1972 Psychological implications of articulation disorders in cleft palate children. Cleft Palate Journal 9: 294–303

McWilliams B J, Paradise L 1973 Educational, occupational, and marital status of Cleft Palate adults. Cleft Palate Journal 10: 223–229

Means B, Irwin J 1954 An analysis of certain measures of intelligence and hearing in a sample of the Wisconsin cleft palate population. Cleft Palate Newsletter 4: 2, 4

Morris H 1962 Communication skills of children with cleft lip and palates. Journal of Speech and Hearing Research 5: 79–90

Munson S, May A 1955 Are cleft palate persons of subnormal intelligence? Education Research Journal 48: 617–622

Musgrave R, McWilliams B J, Matthews H 1975 A review of the results of two different surgical procedures for the repair of clefts of the soft palate only. Cleft Palate Journal 12: 281–290

Nation J 1970 Determinants of vocabulary development. Cleft Palate Journal 7: 645–662

Palmer J, Adams M 1962 The oral image of children with cleft lips and palates. Cleft Palate Bulletin 12: 72–76

Peter J, Chinsky R 1974a Sociological aspects of cleft palate adults: I Marriage. Cleft Palate Journal 11: 295–309

Peter J, Chinsky R 1974b Sociological aspects of cleft palate adults: II Education. Cleft Palate Journal 11: 433–449

Peter J, Chinsky R, Fisher M 1975a Sociological aspects of cleft palate adults: III Vocational and economic aspects. Cleft Palate Journal 12: 193–199

Peter J, Chinsky R, Fisher M 1975b Sociological aspects of cleft palate adults: IV Social integration. Cleft Palate Journal 12: 304–310

Phillips B, Harrison R 1969 language skills in preschool cleft palate children. Cleft Palate Journal 6: 108–119

Plotkin R, Wirls C, Finney B 1970 Developmental evaluation of the cleft infant. Paper presented to the American Cleft Palate Association, Portland, Oregon

Rattner L, Carter N, Pelkey L 1958 Intelligence quotient of children with congenital cleft palate. Dental Research Journal 37: 79

Richman L 1976 Behaviour and achievement of cleft palate children. Cleft Palate Journal 13: 4–10

Richman L 1978a The effects of facial disfigurement on teachers' perception of ability in cleft palate children. Cleft Palate Journal 15: 155–160

Richman L 1978b Parents and teachers: differing views of behaviour of cleft palate children. Cleft Palate Journal 15: 360–368

Ruess A 1965 A comparative study of cleft palate children and their siblings. Journal of Clinical Psychology 21: 354–360

Ruess A 1968 Convergent psychosocial factors in the cleft palate clinic. In: Lencione R (ed) Cleft palate habilitation. Syracuse University Press, Syracuse, p 53–70

Sidney R, Matthews J 1956 An evaluation of the social adjustment of a group of cleft palate children. Cleft Palate Bulletin 6: 10

Smith R, McWilliams B J 1966 Creative thinking abilities of cleft palate children. Cleft Palate Journal 3: 275–283

Smith R, McWilliams B J 1969 Psycholinguistic considerations in the management of cleft palate children. Journal of Speech and Hearing Disorders 33: 26–33

Spriestersbach D 1961 Evaluation of a technique for investigating the psychosocial aspects of the cleft palate problem. In: Pruzansky S (ed) Congenital anomalies of the face and associated structures. Thomas, Springfield, Illinois, 345–362

Spriestersbach D 1973 Psychosocial aspects of the cleft palate problem. University of Iowa Press, Iowa, vol 1

Spriestersbach D, Dickson D, Frazer F, Horowitz S, McWilliams B J, Paradise J, Randall P 1973 Clinical research in cleft lip and cleft palate: The state of the art. Cleft Palate Journal 10: 113–165

Starr P, Chinsky R, Canter H, Meier J 1977 Mental, motor, and social behaviour of infants with cleft lip and/or cleft palate. Cleft Palate Journal 14: 140–147

Tisza V, Silvertone B, Rosenblum O, Hanlon N 1958 Psychiatric observations of children with cleft palates. American Journal of Orthopsychiatry 28: 416–423

Tisza V, Gumpertz E 1962 The parents' reactions to the birth and early care of children with cleft palate. Pediatrics 30: 86–90

Tisza V, Irwin E, Zabarenko L 1969 A psychiatric interpretation of children's creative dramatic stories. Cleft Palate Journal 6: 228–234

Van Demark D, Van Demark A 1970 Speech and sociovocational aspects of individuals with cleft palate. Cleft Palate Journal 7: 284–299

Watson C 1964 Personality adjustment in boys with cleft lips and palates. Cleft Palate Journal 1: 130–138

Weachter E 1959 Concerns of parents related to the birth of a child with a cleft of the lip and palate and implications for nurses. MA Thesis, University of Chicago, Chicago

Wirls C 1971 Psychosocial aspects of cleft lip and palate. In: Grabb W, Rosenstein S, Bzoch K (eds) Cleft lip and palate: Surgical, dental and speech aspects. Little, Brown, Boston, ch 8

Wirls C, Plotkin R 1971 A comparison of children with cleft palate and their siblings on projective test personality factors. Cleft Palate Journal 8: 399–408

11

Management of the neonate

When a child is born with a cleft palate the medical and nursing attendants are faced with two kinds of problem. There are the hazards affecting the baby itself, which may even threaten its life, in particular there is the possibility of neonatal respiratory obstruction and the much more frequent occurrence of difficulty with feeding. Quite distinct from the need to manage these physical problems is the importance of recognizing the distress and bewilderment of the parents, and of spending time explaining to them the nature of the deformity and the plans for treatment.

We should first consider the possible problems which the cleft palate baby faces as soon as he is born.

NEONATAL RESPIRATORY OBSTRUCTION

Most babies with a cleft palate have no difficulty in breathing, but there is a group of infants born with a very small and posteriorly displaced mandible and a tongue which falls backwards, which can cause a severe and potentially lethal obstruction to the airway. Attention was first focused on this association of micrognathia, glossoptosis, neonatal respiratory obstruction and (frequently) cleft palate by Pierre Robin in 1923, and it has come to be known as the *Pierre Robin syndrome* (Fig. 11.1). Recently the use of the term 'syndrome' for this condition has been questioned, and the name *The Robin Anomalad* has been coined to describe it. It is already being used in a number of publications, but it seems unduly pedantic as the common co-existence of the signs and symptoms fulfil the usual definition of a syndrome, and the name 'Pierre Robin syndrome' is universally recognized.

Whether a syndrome or an anomalad, it is important to recognize that the condition Pierre Robin described includes neonatal respiratory obstruction, and that the label should not be attached to a child with a small lower jaw and a cleft palate who breathes without difficulty.

Aetiology
In most cases the deformity is probably due to a failure or delay of the neck of the embryo to extend as it normally does during the 7th week, and this may in turn be because a lack of amniotic fluid (oligohydramnios) constricts the space available for the embryo. The lower jaw is crushed against the chest and there

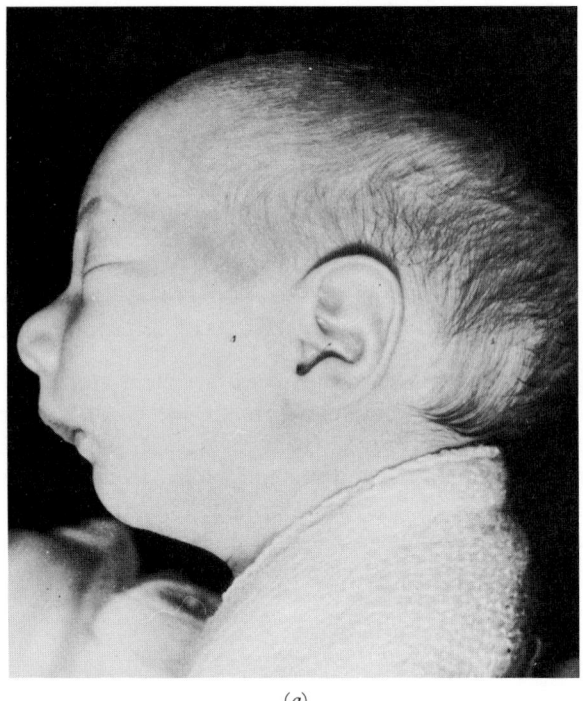

(a)

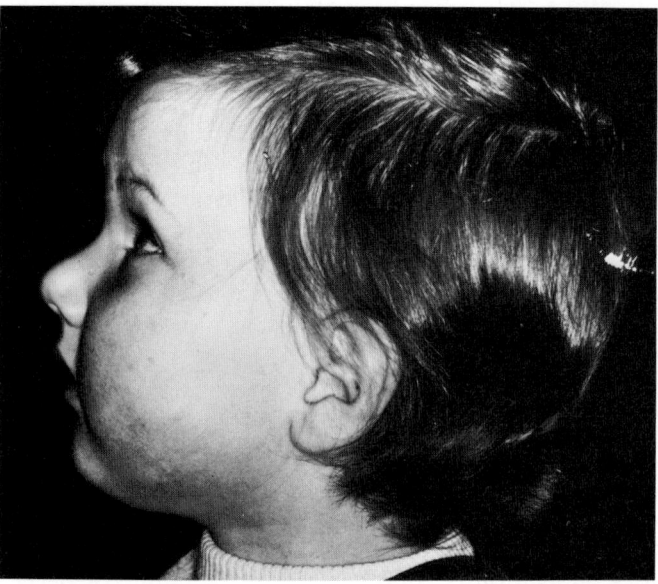

(b)

Fig. 11.1 The Pierre Robin syndrome. (a) Baby aged 1 day. (b) Same child aged 20 months, showing growth of mandible

is no room for the tongue to descend from between the palatal shelves, which therefore cannot come together and fuse. The extent of the cleft of the secondary palate depends on how great is the delay in neck extension. There is a small group of patients in whom the features of the Pierre Robin syndrome are associated with other defects of the respiratory tract and who have a poor prognosis. The aetiology of the anomalies in these patients cannot be explained in this simple mechanistic way.

Clinical features

The muscular control of the tongue depends on its anterior attachment to the mandible, and when the latter is very small the tongue tends to fall back and obstruct the pharyngeal airway. At worst, the obstruction may be complete and immediate measures may be required to save the baby's life. More commonly, the airway can be maintained with difficulty when the baby is awake, but as soon as he falls asleep the tongue falls back and blocks the pharynx. Under these circumstances the baby cannot rest, feeding is almost impossible and death from exhaustion can easily occur.

Management

Because of the potentially lethal result, treatment of the respiratory obstruction is urgent. Placing the baby face-down will often allow the tongue to fall forward and clear the pharyngeal airway. This method should be tried first, but then there is difficulty keeping the nasal airway open. A tube of stockinette taped around the baby's head and suspended to allow the face to hang just above the bed can be useful.

In our experience a frame which allows nursing in the prone position, is almost always effective in overcoming the obstruction (Fig. 11.2). This frame has been adapted by Dr G. B. Hopkin of the Department of Orthodontics, University of Edinburgh, from that described by Bromley & Burston in 1966. It can be made in almost any hospital workshop and avoids the need for the special plaster cradle which is called for in the original design. Instructions on how to make this frame are given in the Appendix.

It is not usually necessary to nurse the infant in the frame for the whole time, and it may be possible to allow him out for one hour in three. However, the frame may be needed for two or three months.

We have already mentioned the feeding difficulties suffered by the baby with the Pierre Robin syndrome. Bottle feeding should be attempted with the baby in the three-quarter prone position with the head turned to the side. The nurse's thumb should be behind the angle of the mandible, holding it forward. It is important that bottle feeding should be tried, so that the baby's normal sucking and feeding mechanism can develop. However, if there are signs of aspiration the bottle should be abandoned. A nasogastric tube may have to be passed, and McEvitt (1973) has described how this may improve respiration by holding the tongue forward and creating an airway on either side of the tube.

If these methods are inadequate, a stitch passed through the tongue as far back as possible and pulled forward to be taped to the baby's chin will usually give temporary relief from airway obstruction, or a towel clip can be used in

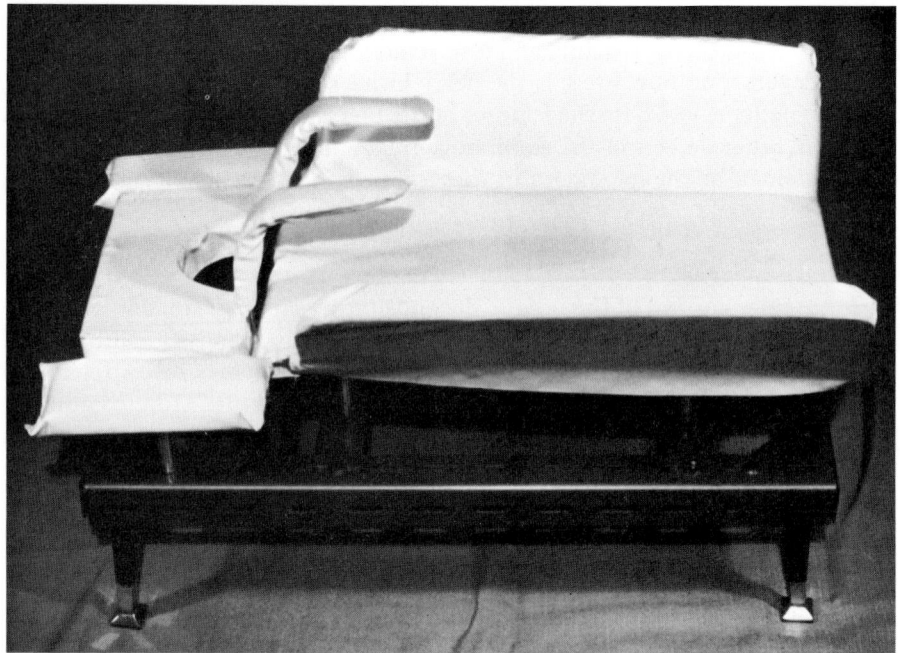

(a)

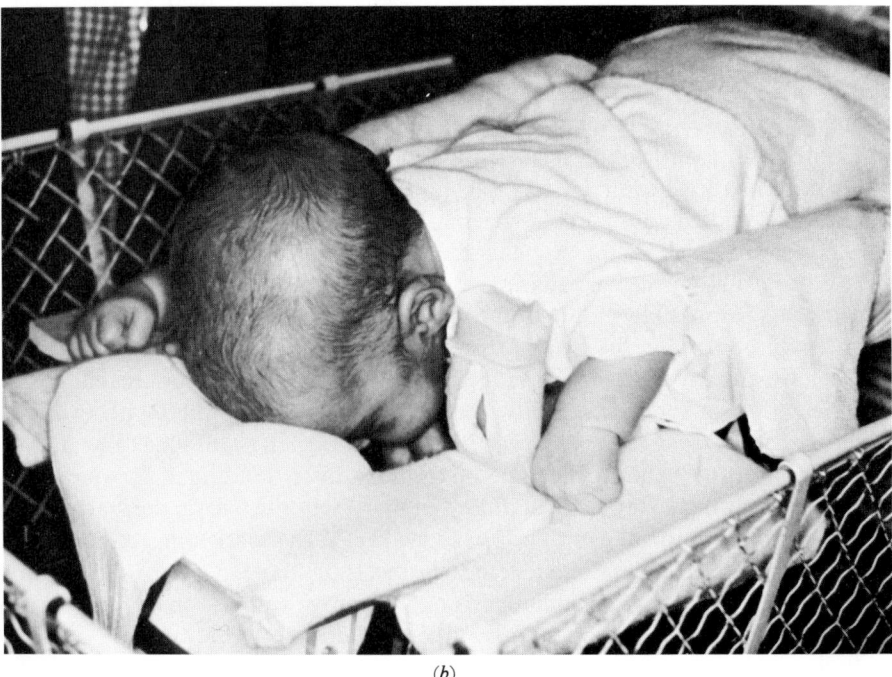

(b)

Fig. 11.2 Hopkin's modification of the Burston frame for Pierre Robin syndrome. (a) The frame, made to Hopkin's specifications. (b) A baby being nursed in the frame. (Photographs by courtesy of Dr G B Hopkin, Department of Orthodontics, University of Edinburgh)

the same way. However, both controls usually pull out after a day or two, and if the face-down position still does not clear the airway some surgical procedure will have to be considered.

Beverley Douglas in 1946 popularized an operation to hold the tongue forward by stitching it to the lower lip, and the technique has been improved by Routledge (1960) and further modified by Randall (1964) (Fig. 11.3). This is probably the most effective surgical method of treatment. Routledge, in his excellent paper, stressed that in the severe case surgery should not be delayed.

Most patients can be managed successfully by one of the methods outlined above. Occasionally a tracheostomy may be required and the condition can prove fatal even with the best care. This is especially likely when it is associated with other anomalies of the upper respiratory tract. Cor pulmonale has been reported

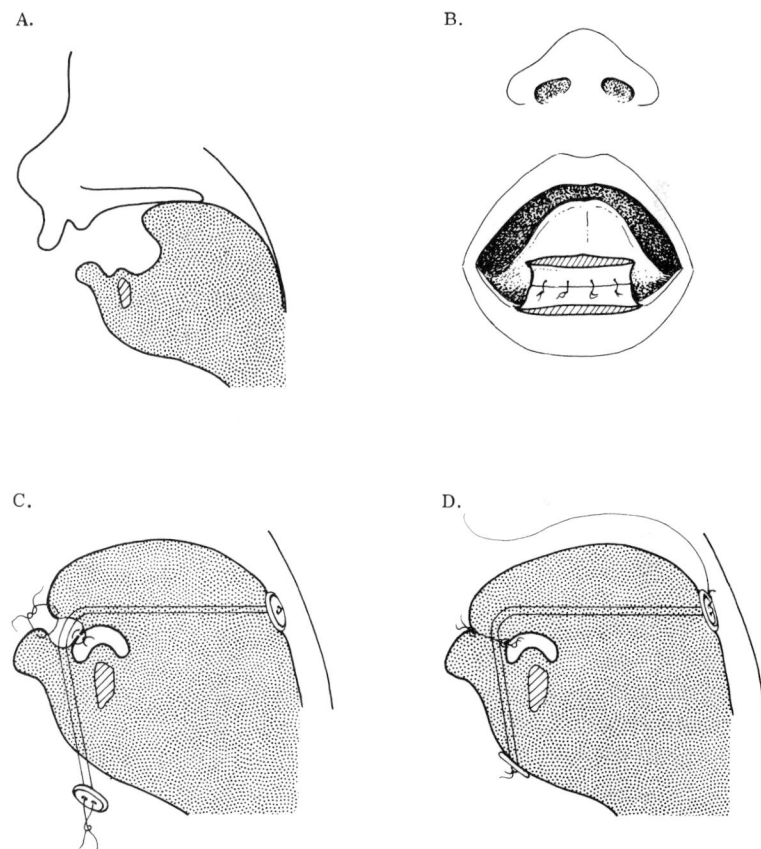

Fig. 11.3 Randall's modification of Routledge's operation for Pierre Robin syndrome. (a) Sagittal section showing tongue falling back to obstruct airway. (b) Anterior view showing horizontal incisions in lower lip and below tongue tip; inferior wound margins sutured together with chromic catgut. (c) Sagittal section showing heavy silk tension suture passing from button at base of tongue, through tongue and lip incisions to be tied through a button below the chin; suture through upper margins of incisions. In addition, tongue and lip muscles are approximated with two 3–0 chromic catgut sutures (not shown here). (d) All sutures tied and the operation completed. Tongue held forward and airway clear. Note anchoring suture to allow retrieval of button when tension suture is removed at 7 to 10 days

as a complication of the chronic airway obstruction (Cogswell & Easton, 1974).

In most cases the mandible grows and the respiratory distress resolves after several months. Often by the age of 2 or 3 years the jaw is of normal size. However, it sometimes remains small and the respiratory difficulties may persist for a long time. When they have settled, treatment can stop and any surgical procedure can be reversed. The small mandible may mean that surgical closure of the cleft has to be delayed. There may be technical problems of access into the small mouth and closure can result in a recurrence of airway obstruction. Holdsworth (1963) took the opposite view and suggested that the Pierre Robin syndrome was an indication for early closure of the palate, as this held the tongue forward and cleared the pharynx, but early closure has not been our practice.

FEEDING

Almost all babies with anything other than the most minor cleft will have some difficulties in feeding, and before expert help became widely available many died from the effects of malnutrition. Fortunately, nearly all centres now have the advice of experts available, and in the developed countries undernourished babies with clefts should hardly ever be seen. The source of advice varies in different places: it may be from the paediatrician, the nurse, or sometimes even the speech therapist. The important purpose is to maintain close contact with mother and child until a good feeding pattern is established, and even with such help it is occasionally necessary for the baby to be readmitted to hospital when feeding takes so long that mother and baby become exhausted. Details of the feeding regime used in the authors' service are given later in this chapter.

COUNSELLING

It is very desirable that the parents of a baby with a cleft palate meet one of the members of the cleft palate team at the earliest opportunity so that an authoritative account of the plans for management can be given and problems discussed. We feel that if possible this team member should be the surgeon, and in our service, where almost all the babies are born in readily accessible hospitals, the surgeon and where necessary the orthodontist see the parents within the first 48 hours after their baby's birth. In other circumstances, where the birth may take place far from the cleft palate centre, the local paediatric staff should be familiar with the regime of treatment favoured by the centre to which the child is referred, so that conflicting advice is not given. Referral to the centre should be as early as possible.

A great deal of what is said at this first interview will be forgotten. Printed handouts can be given to the parents, but it is more important that they are seen regularly and that personal support and advice is provided. The authors are fortunate in working in a centre which has two specialist paediatric nurses who are integral members of the cleft palate team and who provide a home-care service, visiting and keeping in constant touch with the families of cleft palate babies, forming an invaluable link with other members of the team. Other centres have similar arrangements adapted to their particular circumstances.

THE ROLE OF THE NURSE

The role of the nurse in the home management of an infant with cleft lip and palate is as a part of the caring team, which consists of parents, plastic surgeon, orthodontist and nurse. She is mainly adviser, support and go-between for the parents during a time of anxiety and stress.

The initial reaction of the parents when they first see their baby is often of fear, guilt, and revulsion which they are unable to express, and it is very important that contact with the caring team is made as early as possible after the birth of the baby. The mother who is able to look after her baby from the start appears to adjust more easily at home, and sensible practical advice at this stage is vital.

While in hospital, the baby should be examined by the plastic surgeon and orthodontist to assess the extent of the defect, discuss the programme of treatment with the parents and fit the infant with a presurgical orthopaedic appliance if this is included in the regime. Ideally, the home-care nurse should also meet the mother in hospital and explain that she will be available to help once mother and the baby go home.

The mother should be encouraged and helped to feed and care for the baby as early as possible, but a routine will not be established until the family settle in at home and adjust to their new problems.

The daily care of the infant includes care of the nose, mouth and facial skin, and cleaning of the splint at each feed time. The extra time spent on the actual feed can be very exhausting for the mother, and back-up domestic help in the early days should be arranged if possible.

Once the routine is established, feeding will take little longer than normal, but trial and error in the early stages when the mother is first home can add to pressures and anxieties already mounting, and the nurse must be prepared to give as much time as possible to the first few visits, which should start as soon as possible after discharge home. A good listening ear and encouragement to voice fears can be helpful, and reassurance on the mother's own capabilities and the baby's ultimate state should be part of each visit. Relatives, friends and neighbours are always ready with advice and criticism, and the family can be very hurt by comments and old wives' tales. Photographs of similarly affected babies before and after surgery are often helpful, and careful introduction to other parents can be very reassuring, though it is usually wise to join in the interview.

Practical support for the mother ensures that she understands why the programme of care is arranged and exactly what part she plays in the team.

The day of discharge home can be very traumatic for the parents. This is often the first meeting with family and inquisitive friends, and cruel statements can undermine parents who are already anxious and saddened by their baby's condition. An obvious defect is much more difficult to live with than one which can be covered by pretty clothes, even though the end result may be so much more hopeful. Constant reassurance about surgery and results of good early care is essential, but the nurse must be careful not to make statements which she cannot substantiate.

Before the baby is discharged, the requisites for his care are listed, and a check should be made to ensure that the mother has all necessary articles. Teats should be checked and a source of supply arranged. Bottles must match teats—some fit narrow-necked bottles only and it can be difficult to acquire these at short notice. A box or tray with the articles required for pre- and post-feed care can be topped up daily, and the addition of a small cup (or bowl) and teaspoon to the bottle sterilizer is necessary for the sterile water used to clean the mouth at the end of each feed. Requisites in the box are:

Cotton buds
Vaseline
Baby oil
Soft toothbrush
6 mm ($\frac{1}{4}$ in) dressmaker's tape for plate
12.5 mm ($\frac{1}{2}$ in) adhesive tape
5 cm (2 in) Elastoplast
Tissues

Teats required for the infant vary, but a long teat with a large hole or a cross slit which allows the milk to flow only when sucked is usually found most satisfactory (Fig. 11.4). The baby with a cleft palate only may manage well with a flange teat, the flange filling the cleft and acting as a temporary palate. Some mothers manage to breast-feed successfully, and those who wish to do so should be encouraged to try. They need to be highly motivated and given a great deal of support, but if they succeed even for a short time it can be of great psychological help. With severe defects it can be impossible for the baby to fix.

Feeding time should be as relaxed and happy as with any baby, and careful organization is necessary. The baby tray should be to hand, and also the feed at the required temperature, a cup with boiled water and a teaspoon.

If an orthopaedic splint is worn, the baby should have his splint removed immediately before the feed and the plate washed under running water and the tapes changed if necessary. The nostrils should also be cleaned. The plate is then replaced and the feed given. Feeding by bottle rather than spoon is much more natural for the baby and encourages the biting action of the lower lip and jaw function and development. Initially this may take much longer than the mother expects, and care must be taken not to overtire the very small infant. A routine is usually established quite quickly, and as the baby gets stronger he should feed in the normal length of time. When the feed is finished, a small amount (2 to 3 teaspoonsful) of sterile water is given to clean the mouth and plate and the lips are well lubricated with Vaseline. Tapes are checked to see that they are dry and clean and firmly attached to the Elastoplast base on the cheeks. If the baby has pressure strapping externally over the lip it is very important to check that it is clean and dry and not rubbing on the face.

Daily care of the mouth and face are best done at bath time, and include thorough cleaning of the nose and mouth with cotton buds, making sure that all the hidden corners are checked. Thrush infection can be a problem, and careful inspection and, if necessary, treatment should be carried out. The lips should again be well lubricated and the skin of the face observed for dry or

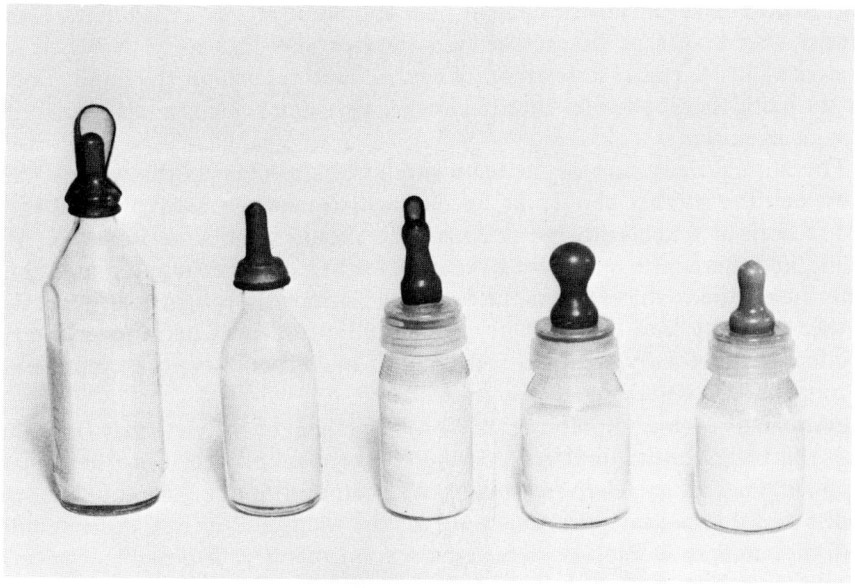

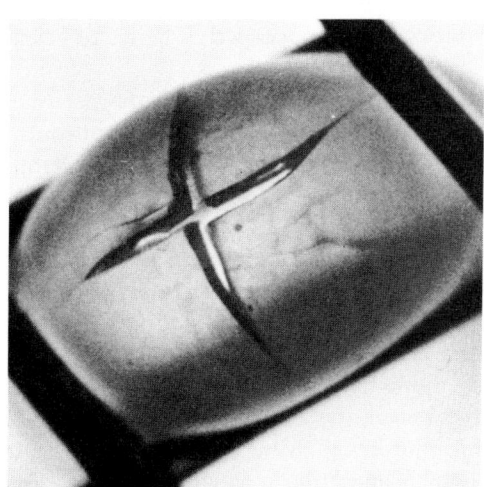

Fig. 11.4 (a) A selection of teats and bottles which can be used for feeding babies with cleft palate. (b) Cross slit cut with scissors in the end of the teat

wet irritation or sore areas. When a splint is being worn, the foundation plaster on the baby's cheeks should only be removed when it is soiled; olive oil will usually aid removal without damage to the skin. Sometimes this plaster will last for 7 to 10 days, but each baby reacts in his own way. If there is any skin irritation, a little hat can be worn and longer tapes applied to the plate and tied around the head to enable it to be kept in position. Trial and error will produce an effective solution, and parents often come up with the ideal answer.

The area round the folds of the neck should also be carefully washed and dried as the baby often dribbles excessive saliva. Any skin which does not respond quickly to normal care should be referred to the family doctor, as removal of the plate for a prolonged spell can delay progress and surgery.

Pressure areas from an orthopaedic plate should be referred back to the ortho-dontist, and cracks or fissures around the lips should also be reported and treated. Colds or runny noses require control, and referral to the family doctor for antibiotic therapy to prevent ear damage, with later hearing and speech prob-lems, is essential.

The normal daily care of the baby should be the same as that of any other baby, and the mother should be encouraged to take the baby out and about and to keep in touch with her friends. She should attend the infant Welfare Clinic, and there is no reason why the milk feeding and weaning regime should differ from other babies' unless the baby has additional problems. It is not wise to take the baby into crowded places or public transport because of the risk of infection, especially preoperatively, and to avoid this transport to clinics and hospital should be arranged when possible.

Preoperative clinic appointments for management of the cleft may be mainly with the orthodontist, and records will be kept of progress and new plates supplied if necessary. Help to attend clinics can usefully be given by voluntary bodies and this can save precious time for the mother. Meeting other families with the same, or worse, problems is also good therapy. If possible, the nurse should attend the clinics, and the exchange of ideas and information at these sessions can be of the utmost importance to all concerned. The more relaxed the meeting, the better.

Preparation of the family for the repair of the cleft lip and of the palate can be started at early visits, with discussion about hospital admission and routine, the feasibility of the mother living in and the procedures which will happen to the baby. Prior understanding of ward routine and other types of patients that may be met, especially if the ward also contains a burns and scalds unit, can allay fears and reassure the mother that the change of routine will not have a lasting effect on a well-established baby. The fact that postoperatively the baby will probably have arm splints, intravenous infusion, nasal pack and tilted bed is also useful information for the mother. Preoperative nasal and throat swabs taken at home can ensure that the baby is not admitted with infection, and that admission is therefore shortly before the day of surgery. The mother should know that it is not unusual for infection to be present and operation temporarily postponed. The age at which operation is performed varies from surgeon to surgeon, as well as depending on the orthodontic treatment, and infection at home can also influence this aspect to a large extent. It is therefore very important that no one gives a fixed age or weight for surgery, and that the parents are always told that delay or cancellation is possible. Contact should be kept with the parents while the baby is in hospital, and communication with ward staff can be very helpful. The reaction of the parents when they see their baby after operation is often of surprise and sometimes slight disappointment, but these initial feelings are usually quickly intermingled with relief and delight. The hospital stay is normally fairly short. After discharge the baby will have his arms in splints until seen by the surgeon as an outpatient, and the normal feeding pattern will be reintroduced as soon as possible. Visits to the orthodont-ist and hospital will now be less frequent, but the nurse should keep in close contact with the family until surgical treatment is complete.

Involvement with a family coping with this problem is very rewarding. It is a privilege to share in the care of such a baby and in the pleasure as each stage of treatment is satisfactorily completed.

REFERENCES

Bromley D, Burston W R 1966 The Pierre Robin syndrome. Nursing Times Dec 30
Cogswell J J, Easton D M 1974 Cor pulmonale in the Pierre Robin syndrome. Archives of Diseases of Childhood 49: 11
Douglas B 1946 The treatment of micrognathia associated with obstruction by a plastic procedure. Plastic and Reconstructive Surgery 1: 300
Holdsworth W G 1963 Cleft lip and palate. Heinemann, London
McEvitt W G 1973 Treatment of respiratory obstruction in micrognathia by use of a nasogastric tube. Plastic and Reconstructive Surgery 52: 138
Randall P 1964 In: Converse J M (ed) Reconstructive plastic surgery. Saunders, Philadelphia, p 1458
Robin P 1923 Backward lowering of the root of the tongue causing respiratory disturbances. Bulletin de l'Académie de Médecine 89: 37
Routledge R T 1960 The Pierre Robin syndrome; a surgical emergency in the neonatal period. British Journal of Plastic Surgery 13: 204

12

Primary surgery

INTRODUCTION

A child with a cleft of the palate cannot speak normally, is likely to suffer from earache and deafness, and has the embarrassment of food and drink coming down his nose. If the cleft involves the primary palate, and in particular the lip, he also has a hideous visible deformity. The aim of treatment is to make this child anatomically and functionally as nearly normal as possible, and the basis of treatment is the surgical closure of the cleft.

The pioneers of cleft palate surgery aimed no further than getting the cleft closed, and were the deformity simply a cleft in otherwise normal tissues this would have been adequate. In reality the problem is much more complicated. Not only is there a cleft, but there is also to a greater or lesser extent a deficiency of tissue. Intrauterine growth of the involved tissues, in which the normal constraints and attachments have been disturbed, gives rise to distortions and displacements of these structures from their normal positions, which add to the difficulties of successful treatment. The amount by which postnatal growth is inhibited and distorted if the cleft is untreated, and the influence of different methods of surgical treatment on growth are matters of argument about which research has not yet been able to provide all the answers. (The reader will find a fuller discussion of facial growth in Chapter 7.) The assessment and recording of cleft palate speech remains subjective and as a result there is still no consistent evidence to suggest that any one operative procedure gives better speech than another.

THE CHOICE OF A TREATMENT REGIME

There are two basic areas of disagreement: the timing of surgery and how radical that surgery should be. There is considerable evidence that the child has a better chance of speaking normally if his cleft is closed early, but operations seem to distort the developing maxilla and the earlier they are carried out the worse the effect. This is particularly true of operations designed to close the bony cleft of the alveolus and hard palate. As a result, some people feel that closure, particularly of the hard palate, is best delayed until growth is almost completed.

Operative techniques are now based on a much sounder appreciation of functional anatomy and pathology than they once were, so that the gross deformities of the maxilla that used to be seen should no longer occur. Nevertheless, the arguments continue over which operation produces the best speech results or causes the least disturbance of growth. Unfortunately there is a lack of controlled trials in which two or more methods of treatment have been scientifically compared in a single centre, and in which a detailed comparison of both speech results and growth has been reported.

Before one can come to a decision as to which treatment regime will give the best chance of both good speech and good appearance, it is important to consider the various factors which are known to contribute to poor results.

Factors related to poor speech

It is significant that if one takes the subjective nature of speech assessment into account, in almost every series of cleft patients about 20 per cent have unsatisfactory speech no matter what type of operation they have had. There are a number of factors which are likely to result in a patient speaking poorly, over which the nature of the treatment will have little or no influence. For example, Drillien and her colleagues (1966) have demonstrated that children of low intelligence and those whose parents are uninterested in their progress tend to speak poorly. The choice of surgical regime is unlikely to influence these children to speak more normally.

Deaf children with clefts speak less well than those with good hearing. Several studies have suggested that early closure of the palate reduces the incidence of middle ear disease, which is so commonly associated with cleft palate and which can lead to deafness (see Chapter 9). However, there is no evidence that one type of operation is any better than another in this respect, and every published series includes a proportion of children whose poor speech is associated with deafness. Whatever surgical regime is chosen, a close watch must be kept on the patient's hearing and active steps taken to deal with middle ear disease.

Patients with complete clefts of the secondary palate have been shown by Glover (1961) and others to run a high risk of poor speech. Many of these clefts are associated with a greater tissue deficiency than any other type. The cleft in the hard palate may be wide and horseshoe-shaped and the muscles of the soft palate very underdeveloped. Whatever method of closure is chosen, the tissue that is available must be used to stretch across the cleft and the soft palate is likely to be short and poorly mobile. There must be a great variation in the degree of hypoplasia in other types of cleft also, and this will influence the results of surgery quite independently of the choice of operation.

The inevitable incidence of children with low intelligence, poor homes, deafness and severe tissue deficiency in any cleft palate population will ensure that no one operation will allow all patients to achieve perfect speech.

If we now attempt to set down those variations in operative treatment which are known to contribute to poor speech results, we face problems. Almost the only fact which is generally accepted is that if the cleft palate is left untouched until after the age of 2 years, the likelihood of the patient having good speech is reduced. By this age faulty speech patterns have become established which are difficult to change postoperatively. There is no consensus on whether closure of the soft palate before 2 years and delayed closure of the hard palate gives speech inferior to that after a complete palate closure before 2 years. While there is general agreement that an operation producing a short, poorly mobile soft palate is unlikely to result in good speech, such palates can be found after any operation. Many people feel that the von Langenbeck procedure produces an excessive number of palates of this type, but it still has its champions who argue to the contrary. These arguments will be considered further in the coming pages.

Factors relating to poor growth of the maxilla

The growth of the maxilla of the cleft palate patient is influenced by one important factor which is quite independent of surgical treatment. This is the primary deficiency of tissue. A cleft is not a fissure in otherwise normal tissues. There is always, to a greater or lesser extent, a hypoplasia of tissue adjacent to the cleft and this tissue has a reduced growth potential. This is best seen in the unrepaired cleft in the adult. Several series of such clefts have been published from developing countries, and in general these patients show a good development of the maxilla and alveolar arch without the collapse often associated with operated clefts. However, they retain a deficiency of tissue in the line of the cleft which may be very great. The soft palate elements are short, the cleft of the secondary palate often wide and the vertical height of the maxilla on each side of the alveolar cleft is reduced. In addition, there are the distortions which one would expect from growth unrestrained by normal bony and muscular attachments.

All operations designed to close the cleft involve the union of the two halves of the soft palate and, if the cleft is a complete one, the two halves of the lip. These procedures create (with an efficiency depending on the nature of the operation) the normal muscular union between the two elements of the maxilla and the muscular pull causes these elements to be drawn together. If there is a great deficiency of tissue, the resulting narrowing of the cleft will produce an abnormal medial displacement of the lateral element (or elements) of the maxilla and 'alveolar collapse' without the operation interfering with growth in any way. There is general agreement that lip and soft palate should be closed early (the first for the sake of appearance and the second for speech development). Primary bone grafting to stabilize the arch has been shown to interfere with growth. As a result, there is no surgical regime which can prevent this collapse, and its effects can only be overcome by later orthodontic treatment.

Closure of the cleft in the alveolus and hard palate involves, in one way or another, mobilizing tissue from the maxilla on each side of the cleft and displacing it across the cleft to be sutured to tissue from the other side. This almost inevitably produces raw areas laterally, which are usually left to epithelialize. Techniques of closing the soft palate often involve quite extensive dissection of soft tissues lateral to it. The scarring produced by all these manœuvres has been blamed for many of the deformities seen in patients who have had their clefts repaired, and regimes have been designed to minimize growth disturbance from these causes.

At the present time it is not possible to say with certainty which is the best operation for closing a cleft palate, or when it should be done. The choice of treatment must depend on the facilities available in a particular centre, on local and national circumstances and on the philosophy of the surgeon; whether he feels he should strive for the best possible speech in his patients, at the possible sacrifice of appearance, or whether, in the attempt to give his patient a normal appearance in adult life he should run a higher risk of giving him poor speech. Our own feeling is that if a choice has to be made then speech should take priority over appearance. However, we do not yet know enough to be sure whether this dilemma is a real one or if one of the many procedures advocated at the present time may prove to be better than all others both for speech and for appearance.

The arguments for the different regimes of surgical treatment will be developed in the following pages, the most commonly used techniques described, and an attempt made to place them in perspective.

TIMING OF SURGERY

Primary palate

A cleft of the lip, with or without a cleft palate, is a grotesque deformity and there is a school of thought which states that it should be closed in the neonatal period so that the parents do not have to suffer the distress of looking after a baby stigmatized in this way. This can be done under either local or general anaesthesia and a quick and simple procedure is usually carried out.

In South Africa, Davies (1970) carried out a complete closure of lip, alveolus and palate in one operation in the neonatal period. This is a surgical *tour de force* which most surgeons would not care to emulate, but it solves the particular problem of dealing with babies who will not be brought back for treatment or follow-up after their mother's discharge from the maternity home. Other surgeons, in similar circumstances, may not be prepared to close the whole of a complete cleft at once, but operate on the palate first. The parents are more likely to bring the child back for correction of the visible deformity of the lip than for an unrepaired palate which is hidden.

However, where circumstances permit, the majority of surgeons prefer to wait until the child is older—usually between 3 and 6 months—before operating, as they feel that they can spend more time and get a better result in the larger and more developed lip tissue. In addition, many feel that it is better for the parents to have to spend some weeks coming to terms with their child's deformity, as this will prepare them to accept the various problems which may arise during childhood and which will require treatment.

In those centres which favour presurgical oral orthopaedics the timing of surgery to the lip and alveolus is dependent on the time it takes the orthodontist to move the segments of the alveolar arch into the proper alignment. This can usually be done by 3 or 4 months, but may sometimes take longer.

Alveolus

Most surgeons close the alveolar cleft at the same time as they close the lip. There is no doubt that it is easier to close at this stage when the cleft is wide open, and it may be very difficult after lip closure when the pull of the united muscles has drawn the two halves of the maxilla together so that they abut each other. Nevertheless, the people who feel that early operation on this bony part of the cleft may interfere with growth leave the alveolus untouched at the primary operation.

Secondary palate

Veau in 1927 showed that children whose palatal clefts were closed after the age of 2 years had very much poorer speech than those who were operated upon before that age. There have been many other studies since that time which have confirmed his findings. The majority of British and American surgeons, and many elsewhere in the world, aim to close the whole palate before the second birthday, and some before the first.

Unfortunately, as we have already indicated, there are other problems which have to be considered, particularly that of growth, which makes many people feel that no surgery should be performed on bony structures before growth is almost completed. In the early 1920s Sir Harold Gillies became appalled at the terrible deformities which he found in adults who had had cleft palate repair as children. The operations then in vogue were very traumatic, particularly those of Brophy, who crushed the two halves of the maxilla together with wire, and Arbuthnot Lane, who turned over huge flaps of mucosa, leaving extensive raw areas which healed by the contraction of scar tissue.

Gillies & Fry (1921) developed an operation in which they closed only the soft palate and left the cleft hard palate to be filled in by an obturator, and in this way avoided the maxillary collapse. They subsequently abandoned this practice, which condemned the patient to wear an obturator for the rest of his life, but remained very concerned about the effect of early surgery on growth and suggested that it would best be delayed until the age of 4 or 5 years.

In 1949 Graber published a study of facial growth in children with cleft lip and palate in which he concluded that surgery was the major cause of deformity in these children. His paper stimulated a controversy which still rages. In spite of many subsequent investigations into the facial growth of normal children and cleft patients after a variety of operations, and experimental studies of growth after different types of surgical interference in animals, there is still no agreement. Those surgeons who advocate early surgery in the interests of speech believe that modern, less traumatic operations carried out skilfully do not cause significant deformity, but only minor contractions. Others, such as Slaughter & Brodie of Chicago (1949, 1971), have disputed this, and advocated closure of the soft palate alone at some time during the first two years of life, delaying hard palate closure until the age of 4 or 5 years, when 80 per cent of transverse maxillary growth has taken place. Some, like Schweckendieck of Marburg, even wait until the child is 12 to 14 years old, when maxillary growth is virtually completed. Schweckendieck has recently published (1978) a series of over 250 cases treated in this way, with a 25-year follow-up of patients, none of whom have apparently got any maxillary deformity. These surgeons accept that many of their patients will have to wear obturators to allow them to speak satisfactorily until the time comes for hard palate closure, and some suggest that the speech problems which their patients encounter are simpler to correct than those resulting from collapse of the maxilla (Hotz et al 1978). At the present time there does not seem to be any immediate likelihood of these two views being reconciled.

OPERATIVE TECHNIQUES

One of the great difficulties in trying to judge the merits of the arguments of those who advocate early or late surgery of the cleft palate is that their results are likely to be influenced as much by the type of operation to which their patients have been submitted as by its timing. There is, of course, also the influence of the skill of the individual surgeon. There are many different surgical techniques in use at the present time, all of which seem to those who use them to give satisfactory results, and the difficulties of comparing the results of one with another are such that it is uncommon to find a surgeon abandoning his well-tried method to take up an alternative one. It is regrettably rare to find a scientifically controlled comparison of two techniques in the same centre, and it is only when this has been done that general acceptance of an advance in treatment can take place.

In the following section we will attempt to review in an orderly manner the most widely used approaches to closing the cleft, starting with the primary palate.

Primary palate

(a) Cleft lip

A detailed account of the bewildering number of procedures designed to close the cleft lip is beyond the scope of this book, in which we are principally concerned with clefts of the palate. However, as the two deformities are so intimately related, and as a cleft of the lip has a great influence on the behaviour of a cleft palate, some consideration must be given to it.

The history of cleft lip repair is of a steady improvement in the cosmetic result, as surgeons have gradually come to appreciate the true nature of the defect. The recognition that, in the unilateral cleft, elements of the lip such as most of the cupid's bow and philtrum are already present and should be preserved, and the development of operations in which almost none of the precious tissue is thrown away, have resulted in lips that look far more natural. The nasal deformity which always co-exists with the cleft lip is now more effectively dealt with than ever before, although there is still argument about how much of the deformity should be treated at the primary operation.

One of the most important advances in the surgery of the cleft lip in the last few years has been the recognition that the muscle of the cleft lip runs parallel to the free margins of the cleft and is abnormally attached to the edge of the piriform forsa. (In the bilateral cleft the muscle in each lateral element of the lip runs in this way, and there is no muscle in the prolabium—Fig. 12.1.) Unless the muscle is freed and rotated across the cleft during the repair, the lip, which may look excellent at rest, will be noticeably abnormal during movement and the muscle bundles will bulge unnaturally on each side. In this respect the lip resembles the soft palate, and the importance of muscle mobilization is the same.

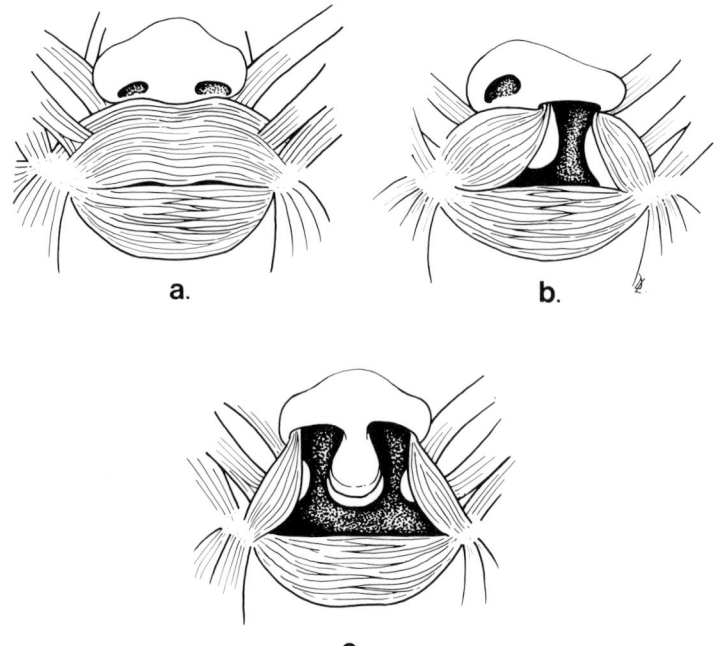

Fig. 12.1 The configuration of the orbicularis oris muscle. (a) Normal. (b) Unilateral cleft lip. The orbicularis oris muscle runs parallel to the edges of the cleft and inserts into the margins of the piriform fossa. (c) Bilateral cleft lip. There is no muscle in the prolabium

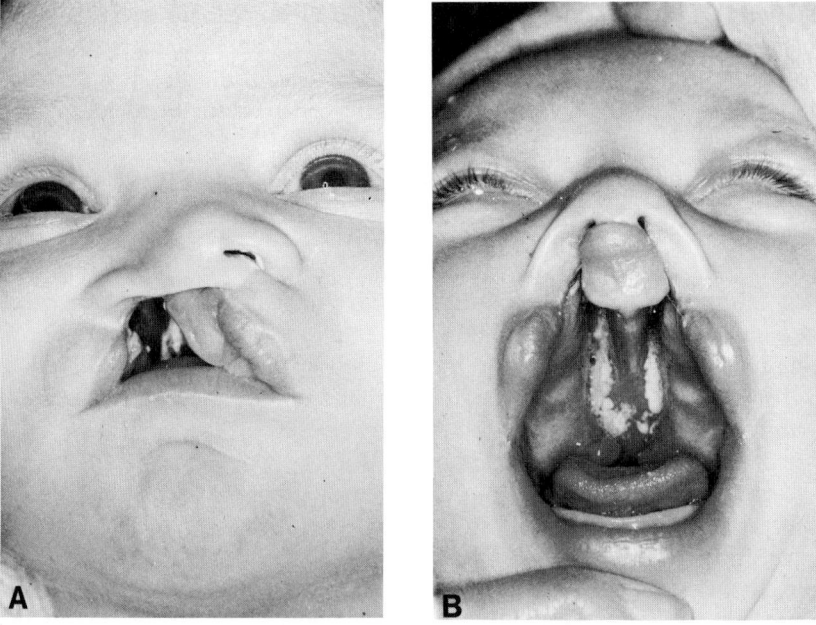

Fig. 12.2 Displacements of the elements of the alveolar arch in complete clefts. (a) Unilateral cleft. Note the wide gap between the two parts of the alveolus. (b) Bilateral cleft. Note how the prolabium and premaxilla are suspended from the tip of the nose and the lateral elements of the maxilla lie far behind them

Reconstitution of the muscle sphincter around the mouth not only allows the lip to function more naturally; if there is a complete cleft of lip, alveolus and palate then the muscle pull across the repaired lip draws the two halves of the maxilla together anteriorly and narrows the alveolar cleft and the anterior part of the cleft palate. We have already pointed out that if the cleft is associated with a significant deficiency of tissue this can by itself cause maxillary collapse without in any way interfering with growth.

In many infants born with a complete cleft of lip and palate the two halves of the maxilla are displaced laterally, making the cleft very wide and surgical

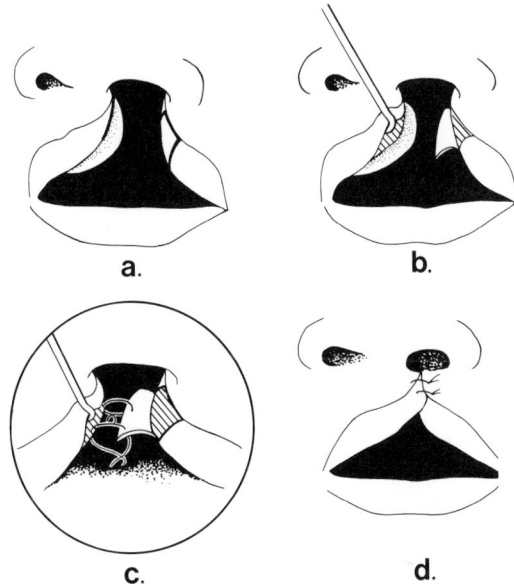

Fig. 12.3 The lip adhesion operation (after Millard). (a) Incisions marked. The medial element of the lip is elevated from the maxilla enough to allow it to advance laterally to meet the lateral element. (b) A mucosal flap is raised from the lateral element. (c) The lateral flap is sutured to the posterior edge of the raw area on the medial lip. (d) The muscles are sutured separately and finally mucosa is stitched to skin

closure very difficult. In the complete bilateral cleft the prolabium and premaxilla are suspended from the tip of the nose and the lateral elements can be collapsed inwards far behind them (Fig. 12.2). The definitive closure of the lip can be made easier, and therefore better, by narrowing the cleft preoperatively. This narrowing can be achieved either by the fitting of a series of presurgical orthopaedic splints by the orthodontist (see Chapter 13) or by a simple preliminary operation known as a *lip adhesion* carried out in the first few weeks of life. Such a procedure has been popularized by Randall and Graham, and modified by Millard (1976) so that it does not interfere with tissues which will be needed in the definitive lip closure (Fig. 12.3). The muscles are exposed in the opposing margins of the upper half of the cleft. They are sutured together across the cleft after minimal undermining, so converting the complete cleft into what is, in effect, an incomplete cleft. In the bilateral cleft an adhesion can be done first on one side and then on the other. The two halves of the maxilla are drawn together by the pull of the united lip, and a protruding premaxilla can be tilted back. Presurgical orthopaedics should produce a similar effect in a more controlled but time-consuming way, and moreover can expand a collapsed lateral segment, which an adhesion cannot do. When the time comes for the definitive operation the available tissue does not have to be stretched across a wide gap, and the surgeon can concentrate on using it to the best advantage in constructing the features of the normal lip and nose.

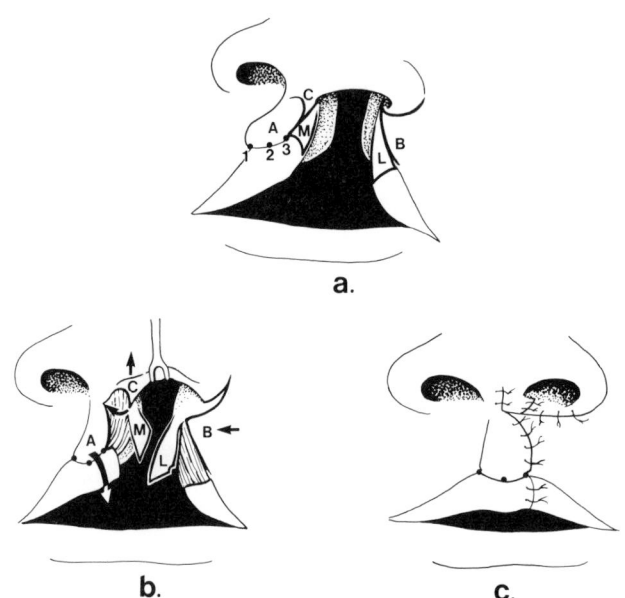

Fig. 12.4 Millard's rotation advancement operation for unilateral cleft lip. (a) The peak of the Cupid's bow on the non-cleft side (1) and the mid-line (2) can be identified and marked. Point 3 lies an equal distance from point 2, and represents the peak of the Cupid's bow on the cleft side. The first incision passes from point 3 parallel to the cleft and then curves under the base of the columella and must not go further than the philtral ridge on the non-cleft side. It cuts through the whole thickness of the lip and if necessary can be extended by a back cut. The incision at point 3 is completed by cutting through the free margin at right angles to the edge of the cleft. This frees flap A (the rotation flap). Flaps C and M are freed by an incision along the mucocutaneous junction continued along the membranous septum. On the lateral lip element flap B (the advancement flap) and flap L are created by the incisions shown. The length of the incision along the mucocutaneous junction should equal the length of the incision delineating flap A and can be adjusted later in the operation if necessary. (b) Flap A rotates downwards to bring the Cupid's bow into the horizontal position. If rotation is inadequate it can be increased by a back cut as indicated in (a) above. Flap B advances into the triangular defect left in the upper part of the lip. Muscle is freed from its attachment to the piriform margin and rotated downwards towards the horizontal position. Flap C advances upwards to lengthen the cleft side of the columella. Flaps M and L can be used in various ways, to construct the nasal floor, provide extra lining for the nostril or close the alveolar cleft. A small 'white roll' flap is raised from the lateral element at the mucocutaneous junction to fit into an incision on the medial element and break up the line of the scar at this point. (c) The flaps are sutured into position. Closure is in layers, particular attention being paid to suturing the muscle in its correct alignment. The contour of the free margin can be adjusted by excision of excess mucosa and transposition of mucosal flaps to augment deficiencies

Unilateral cleft lip

To illustrate the principles of modern unilateral cleft lip repair we have chosen Millard's Rotation Advancement operation, which he first described in 1955 and has been refining ever since. In its latest form the operation is expounded in great detail in Millard's book 'Cleft Craft' (1976). It is only one of a number of procedures in use at the present time, but it is gaining in popularity around the world for many reasons. It is relatively simple to plan and does not involve complicated markings and measurements (Fig. 12.4). It is a 'cut as you go' method, so that at no point in the operation has an irrevocable step been taken, and adjustments can be made up to the very end of the procedure. It allows as much correction of the nasal deformity as the surgeon feels is wise to carry out at the primary operation. Any tightness is high up under the nose in the normal position, and the free margin of the lip remains pleasingly full. The two-thirds of the cupid's bow and philtrum which are already present are preserved and rotated into their normal positions, fixed there by the advancement flap from the lateral side, which moves across above the downwardly rotated medial flap. In doing so, this advancement flap draws the splayed out alar base into its correct position. Even the little 'C' flap can be slid upwards to lengthen the deficient cleft side of the columella. Most important of all, the operation can be carried out in such a way that no tissue whatever need be discarded. Every piece of tissue seems to fall so naturally into its proper place that one feels that the operation must be 'right'. Yet two criticisms can be levelled at it. The first criticism is that in complete clefts the free margin of the cleft side of the lip can be too short (from cupid's bow to the angle of the mouth) if the lateral element of the lip is small. The other is that some people feel that the operation does not adequately rotate the abnormally situated muscle bundles into a horizontal position. However, wider mobilization and rotation of the muscle can be carried out through the same incisions if so desired.

Bilateral cleft lip

The bilateral cleft lip is a much more severe deformity than the unilateral. The absence of muscle in the prolabium, the lack of any vestige of a Cupid's bow or philtrum, the missing columella and the fact that the deficiency of tissue is in general greater, make the challenge of surgical repair much more difficult.

When the bilateral cleft is complete, the projection of the prolabium and premaxilla and inward collapse of the lateral elements behind them add to the surgeon's problems. Lip adhesions can help him by tilting the premaxilla backwards, and presurgical orthopaedics can often add expansion of the lateral elements so allowing the premaxilla to fit between them. Correct alignment of the alveolar arch brings the lip elements closer together. (In the incomplete cleft the bony deformity is less severe and surgical closure is easier.) The practice of surgically retropositioning the protruding premaxilla has fallen into disrepute because of the disastrous effect it can have on growth, but some surgeons still do it on occasion, taking care to avoid damage to the growth centre of the vomerine–prevomerine suture. However, if the premaxilla is not interfered with, cephalometric studies show that it projects relatively less as the face grows and the lateral maxillary segments grow forward. By the time growth is complete, the profile may be fairly normal. In contrast, the patient whose premaxilla has been surgically set back, or who has lost the teeth from it, often reaches adult life with a small, retrusive premaxilla and severe deformity. As a result, we feel that surgical setting back of the premaxilla should be avoided.

Closure of the lip can be carried out in one stage or in two. There is a choice of techniques, and no one technique has pre-eminence at the present time. An important point to remember when one is making a choice is that the prolabium,

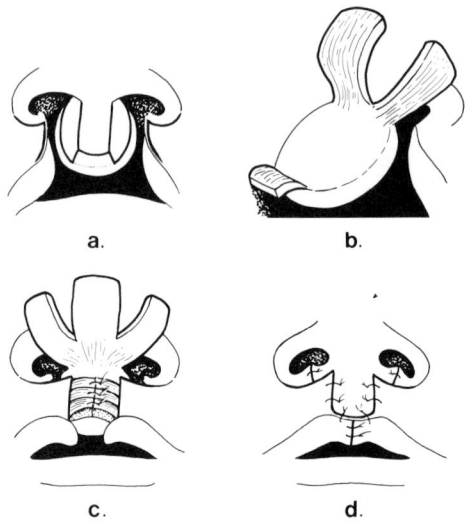

Fig. 12.5 Millard's method of bilateral cleft lip repair: first stage

(a) The incisions marked out. The prolabium is divided into three flaps, based superiorly. The central flap is shaped to resemble a philtrum and the lateral ones are to be banked to lengthen the columella at the second stage. The vermilion of the prolabium, based on its attachment to the premaxilla, is separated from the philtral flap. The flaps on the lateral elements resemble the advancement flap in the rotation advancement procedure, and the incisions along the mucocutaneous junctions are the same length as the philtral flap.

(b) The prolabial flaps have been raised. The prolabial vermilion is shown turned down, but will be turned up to line the raw area on the front of the premaxilla and help form a buccal sulcus.

(c) The mucosa and muscle of the lateral elements have been advanced in front of the premaxilla and sutured together. Vermilion flaps from the lateral elements are turned down.

(d) The philtral flap has been laid back over the approximated muscles and sutured to the skin of the lateral elements. The vermilion flaps have been approximated with a slight excess to form a mid-line tubercle in the free margin. The two lateral prolabial flaps are being banked in the floor of the nose where they form little mounds. Alternatively, they can be inserted between alar base and lateral lip element, where they do not obstruct the airway.

even if it seems very small, stretches greatly after it is united to the rest of the lip, so that no technique should be chosen which introduces skin from the lateral elements below the prolabium. This results in a lip which is too tight and too long. The vermilion of the prolabium is of a different quality from that of the rest of the lip, and should be hidden, or it remains as an obvious blemish.

Many surgeons recommend closure of one side of a bilateral cleft lip at a time, and a variety of techniques are available. If the premaxilla and prolabium lie far in front of the lateral lip elements then it may be very difficult to close both sides of the lip at once, and the use of a staged technique may be essential.

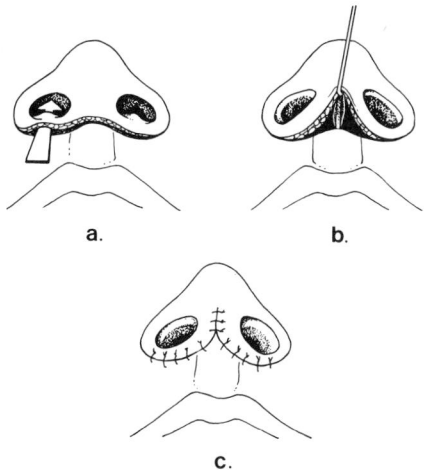

Fig. 12.6 Second stage of Millard's bilateral cleft lip repair: columellar lengthening. (a) The banked flaps and nostril sills are separated from the lip and from the floor of the nose posteriorly by parallel incisions so that they remain attached medially to the columella and laterally to the alar bases. The columella is also freed from the lip and from the septum. (b) The bipedicled flaps so formed are rotated medially into the columella and sutured together. The columella is lengthened and the tip of the nose raised. (c) Incisions sutured. This procedure resembles that described by Cronin. If the flaps are banked below the nostril floors they can be freed so that they retain only a medial attachment to the columella and then advanced as before to lengthen the columella

Unfortunately it is difficult to get good muscle union across the mid-line if one side is done before the other, and it is not always easy to achieve symmetry.

Millard's technique (Fig. 12.5) closes the lip in one stage, leaves a prolabial element which looks much more like a philtrum than the other methods, and brings muscle across behind the prolabium. At the second stage the 'banked' forked flap is used to lengthen the columella (Fig. 12.6). It produces excellent early results, but fears have been expressed that the pull of the muscle might cause recession of the premaxilla. Time will tell if this is true.

(b) Alveolar cleft
A cleft in the alveolus does not occur in the absence of a cleft lip, and together they represent a complete cleft of the primary palate. They are also frequently associated with a complete cleft of the secondary palate, but occasionally a complete unilateral or bilateral cleft of the primary palate is found with the secondary palate intact behind it. In the more usual situation where the two halves of the maxilla are completely separated they drift apart and are subject to distortion from a variety of forces. The surgeon has to ask himself and his orthodontic colleagues what effect the closure of the alveolar cleft may have on the maxillary distortion, what is the best age to perform the closure, and whether he should attempt to produce bony union across the cleft alveolus.

Older techniques of lip repair very often ignored the problem of the cleft alveolus, but once the pull of the repaired lip has drawn the margins of the cleft together closure of the alveolus can be difficult. Consequently many patients were left with oronasal fistulae between the repaired lip and the repaired secondary palate. These can be a great nuisance, allowing particles of food and drink to escape into the nose and having a significant effect on speech. These fistulae may be left by some surgeons as part of a deliberate policy to avoid interfering with bony structures during the growth period, and can be closed once growth has been complete.

Closure of the alveolar cleft with the cleft lip

Although at birth the separated elements of the maxilla are often far apart, we have already seen how they can be brought together by lip adhesion or preoperative orthopaedics. The latter treatment can also overcome the frequent inward collapse of the lesser segment and approximate the opposing ends of the cleft alveolus in a controlled manner. At the time of closure of the cleft lip it is usually possible to close the cleft in the alveolus without difficulty, together with a greater or lesser part of the hard palate. Such a closure can be carried out in one layer, by elevating the septal mucoperichondrium and suturing it to the mucosa of the side wall of the nose (Fig. 12.7). This is usually enough to achieve closure, but the raw undersurface will contract and drag the edges of the cleft together, and this may contribute to the collapse of the alveolar arch. Veau (1938) described a flap of palatal mucoperiosteum, based posteriorly, which he swung across the cleft to reinforce the nasal closure behind the alveolus, but it cannot reach forward into the critical area of the alveolar cleft (Fig. 12.8). A two-layer closure in this area can be obtained by bringing in a flap of lip mucosa as de-

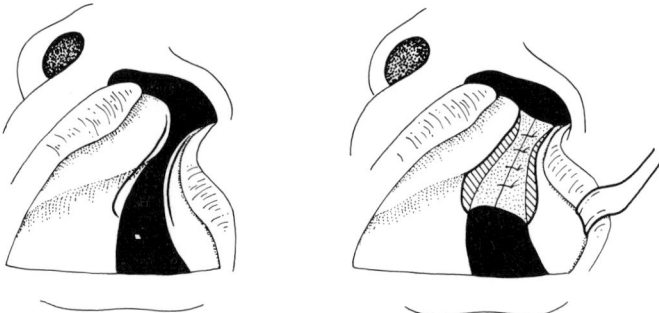

Fig. 12.7 Single layer closure of cleft alveolus and nasal floor. Incisions are made at junction of oral and nasal mucosa on each side of the cleft. Nasal mucosal flaps are then elevated from septum (cartilage anteriorly and vomer posteriorly) and lateral wall of nose and sutured together.

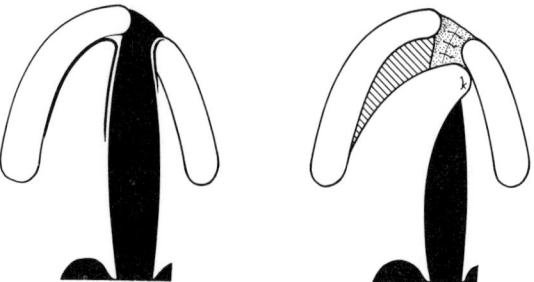

Fig. 12.8 Veau mucoperiosteal flap for closure of oral aspect of anterior palate cleft. Shown in association with nasal mucosal closure of alveolar cleft. Incisions are made and the mucoperiosteal flap elevated and transposed across cleft

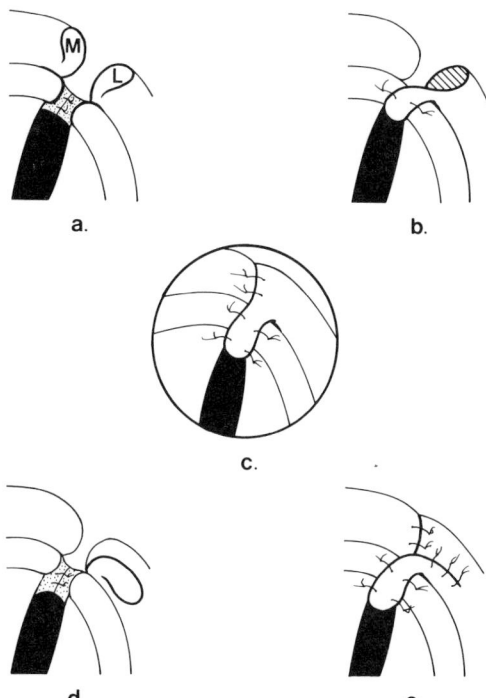

Fig. 12.9 Muir and Burian flaps for two-layer closure of alveolar cleft. The Muir flap uses mucosa from the margin of the cleft lip, from where it can be better spared than the buccal mucosal flaps of Burian. (a) Flaps marked at cleft margins (see Fig. 12.4). Muir described the use of flap L but flap M can be used as an alternative. (b) Flap L transposed to reinforce nasal closure. (c) Closure completed. (d) Burian flap marked on buccal mucosa of lateral lip element. (e) Burian flap transposed to reinforce nasal closure.

scribed by Muir (1966) or Burian (1968) (Fig. 12.9). Muir's flap makes use of tissue which would otherwise be discarded, and both procedures can help to prevent or reduce the alveolar collapse by providing a soft tissue bridge between the bone ends. No bone is laid down in this bridge, but this may be an advantage, as the following section shows.

Primary bone grafting
In the 1950s it was argued by Nordin, Johansson and others that if the alveolar cleft could be closed and stabilized by bone grafting at the primary operation, later collapse would be prevented. Many eminent surgeons took up this apparently promising technique, but after careful assessment of their results over the next ten years most of them abandoned it. They found that, contrary to expectations, there was more maxillary collapse after primary bone grafting than without it. It has been suggested that if the graft produces solid bony union across the cleft, with no sutures or growth centre, this tethers the halves of the maxilla together and prevents their normal growth. There is considerable experimental evidence to support this suggestion.

Periosteal flap
Skoog (1965), in an attempt to achieve bony union across the cleft without having to take bone from elsewhere, developed a method of using a flap of perio-

steum taken from the anterior surface of the maxilla to close the cleft (Fig. 12.10). Not only was he able to show evidence of new bone filling in the cleft, but he claimed that this technique did not interfere with growth of the maxilla. He produced experimental evidence that confirmed these findings in rabbits. The majority of surgeons, while recognizing the ingenuity of the procedure and the excellence of Skoog's published results, await the publication of a longer-term follow-up of clinical results before they accept that it has significant advantages in humans.

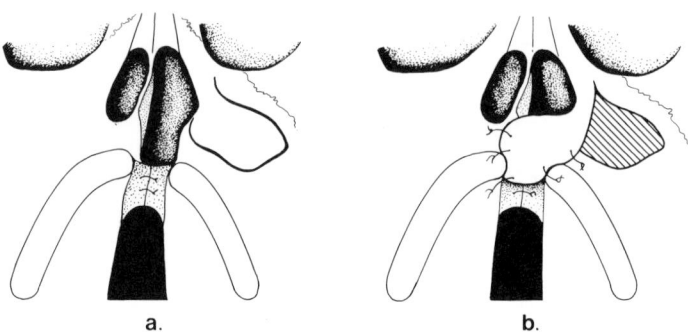

a.   b.

Fig. 12.10 Skoog periosteoplasty. (a) Nasal mucosal flaps closing nasal aspect of alveolar cleft. Periosteal flap marked on anterior aspect of maxilla. (b) Periosteal flap transposed to cover anterior and inferior aspects of alveolar cleft. Surgicel can be packed into the cavity between the flaps

Ritsilä and his colleagues (1973) have advocated the use of a free graft of tibial periosteum to achieve the same ends as the periosteal flap without endangering the growth of the anterior surface of the maxilla. However, it does not seem justifiable to inflict a distant scar on the leg of a baby without strong evidence that a good result cannot be achieved without it.

Closure of the secondary palate

We have already discussed the arguments over whether to close the whole of the secondary palate at one procedure or to close the hard and soft palate at different times.

We will first consider those procedures which achieve complete closure in one operation.

The von Langenbeck operation

Von Langenbeck (1861) was the first surgeon to devise a reliable method of closing the cleft palate, and his operation is still widely practised, with modifications, to this day (Fig. 12.11). The mucous membrane of the hard palate is densely adherent to the underlying periosteum and in this procedure the two are stripped off the bone as a single strong and thick layer. The edges of the cleft are pared and the soft tissues of the two halves of the palate—that is, muco-periosteum anteriorly and soft palate posteriorly—are slid towards each other and stitched together in the mid-line. To allow this to happen, release incisions have to be made on each side and these run just inside the alveolar process from the region of the canine anteriorly, curving round the maxillary tuberosity, to

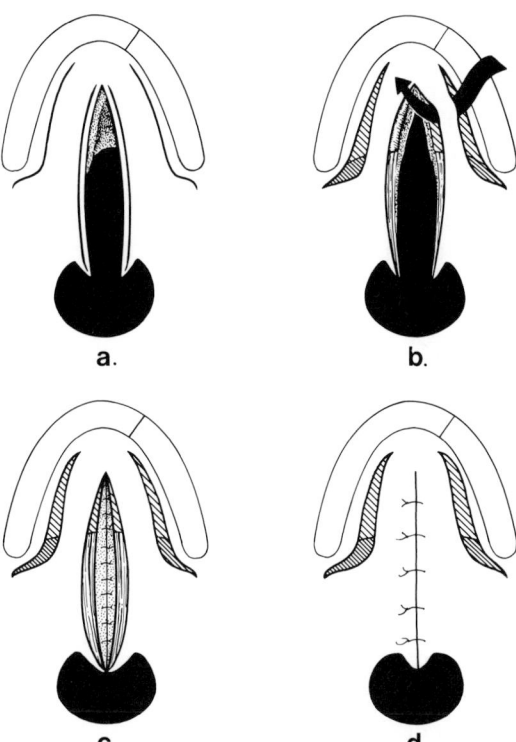

Fig. 12.11 The Langenbeck operation for closure of the secondary palate. (a) The margins of the cleft have been pared and the release incisions have been made medial to the alveolar processes, curving behind the maxillary tuberosities. (b) Mucoperiosteum stripped from the oral surface of the hard palate. The arrow on the right of the diagram indicates how the mucoperiosteum is raised as a bipedicled flap. The nasal mucosa on the upper surface of the hard palate and, if necessary, the septum is mobilized far enough to allow it to meet across the cleft. (c) Appearance after suturing the nasal layer. (d) Closure of the cleft completed. Raw areas are left on each side, exposing the bare bone of the hard palate anteriorly

end just behind the region of the pterygoid hamulus. The mucoperiosteum is then elevated from the bone as a bipedicled flap, attached anteriorly and posteriorly, and dissection is carried out through the posterior ends of the release incisions to relax the soft palate. This is described in greater detail in relation to the push-back operation. After this dissection has been completed, the mucoperiosteal flaps of the hard palate and the two halves of the soft palate can be approximated in the mid-line without tension.

Scarring of the palate. The medial displacement of the palatal tissue in the von Langenbeck procedure leaves raw areas on each side. Over the hard palate bare bone is exposed. Epithelialization takes place quickly and healing is usually complete within two weeks, but some scar tissue is inevitably formed. This scar tissue has been blamed for tethering and restricting the growing palatal bones, and for pulling medially the teeth to which it is related. There is no question that it must have some effect, but the extent to which it can be blamed for secondary deformities in man is not clear. Many experimental studies have been published which confirm distorted growth if raw areas are left in relation to the teeth, e.g. that of Kremenak and his colleagues (1970). Care should therefore be taken not to make the lateral release incisions too far lateral, but as the operation is usually done before the teeth have erupted accurate measurements are impossible and careful judgement is needed.

There are two main criticisms levelled against the von Langenbeck operation. The first criticism is that if the cleft involves the primary palate a fistula must be left anteriorly, behind the alveolus, unless this area has been closed with the lip. The other is that the procedure does nothing to lengthen the palate, which is almost always short. It is therefore very common for patients who have been operated upon by this method to have abnormal nasal escape during speech, and hypernasality. Schoenborn, who was a pupil of von Langenbeck, was probably the first to record his dissatisfaction with the operation in 1876, and he devised the posterior pharyngeal flap operation in an attempt to improve his speech results. Many years later Veau, who was a pioneer in the careful recording and reporting of the speech of his patients, reported that none of his patients spoke normally after a von Langenbeck operation. He developed a 'push-back' operation to lengthen the palate, and obtained very much better speech results (Veau 1931).

In spite of these attacks, the von Langenbeck palate repair still has champions, as it is simple, it leaves smaller raw areas than any of the push-back procedures and probably interferes less with forward growth of the maxilla. Lindsay and his colleagues in Toronto are powerful advocates of the operation and in their series they reported (Lindsay 1971) not only better occlusion but, surprisingly, better speech results when their patients were 4 years old than after a push-back procedure. Unfortunately other groups have published results which confirm the earlier workers' experience that push-back operations give better speech (McEvitt 1971; Musgrave et al 1975; Krause et al 1976). Bishara et al (1976) found no difference in anteroposterior and vertical maxillary growth between the two methods. As always, the different results reported from different centres when comparing what are apparently the same procedures are very confusing. They can be explained by the presumption that there must be variations in operative technique, that some surgeons are more skilful than others, and that methods and timing of assessment vary from place to place. There is no practical way in which these difficulties can be overcome and the best we can hope for is that gradually the weight of published evidence will make the answers clear. Until then, such controversies will continue.

Push-back operations

Victor Veau's dissatisfaction with the von Langenbeck procedure, and his development of a push-back operation, has already been mentioned. His greatly improved speech results stand up to comparison with figures reported today. His push-back procedure has since been modified by Wardill of Newcastle (1937), Kilner of Oxford (1937) and Wardill's successor Braithwaite (1968), and in its present form, with individual variations, is the most popular method of cleft palate closure in the United Kingdom (Figs 12.12, 13, 14). The operation commences in the same way as the von Langenbeck, with the raising of muco-periosteal flaps, and similar release incisions are made laterally. However, the

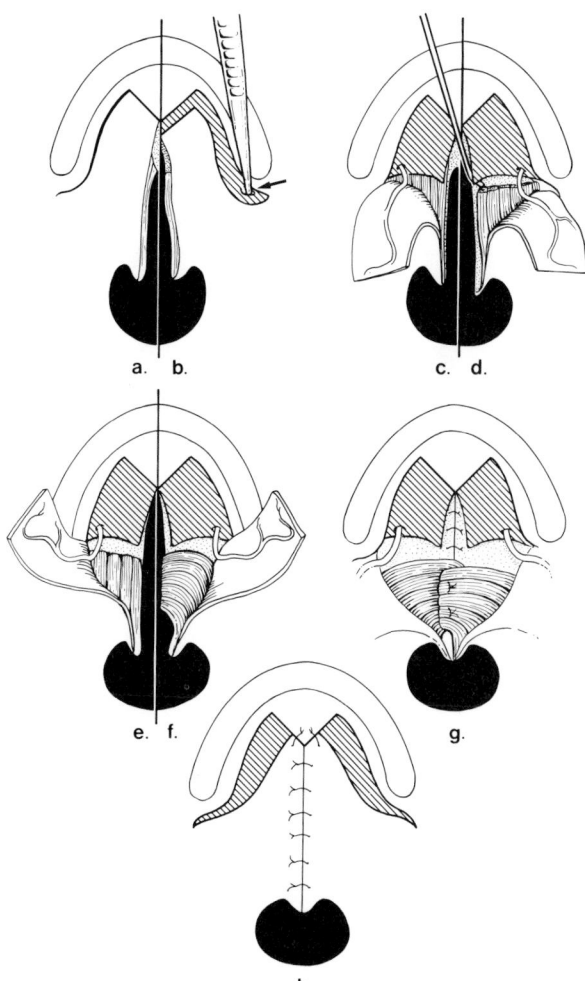

a. b.

c. d.

e. f.

g.

h.

Fig. 12.12 The three-flap Wardill–Kilner push-back operation, modified after Braithwaite. (a) The margins of the soft palate cleft have been pared and the cleft of the hard palate incised along the junction of oral and nasal mucoperiosteum. The lateral incision has been made inside the alveolar ridge from opposite the canine anteriorly to a point just behind the hamulus posteriorly. An oblique incision joins the anterior end of the lateral incision to the cleft margin. (b) The mucoperiosteal flap has been elevated from the hard palate. The point of a pair of forceps is fracturing the pterygoid hamulus by pushing it medially. Deeper blunt dissection at this site strips mucoperiosteum from the side wall of the nose anteriorly and frees the attachment of the superior constrictor to the medial pterygoid plate. (c) The oral mucoperiosteal flap has been turned back showing the greater palatine vessels passing from the greater palatine foramen to the flap. The muscles of the soft palate are seen attached to the back of the hard palate. The mucosa has been elevated from the septum (the vomer) which is attached to the margin of the palate on this side. (d) The muscles have been detached from the back of the hard palate. The nasal mucosa is intact and is being dissected free from the upper surface of the hard palate. The dissector is behind the posterior nasal spine. The soft palate is falling away from the hard and becoming elongated. This is the 'push-back'. (e) The muscle has been freed from the overlying mucosa. (f) The muscle has been freed laterally and has been rotated medially. (g) The two muscle bundles have been overlapped and sutured under slight tension to construct the muscle sling. The nasal mucosa has been sutured. (h) Suturing of the oral layer completed. The tips of the oral mucoperiosteal flaps are sutured to the apex of the anterior flap, indicating the degree of palatal lengthening

anterior ends of the lateral incisions are joined to the margins of the cleft by oblique cuts which produce three flaps in the incomplete cleft or four in the complete cleft. The palate can be lengthened by freeing the two posterior muco-periosteal flaps so that they can be slid backwards. This involves freeing the aponeurotic and muscular attachments of the soft palate from the back of the hard palate, and undermining the nasal mucosa as far as possible from the upper surface of the hard palate. The mucoperiosteal flaps remain tethered by their vascular pedicles, the greater palatine vessels, as they emerge from the greater

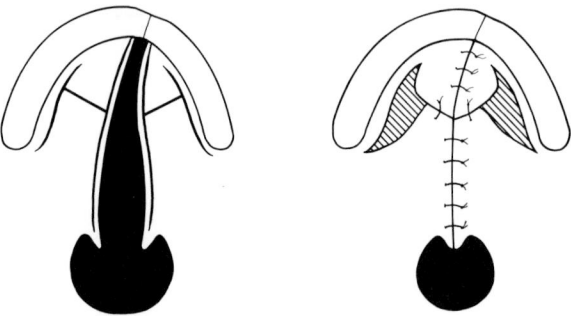

Fig. 12.13 Four-flap modification of Wardill–Kilner operation for closure of unilateral clefts extending forward to the alveolus. (a) Incisions. (b) Closure completed

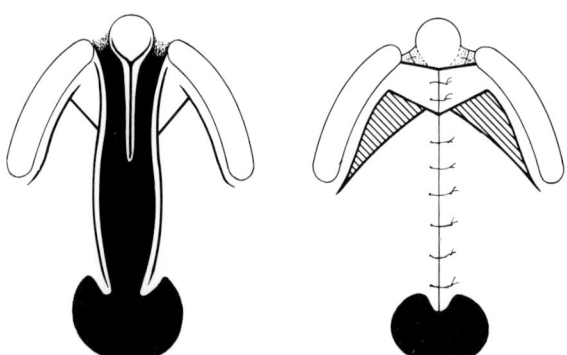

Fig. 12.14 Four-flap modification of Wardill-Kilner operation for closure of bilateral clefts. Bilateral vomer flaps are used for the nasal closure. (a) Incisions. (b) Closure completed

palatine foramina. These pedicles may be lengthened a little by teasing them out of the foramina, or a better push-back can be obtained by removing the bone from behind the foramina to allow the vessels to fall backwards. Alternatively, some surgeons divide the vascular pedicles, thereby freeing the flaps even more. Many reservations have been expressed regarding this last manœuvre, but those who practise it claim they have no trouble with necrosis of the flaps and no more fistulae than they get when preserving the vessels. Bishara (1974) has shown no difference in maxillary growth between patients with and without division of their greater palatine vessels.

Fracture of the hamulus. Mobilization of the soft palate must be carried out, not only to allow it to slide backwards, but also to allow the two halves to move medially and be sutured in the mid-line. After freeing the nasal mucosa from the upper surface of the hard palate, it is further freed from the lateral wall of the nose and pushed medially, opening up a space lateral to the soft palate and allowing the halves of the palate to approach each other. The pterygoid hamulus is exposed and may be fractured to relax the tensor palati, which passes round it, and make it easier to close the soft palate. This manœuvre was first described by Billroth in 1889 and is carried out as part of many operations. It is frowned upon by some (e.g. Kriens, 1970) on the grounds that it interferes with normal function of the tensor palati, but Thomson & Harwood Nash (1972) have shown by X-ray studies that the hamulus returns to its normal position in a few months.

It is not usually necessary to fracture the hamulus if a thorough mobilization of the muscles medial to it is carried out (see below), but if the cleft is very wide and closure is difficult it can probably be done without danger.

Formation of the levator sling. Once the two halves of the palate have been fully mobilized they can be sutured together in layers without tension in their lengthened condition. This is how the standard Wardill–Kilner procedure was completed, but Braithwaite and Maurice in 1968 pointed out the importance not only of freeing the levator palati and other muscles from their abnormal attachments to the back of the hard palate but also of rotating them medially so that they can be sutured together to form the muscle slings (Fig. 12.12e, f). Only if this is done can the muscles function in the normal way. Braithwaite also advised wide mobilization of the superior constrictor, detaching it from the medial pterygoid lamina so that when the levator muscles were overlapped and sutured together under some tension the constrictor was pulled in as well. This produced a side-to-side narrowing, or isthmus, of the pharynx at the level of the soft palate.

The formation of the muscle sling in this way is now widely accepted as a very important step in the closure of the soft palate. However, if it is to be successful in improving the mobility of the soft palate it is essential that the surgeon frees the whole of each muscle bundle from the hard palate and sutures them together under tension, preferably with some overlap. If the muscles are too lax then the palate will not move backwards when they contract.

Closure. Suturing of the palate is usually carried out in the child with interrupted chromic catgut sutures, using 4–0 for the nasal layer and 3–0 for the oral. However, some surgeons prefer silk. Once the oral mucoperiosteal flaps and the soft palate have been properly mobilized they will fall together without tension. Closure must begin with the nasal layer of mucoperiosteum. In the unilateral cleft the septum is attached to the palatal shelf on the non-cleft side, and the cleft can be bridged by elevating the septal mucoperiosteum from the underlying bone (the vomer) through the incision that has already been made along the cleft margin. The superiorly based vomer flap that is raised in this way can be swung across the cleft and sutured to the nasal mucosa on the opposite free margin of the cleft. Elevation of the vomer flap should not be more extensive than is necessary to close the nasal layer without tension, as it is possible that this procedure may interfere with growth of the vomer.

In the bilateral cleft the vomer hangs suspended from the roof of the nose with its free edge lying between the two palatal shelves. Although it is often hypoplastic, an incision along the free margin allows elevation of mucoperiosteal flaps from both sides which can be sutured, as in the unilateral cleft, to the margins of the nasal mucoperiosteum elevated from the palatal shelves on each side (Fig. 12.14).

At the posterior end of the vomer, near the junction of hard and soft palates, it can sometimes be quite difficult to bring the nasal mucoperiosteum of the palate together without tension if the cleft is a wide one. However, the thorough mobilization of this nasal mucoperiosteum which should have been carried out usually allows it to be closed successfully. The closure at this point can be made more secure if, after passing the suture through both flaps of nasal mucoperiosteum, it is left untied and its ends long. Later the ends are crossed and brought out through the oral mucoperiosteal flaps, to be tied on the oral side. This approximates oral and nasal layers and eliminates any dead space between them.

Closure continues with the nasal mucosa of the soft palate, and the sutures here should pass through the muscle and reinforce the muscle sling. Vertical mattress sutures and good overlapping of the muscles may help to avoid the mid-line groove which is often seen endoscopically on the dorsal surface of the repaired palate, and which can contribute to palatal incompetence. The mobilized muscles are sutured under slight tension with one or two mattress sutures. Once the tip of the uvula has been reached, suturing proceeds forwards along the oral side of the cleft. At the junction of the soft and hard palates the ends of the suture on the nasal side, which have been left untied and long, are crossed and passed through the oral mucoperiosteum and tied.

If the anterior end of the cleft extends to, or near to, the incisive foramen then there will be two anterior flaps of oral mucoperiosteum. These must be mobilized enough to allow them to be sutured together and the anterior ends of the posterior flaps are approximated to them (Figs. 12.13 and 12.14). Because of the push-back much larger raw areas are left anterolaterally than in the von Langenbeck procedure, but there is no need to pack them and they epithelialize within two weeks.

Lengthening of the nasal mucosa. The Veau–Wardill–Kilner operation cuts through the oral mucoperiosteum and frees the muscles from the back of the hard palate to allow them to fall back, but they remain tethered to an intact nasal mucosa. The amount of palatal lengthening is therefore dependent on how much the nasal mucosa will stretch after it has been freed from the upper surface of the hard palate. A little more lengthening can be obtained by incorporating a Z-plasty in the closure of the nasal layer (Fig. 12.15). This technique was described by Schuchardt (1964), who also lengthened the oral layer with a Z-plasty in his modification of the von Langenbeck operation. It can, of course, also be used in association with a push-back procedure.

In an attempt to gain greater length some surgeons have divided the nasal mucosa transversely just behind the hard palate. The immediate result is spectacular, but following the inevitable laws of healing, if the gap in the nasal mucosa is left raw, scar tissue will form and contract, and as it does so the long palate will be pulled forward again and the advantage be lost.

To overcome this problem many ingenious methods have been devised to fill the raw area. Dorrance (1925) used a skin graft, but it was not very satisfactory, tending to desquamate and produce a foul smell. Cronin (1957) carried

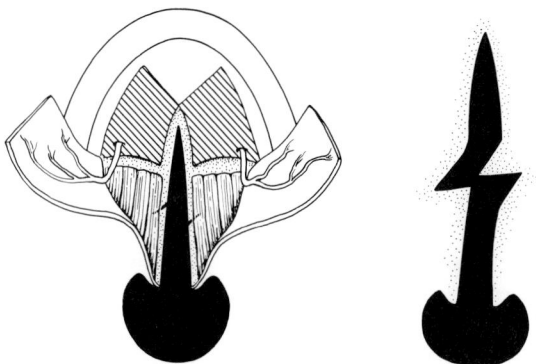

Fig. 12.15 Schuchardt's elongation of the nasal mucosa with a Z-plasty

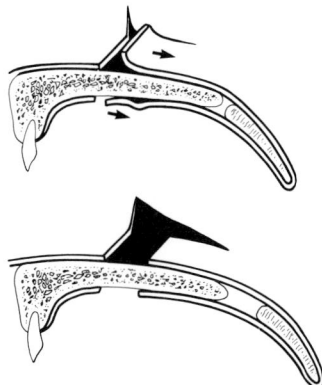

Fig. 12.16 Cronin's technique of elongating the nasal mucosa. It is mobilized and incised using special instruments through the nose. Raw areas on the nasal side lie over bone

out a very thorough mobilization of the nasal floor mucosa using special instruments through the nostrils. He then cut through the mucosa transversely over the hard palate, raising flaps which roughly corresponded with those on the oral side, and which left a raw area over the hard palate after push-back. As on the oral side, the exposed areas of bone epithelialized without the marked scar contraction to be expected in the region of the soft palate (Fig. 12.16). In those patients in whom he particularly wished to lengthen the palate Millard (1962) filled the gap by turning over an island flap of oral mucoperiosteum based on a vascular stalk consisting of one of the greater palatine vascular bundles

(Fig. 12.17). This maintained the length of the palate very well, although Millard pointed out the increased risk of anterior fistula formation if the cleft is wide and there is a shortage of tissue. Unfortunately, recent reports suggest that although the palate is long it does not move very well, and the speech results are disappointing (Lewin et al 1975; Luce et al 1976).

In 1975 Kaplan described the use of a buccal mucosal flap or flaps to close the defect in the nasal mucosa after reconstructing the levator sling (Fig. 12.18). This has the advantage of bringing in tissue from where it can be spared outside

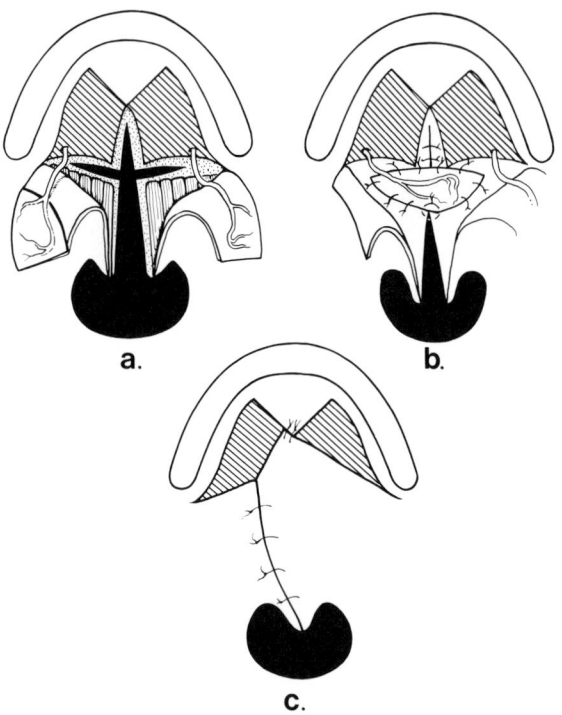

Fig. 12.17 Millard's neurovascular island flap technique of lengthening the nasal layer. (a) Oral mucoperiosteal flaps raised and soft palate mobilized. Transverse incision through nasal mucosa behind posterior edge of hard palate. One neurovascular bundle freed from base of flap and island of mucoperiosteum marked out at tip. (b) Island flap, carried on neurovascular bundle, turned over and sutured into gap in nasal mucosa to augment the push-back. Muscle mobilization and closure of nasal mucosa and muscle can now proceed. (c) Closure completed. The intact mucoperiosteal flap is sutured across the mid-line

the palate, and avoids the extra raw areas over the bony palate produced by Cronin's and Millard's techniques. One would therefore expect fewer problems with maxillary growth, but it is still too soon to know whether this ingenious method will fulfil its promise.

Primary pharyngeal flap. Schoenborn in 1876 was the first to use the posterior pharyngeal flap as a primary procedure. Its use was championed by Burian in Prague, and is still used by his successor, Fara, and by Stark in New York among others. (The operative details of the various types of pharyngeal flaps will be

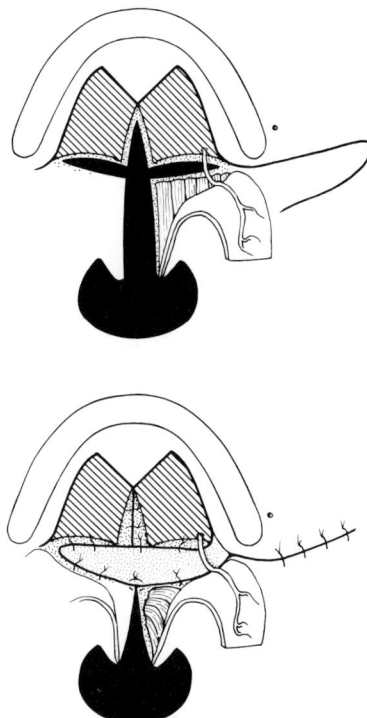

Fig. 12.18 Kaplan's technique for lengthening the nasal layer with a buccal mucosal flap. Mucoperiosteal flaps raised, soft palate mobilized and transverse incision made in nasal mucosa. Mucosal flap outlined. Flap is then raised and transposed deep to the greater palatine neurovascular bundle to fill the defect in the nasal mucosa. Donor site sutured. Closure of the palate can now proceed in the usual way

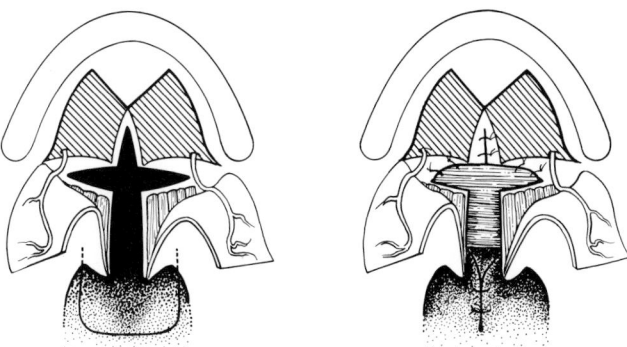

Fig. 12.19 Hönig's technique of lengthening the nasal layer by inserting a superiorly based pharyngeal flap into the defect. Mucoperiosteal flaps raised, soft palate mobilized and transverse incision made in nasal mucosa. Long, superiorly based pharyngeal flap outlined. Pharyngeal flap is then sutured into defect in nasal mucosa. Donor site sutured. Closure can now proceed in the usual way

found in Chapter 17.) The flap may be superiorly based and inserted into the defect in the nasal mucosa behind the hard palate, as described by Hönig (1964), so helping to lengthen the palate (Fig. 12.19). Alternatively, it may be inset more posteriorly into the soft palate in association with a von Langenbeck type of procedure, and act only as an obturator (Stark & De Haan 1960). The proponents of this technique argue that 20 to 30 per cent of patients will suffer from velopharyngeal incompetence after any method of closure of the palate. Many of them will require some form of secondary operation such as a pharyngeal flap to overcome this disability. Stark says that it is impossible to predict which patients will need secondary surgery, but that by using a pharyngeal flap in every primary operation he improves his overall speech results. Although 70 per cent of children may have this added procedure unnecessarily, it has virtually no side effects and is therefore justifiable. Stark & Frileck (1971) have reported that 90 per cent of their patients have acceptable speech. Dalston & Stuteville (1975) showed similar results. In their careful study the pharyngeal flap had been used selectively in those patients with short palates and poor lateral pharyngeal wall movement.

Primary closure of the soft palate alone

The push-back techniques we have been discussing have all been developed in response to the desire of the surgeon to allow more of his patients to speak normally. The proponents of these operations maintain that any increase in deformity that may result from their more radical nature is insignificant when compared with the benefit of improved speech.

The opposite school of thought is exemplified by Blocksma and his colleagues (1975), who stated: 'Since the techniques (of secondary palatopharyngeal surgery) have become such relatively simple procedures it seems needless to create a serious skeletal growth deformity in order to prevent [a] theoretical increase in rhinolalia.' They reported on 107 patients who had had only the soft palate closed between the ages of 18 months and 2 years, and hard palate closure usually after 5 years. None of these children apparently had any maxillary deformity, although half of them needed a pharyngeal flap to overcome velopharyngeal incompetence.

We have already referred to other workers such as Slaughter, Schweckendieck and Hotz who strongly support this view, and we must now consider how soft and hard palate may be closed independently.

The technique of closing the soft palate is often by simple paring of the cleft edges and muscle suture as far forward as possible. This does not accord with the principles of muscle mobilization which we have described, and we believe that soft palate closure should always incorporate dissection of the palatal muscles from the back of the hard palate, wide mobilization and rotation medially to construct the muscle sling.

The technique of soft palate closure originally described by Widmaier (1964) in association with a rather unappealing method of hard palate closure can be adapted to achieve this and lengthen the soft palate (Fig. 12.20). The freeing of the muscle and aponeurosis from the back of the hard palate, and mobilization

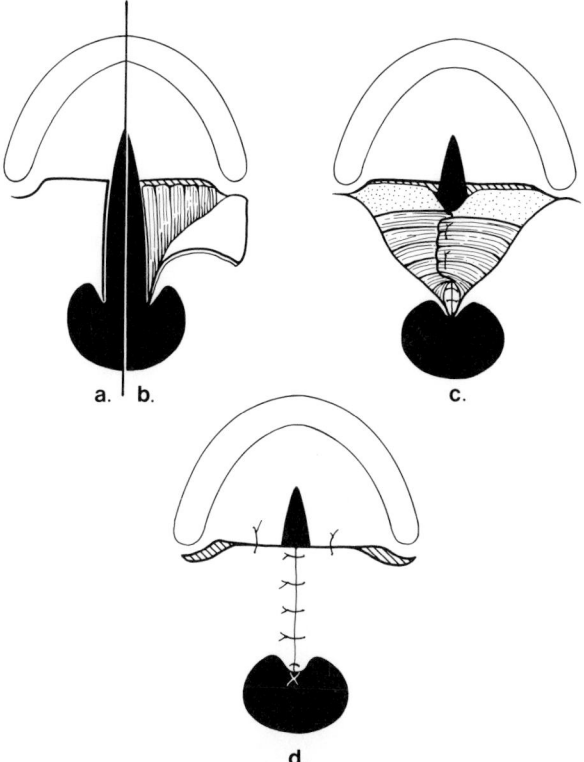

Fig. 12.20 Closure of the soft palate alone after the method of Widmaier. (a) Flap outlined, reaching no further than the posterior edge of the hard palate. (b) Flap elevated to expose muscle which is mobilized in the usual way. (c) After mobilization of the soft palate the muscle has been transposed and it and the nasal mucosa have been sutured. (d) Closure completed. The raw areas lie behind the hard palate

and suture of the muscle and mucosa, is carried out in the way that has already been described (pp. 151, 153).

Closure of the hard palate after previous soft palate repair
The hard palate has been left undisturbed in the procedure which has just been described, and after the soft palate has healed a large fistula is left in front of it. The tension of the muscle sling in the soft palate draws the halves of the maxilla together and narrows this fistula to such an extent that, when the time comes to close it, it may be possible to do so without making any lateral relaxing incisions, but simply by undermining the mucoperiosteum from the free edges of the palate.

This would appear to be a considerable advantage of this method, as the absence of raw areas near the teeth might be expected to reduce the incidence of malocclusion. However, closure of the cleft can only be achieved by allowing the mucoperiosteal flaps to fall away from the bony palate so that there is a considerable dead space between the nasal and oral layers (Fig. 12.21).

Sometimes the palatal shelves are aligned almost vertically, presumably due to tongue pressure, and, if this is so, the oral flaps are quite unsupported and the pressure of the tongue postoperatively can lead to a risk of secondary fistula formation. The author's experience with this technique is limited, and the leading proponents of primary veloplasty give the impression in their publications that hard palate closure with minimal elevation of flaps does not present any problems. Nevertheless, it seems to us to be advisable that relaxing incisions of a von Langenbeck type should be made unless the cleft is very narrow, as these will allow the periosteal flaps to lie against the bone. The long-term use of a dental plate to keep the tongue out of the cleft might allow better alignment of the shelves, but carries its own disadvantages. On the other hand, the use of such a plate for a short time postoperatively when no relaxing incisions have been made should present no problems and might reduce the chance of fistula.

One of the very few randomized controlled trials between two surgical regimes has been carried out using this type of two-stage procedure by Robertson &

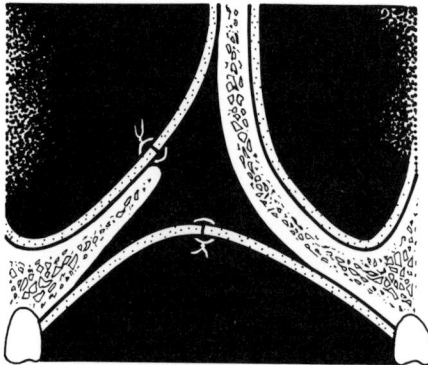

Fig. 12.21 Coronal section through septum and palatal cleft, demonstrating that closure of the cleft without lateral relaxing incisions can only be achieved by allowing the mucoperiosteal flaps to fall away from the bone, leaving a large dead space

Jolleys (1974). They reported on 40 infants with complete unilateral clefts of lip and palate, whom they allocated randomly to two groups. Both groups had lip and soft palate repaired at the age of about 3 months. In one group the hard palate was closed at between 12 and 18 months; in the other closure was delayed until 4 or 5 years. There was no significant difference in occlusion between the groups at 4 or 7 years, and the delayed group had significantly worse speech.

While recognizing that this is only one study among many, it has yet to be matched in scientific method by the advocates of late closure of the hard palate, and strikes a significant blow for one technique of early surgery. However, closure of soft and hard palate in two stages before the age of 2 years has yet to be compared with other methods of early operation. It may produce less malocclusion and maxillary deformity than a push-back procedure, or even a von Langenbeck operation, by reason of the smaller raw areas which are left, and speech may be better than after the von Langenbeck operation because of the mobilization of the muscles and creation of a proper muscle sling in the soft palate. A controlled study comparing these methods would be a valuable contribution to cleft palate surgery.

THE PRE- AND POSTOPERATIVE CARE OF THE CLEFT PALATE PATIENT

The success of surgery to the cleft lip and palate depends not only on the surgeon and his choice of treatment, but on the care that the child must receive while in hospital for the operations. This burden falls largely on the nursing staff, and skilled and devoted nurses are essential in any ward where cleft lip and palate patients are cared for.

When patients are called for operation they must be examined carefully and if there is any sign of an upper respiratory tract infection then the operation must be postponed. This may happen quite often in the winter months.

Because the oral mucosa cannot be properly cleaned preoperatively in the way that the skin can be prepared, it is important to ensure that there are no pathogenic bacteria in the mouth or nasopharynx before embarking on surgery. Bacterial swabs should be taken from nose and throat and sent for culture on the three days before operation. If the patient lives close to the hospital this can be done on an outpatient or domiciliary basis, but if this is not possible then the child will have to be admitted early. The mother should be encouraged to stay with the child, and early admission allows both to get used to the hospital environment. However, it does carry the hazard of introducing hospital organisms into the patient's nasopharynx. The usual organisms found in nose and throat are harmless but if a *Staphylococcus aureus* is grown on culture the child should be started on a course of flucloxacillin, and ampicillin should be given in the presence of haemophilus. If a group-A haemolytic streptococcus is found preoperatively then the operation should be postponed, for there is a serious risk of wound breakdown. A course of penicillin should be started and the child brought to theatre only when cultures are free of the organism. Sometimes it happens that the finding of a group-A streptococcus is not reported until after the operation, and in this case a course of intramuscular penicillin may save the situation. Haemolytic streptococci of other groups are less worrying, and surgery can proceed safely if penicillin is given.

If a presurgical orthopaedic appliance is being worn there may be some superficial mucosal ulceration, in which case the appliance should be removed a few days preoperatively. The lips should be well massaged with Vaseline after feeds, especially at the angles of the mouth, as this helps to reduce the splitting of the mucosa when the mouth is stretched by the gag.

On admission the child should be weighed and his haemoglobin checked. The old maxim of surgery being safe when the child weighs 10 pounds, has a haemoglobin of 10 grams and is 10 weeks old still has much to commend it. It should not be necessary to cross-match blood for a lip operation, but blood replacement is occasionally necessary after palate surgery and it should be available.

If a baby is breast-fed there is no need to change the regime before lip surgery, as breast feeding can safely be continued postoperatively. Bottle feeding in the early postoperative period can damage the lip, and it is safer to use a spoon or cup. If preferred, the mother of a breast-fed baby can express her milk and give it in the same way. After surgery to the palate, a spoon or a cup with a short spout should always be used, and it is wise to get the child used to feeding from these by starting preoperatively. The last feed before the operation should be given four hours beforehand and be followed by some sterile water. A thorough toilet of nostrils and lips should be carried out.

After the child is anaesthetized a throat pack is inserted to prevent blood reaching the larynx. This is removed at the end of the operation and any blood carefully sucked from the pharynx and throat, but there is always some oozing of blood from raw areas. In addition, an operation to close the palate reduces the airway considerably, so careful precautions must be taken to avoid respiratory obstruction in the immediate postoperative period.

When the child returns from the operating theatre he should have had a tongue stitch inserted and taped to the chin so that the tongue can easily be pulled forward if there is any respiratory obstruction. This should be left in place until the patient is fully awake and can conveniently be removed before the first postoperative feed.

The cot or bed in the recovery area should be provided with an oxygen outlet and suction, and a laryngoscope and appropriate endotracheal tubes should be immediately available. The child should be placed in the lateral position with the foot of the cot raised. Restraints should be attached to all four limbs and tied to the cot frame, and elbow splints are also valuable. A trained nurse should remain with the child until he has fully recovered from the anaesthetic; and pulse, respirations and temperature should be recorded. The medical staff should ensure that clear written instructions are given for intravenous fluids if these are being given. Sedation should be given intramuscularly before the child becomes unduly restless with pain, but it must be remembered that if there is any obstruction to the airway the resulting hypoxia will cause restlessness and it will be aggravated by sedation.

Once the child is fully awake and his condition stable he can be sat up in a hiatus hernia chair (or one of the many varieties of plastic baby chair), but it is important that elbow splints are kept on for three weeks postoperatively to prevent thumb or finger sucking and other interference with the operation site. These splints allow much more freedom than wrist restraints, which should not be necessary after the first few hours. However, if the baby is very active after lip repair, and restraints are required, all four limbs should be tethered to the frame of the cot. This can be done very easily with the baby sitting up in a chair in the cot, and is much more humane than having him lying flat on his back. The likelihood of postoperative chest problems is also much reduced.

The first feed can usually be given two or three hours postoperatively, and should be of sterile water or 5 per cent dextrose. The feeds are gradually built up, but should always by followed by a drink of sterile water. Following repair of the hard palate, the breast or bottle are contraindicated as the pressure of the nipple between tongue and the repaired palate during the action of sucking could very easily cause breakdown of the repair. As suggested above, the feed is best given by a spoon or cup with a short spout, taking great care not to damage the suture lines. This is not so critical after repair of the lip or soft palate if the latter is closed independently of the hard palate, but very often the same precautions are taken. Nevertheless, we have seen a number of babies successfully breast-fed immediately after lip repair with no damage to the lip. The older child after palate repair should persist with a sloppy diet for three weeks.

After closure of the cleft lip a pack is usually left in the nostril and there is often a dressing over the suture line. The length of time the nasal pack is left in place varies with the amount of surgery that has been done, but the lip dressing, if present, should usually be removed after 24 hours. Thereafter, suture toilet is carried out regularly after each feed and the suture lines can be smeared with an antibiotic ointment. The sutures are removed between the fourth and seventh day after operation. In the young baby this can often be done with little or no sedation. The older child may be more restless, even with sedation, and rather than risk damaging the repair it is occasionally better to remove the sutures under an anaesthetic such as ketamine.

The suture lines of a cleft palate repair are inaccessible in the infant, and no attempt should be made to insert cotton buds or to carry out wound toilet, as there would be a great risk of damaging the repair. Plentiful drinks, with feeds followed by sterile water, are adequate to keep the mouth clean, and care must be taken to prevent dehydration, as a copious flow of saliva is important. Chromic catgut sutures are absorbed and the exposed knots swallowed when they separate.

Patients are usually discharged about a week after operation and there is no need to inspect the inside of the mouth before this time. The parents should be reassured that any raw areas on the palate, covered by a whitish slough, will heal within two weeks. They should be given written instructions regarding the need for the child to continue to wear elbow splints, to have only sloppy food and frequent drinks until three weeks after surgery. After a lip operation the child's parents should be encouraged to keep the nostrils clean with a cotton bud and to cream and gently massage the lip scar.

Complications

The majority of children recover very quickly from an operation to their lip or palate and are playing and feeding happily after 24 hours. When there are extensive raw areas in the mouth the child may be rather miserable for slightly longer. Unreplaced blood loss can delay recovery and operative blood loss of more than 100 ml in a child under 2 years old should be replaced.

A respiratory tract infection sometimes occurs in spite of the preoperative precautions. This must be treated in the usual way with antibiotics and physiotherapy, but it carries an increased risk of wound breakdown.

In the absence of a haemolytic group-A streptococcus or postoperative respiratory infection, wound breakdown or fistula formation in the palate is very uncommon if proper mobilization of the tissues has been carried out and the suturing done without tension. If such a breakdown does take place, secondary closure should not be attempted immediately. All the scarring and induration should be allowed to settle before anything more is done to the lip or soft palate, and a fistula in the hard palate is best left until the age of 4 or 5 years before secondary closure is attempted.

REFERENCES

Bishara S E, Enemark H, Tharp R F 1976 Cephalometric comparisons of the results of the Wardill–Kilner and von Langenbeck palatoplasties. Cleft Palate Journal 13: 319

Blocksma R, Lenz C A, Mellerstig K E 1975 A conservative program for managing cleft patients. Plastic and Reconstructive Surgery 55: 160

Braithwaite F, Maurice D 1968 The importance of the levator palati muscle in cleft palate closure. British Journal of Plastic Surgery 21: 60

Burian F 1978 The plastic surgery atlas 2. Macmillan, New York

Cronin T D 1957 Method of preventing raw area on nasal surface of soft palate in push-back surgery. Plastic and Reconstructive Surgery 20: 474

Dalston R M, Stuteville O H 1975 A clinical investigation into the efficacy of primary nasopalatal pharyngoplasty. Cleft Palate Journal 12: 177

Davies D 1970 The radical repair of cleft palate deformities. Cleft Palate Journal 7: 550

Dorrance G M 1925 Lengthening the soft palate in cleft palate operations. Annals of Surgery 32: 208

Drillien C M, Ingram T T S, Wilkinson E M 1966 The causes and natural history of cleft lip and palate. Livingstone, Edinburgh

Gillies H D, Fry K 1921 a new principle in the surgical treatment of congenital cleft palate and its mechanical counterpart. British Medical Journal 1: 335

Glover D M 1961 A long-range evaluation of cleft palate repair. Plastic and Reconstructive Surgery 27: 19

Graber T M 1949 Craniofacial morphology in cleft palate and cleft lip deformities. Surgery, Gynaecology and Obstetrics 88: 359

Hönig C A 1964 In: Schuchardt K Treatment of patients with clefts of lip, alveolus and palate. Thieme, Stuttgart, p 207

Hotz M M, Gnoinski W M, Nussbaumer H, Kistler E 1978 Early maxillary orthopaedics in cleft lip and palate cases: Guidelines for surgery. Cleft Palate Journal 15: 405

Kaplan E N 1975 Soft palate repair by levator muscle reconstruction and a buccal mucosal flap. Plastic and Reconstructive Surgery 56: 129

Kilner T P 1937 Cleft lip and palate repair technique. In: Maingot R (ed) postgraduate surgery. Medical publishers, London, vol 3

Krause C J, Tharp R F, Morris H L 1976 A comparative study of results of the von Langenbeck and V–Y push-back palatoplasties. Cleft Palate Journal 13: 11

Kremenak C R Jnr, Huffman W C, Olin W H 1970 Maxillary growth inhibition by mucoperiosteal denudation of palatal shelf bone in non-cleft beagles. Cleft Palate Journal 7: 817

Kriens O B 1970 Fundamental findings for an intravelar veloplasty. Cleft Palate Journal 7: 27

Langenbeck B von 1861 Die Uranoplastik mittels ablösung des mukös-periostalen Gaumenüberzuges. Archiv für klinische Chirurgie 2: 205

Lewin M, Heller J C, Kojak D J 1975 Speech results after Millard island flap repair in cleft palate and other velopharyngeal insufficiencies. Cleft Palate Journal 12: 263

Lindsay W K 1971 von Langenbeck palatorrhaphy. In: Grabb W C, Rosenstein S C, Bzoch K R (eds) Cleft lip and palate. Little Brown, Boston

Luce E A, McClinton M, Hoopes J E 1976 Long-term results of the island flap palatal push-back. Plastic and Reconstructive Surgery 58: 332–339

McEvitt W G 1971 The incidence of persistent rhinolalia following cleft palate repair. Plastic and Reconstructive Surgery 47: 258

Millard D R Jnr 1957 A primary camouflage of the unilateral harelook. In: Transactions of the first international congress of plastic surgeons. Williams and Wilkins, Baltimore

Millard D R Jnr 1962 Wide and/or short cleft palate. Plastic and Reconstructive Surgery 29: 40

Millard D R Jnr 1976 Cleft craft. Little Brown, Boston

Muir I F K 1966 Repair of the cleft alveolus. British Journal of Plastic Surgery 29: 30

Musgrave R H, McWilliams B J, Matthews H P 1975 A review of the results of two different surgical procedures for the repair of clefts of the soft palate only. Cleft Palate Journal 12: 281

Ritsilä V, Alhopuros R R, Rintala A 1973 Free periosteum for bone formation in maxillary clefts. In: Johanson B (ed) second international congress on cleft palate. Copenhagen, abstracts

Robertson N R E, Jolleys A 1974 The timing of hard palate repair. Scandinavian Journal of Plastic and Reconstructive Surgery 8: 49–51

Schoenborn D 1876 Ueber eine neue methode der staphylorrhaphie. Archiv für klinische Chirurgie 19: 527

Schuchardt K 1964 Treatment of patients with clefts of lip, alveolus and palate. In: Second Hamburg international symposium. Thieme, Stuttgart, p 97

Schweckendieck W 1978 Primary veloplasty: Long-term results without maxillary deformity. Cleft Palate Journal 15: 268

Skoog T 1965 The use of periosteal flaps in the repair of the primary palate. Cleft Palate Journal 2: 332

Slaughter W B, Brodie A G 1949 Facial clefts and their surgical management. Plastic and Reconstructive Surgery 4: 311

Slaughter W B, Brodie A G 1971 In: Grabb W C, Rosenstein S W, Bzoch K R (eds) Cleft lip and palate. Little Brown, Boston

Stark R B, De Haan C R 1960 The addition of a pharyngeal flap to primary palatoplasty. Plastic and Reconstructive Surgery 26: 378

Stark R B, Frileck S 1971 In: Grabb W C, Rosenstein S W, Bzoch K R Cleft lip and palate. Little Brown, Boston, ch 27

Thomson H G, Harwood-Nash D 1972 The fate of the infractured hamulus. Plastic and Reconstructive Surgery 50: 354

Veau V 1926–7 Proceedings of the Royal Society of Medicine 10: (3) Sect surg 127

Veau V 1931 Division palatine. Masson, Paris

Veau V 1938 Bec-de-lievre. Masson, Paris, p 184

Wardill W E M 1937 Technique of operation for cleft palate. British Journal of Surgery 25:97

Widmaier W 1964 In: Schuchardt K Treatment of patients with clefts of lip, alveolus and palate. Second Hamburg international symposium. Thieme, Stuttgart, p 87

13

The role of orthodontic treatment

The normal functions of the oral structures are particularly related to the activities of respiration, speech and the ingestion of food. In all these activities, the integrity, form and relationship of the dento-alveolar arches and the palate play an important part. The accepted ideals of form and relationship are not always achieved naturally, and in cleft lip and palate there is usually a potential for gross deformity of the dento-alveolar structures as well as of the basal elements of the upper jaw and palate. Orthodontic treatment for children with cleft lip and palate has as its objectives the alignment of the dento-alveolar and jaw structures to their optimum form and relationships for the achievement of the best possible oral function. The term 'orthodontic treatment', if strictly applied, refers to treatment for the correction of the position of the teeth. Since, in cleft lip and palate it is often possible to modify the position of the basal parts of the jaw, the alternative term 'oral orthopaedic treatment' has come into use in many treatment centres.

Ideally, optimum form and relationships of the jaws would be achieved at an early stage in development, particularly so that speech development could take place in the best possible structural conditions. This can rarely be achieved, since growth and development of the jaws and of the dentition usually brings further aberration of form which it is often not possible to correct until relatively late in the growth phase. Therefore, orthodontic treatment in cleft lip and palate is important at several stages during the growth period if optimum oral conditions are to be achieved by the end of that period. Various aspects of treatment are applied from birth to adolescence, and the purpose of this chapter is to examine the rationale, the success and the practicalities of such treatment. It is convenient to consider the problems posed and the treatment methods employed in four stages of dental development, these being from birth to the primary repair operations, the primary dentition stage, the mixed dentition stage and the permanent dentition stage.

BIRTH TO PRIMARY SURGICAL REPAIR

The presurgical stages of treatment have promoted more discussion and controversy than any other aspect of orthodontic treatment in cleft lip and palate. The problems posed at this stage are essentially those of distortion and separation of the elements of the upper jaw and the concomitant separation of the

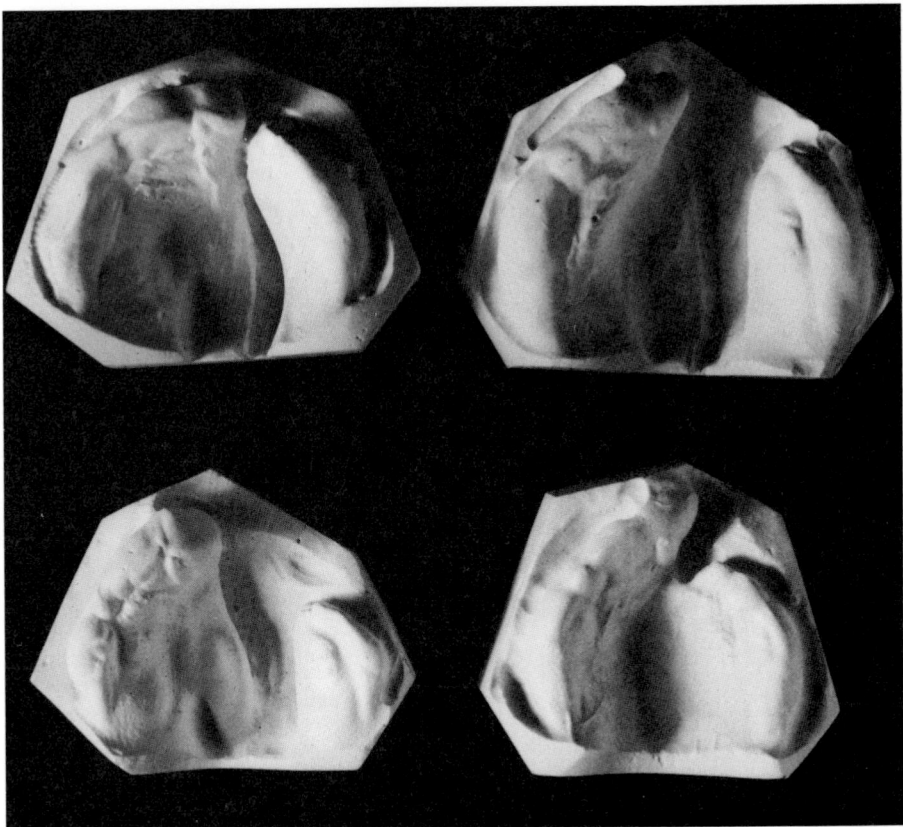

Fig. 13.1 Models of upper jaw of infants with unilateral cleft lip and palate, shortly after birth. (a) (Top left) Narrow complete cleft, little tissue deficiency, no distortion of segments. (b) (Top right) Wide complete cleft with little palatal shelf development, lateral displacement of the maxillary segment and forward rotation of the premaxilla. (c) (Bottom left) Complete cleft with tissue deficiency illustrated by the diminutive maxillary segment which is medially displaced. Wide alveolar defect. (d) (Bottom right) Incomplete cleft involving primary palate, but showing forward rotation of the premaxilla

upper lip segments and distortion of the nasal septum. These problems are particularly marked in complete clefts of the lip and palate but can be present in incomplete clefts (Figs 13.1d and 13.2d). They are not usually present in post-alveolar clefts.

Unilateral clefts
The unilateral cleft presents a variety of conditions at birth. In some infants, the jaw elements are reasonably well aligned (Fig. 13.1a). In others there are varying degrees of distortion. The commonest type of distortion appears to be that in which the smaller segment is displaced laterally, and the premaxillary part of the larger segment is rotated forward and away from the cleft (Fig. 13.1b). There is usually some deviation of the nasal septum associated with the distortion of the premaxilla. Less commonly, the smaller segment is displaced

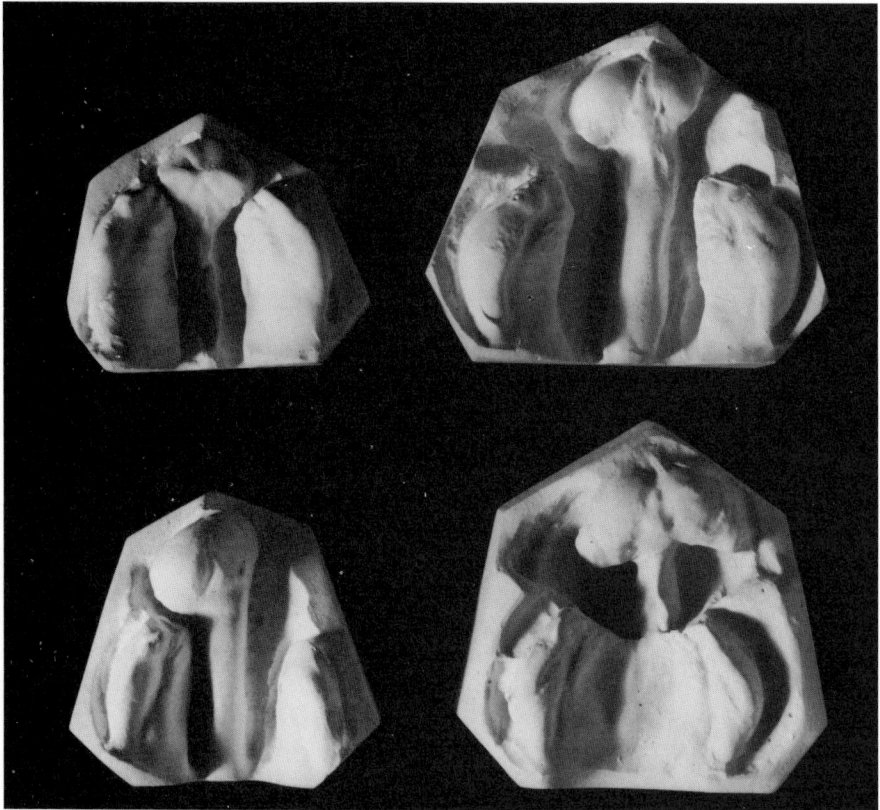

Fig. 13.2 Models of upper jaw of infants with bilateral cleft lip and palate, shortly after birth. (a) (Top left) Narrow complete cleft, with no displacement of the segments. (b) (Top right) Complete cleft with forward displacement of premaxillary segment. Maxillary segments not displaced. (c) (Bottom left) Complete cleft. The premaxillary segment is forward and rotated. The maxillary segments, though small, are not displaced. (d) (Bottom right) Incomplete cleft involving primary palate, with marked forward displacement of the large premaxillary segment

medially (Fig. 13.1c). There are also varying degrees of separation, both between the alveolar segments and between the palatal shelves.

Bilateral clefts
In bilateral clefts, the commonest deviation is a forward position of the premaxillary element relative to the maxillary segments (Fig. 13.2b). This has the effect of separating the prolabium from the lateral elements of the upper lip. In some cases there is also a lateral distortion of the nasal septum (Fig. 13.2c). The position of the maxillary segments may also vary. In some cases they are reasonably positioned in relation to the line of the lower arch, but in others the maxillary segments are displaced medially, leaving insufficient space for the premaxilla to be accommodated between them.

Presurgical alignment of the upper jaw segments
The concept of presurgical alignment has a relatively long history, though the rationale has changed with time. Brophy (1927) claimed that the cleft malforma-

tion is simply a failure of union of well-developed parts, that there is always the correct amount of tissue present, but that the segments need to be adjusted to their correct position so that bony union could occur before soft tissue repair. He therefore repositioned the bony elements, immobilized them with silver wires and awaited bony union before operating on the lip. The results, as far as eventual growth and development was concerned, were apparently poor. Kjellgren (1949) aimed to align the smaller maxillary segment only, and accepted that the lip repair would rotate the premaxillary element into a better position. He illustrated the expansion of the smaller segment with a screw appliance, a movement which would only be necessary in a relatively small proportion of subjects. Presurgical alignment was further developed by the work of McNeil (1954) and of Burston (1958), and the method was developed to include the repositioning of the premaxillary element in both unilateral and bilateral clefts and the closure of the alveolar gap in unilateral clefts to give a reasonable upper arch form.

Presurgical alignment is now practised in many centres throughout the world, though it is by no means universally accepted as an essential part of the management of cleft lip and palate. The present rationale of those advocating its use can perhaps be summed up as providing a threefold benefit. Firstly, by placing the elements of the jaw and lip into their correct relationships and by reducing the width of the palatal cleft it facilitates surgical repair. Secondly, it avoids the major occlusal defects so often seen during later development in cleft lip and palate. Thirdly, it has a social benefit, improving the morale of the parents by providing care and attention at a very early stage. These points, particularly the second, have been disputed.

Methods of presurgical alignment
Methods of presurgical alignment can be discussed from two aspects, though the two are intimately linked. These are: (a) control of the maxillary elements in the lateral dimension; (b) control of the premaxillary element in the sagittal dimension.

Control of the maxillary elements. The aim of control of the maxillary elements should be to achieve an upper arch form which conforms to that of the lower arch. In those subjects where the upper arch is distorted, this should mean either expansion or contraction of the upper arch. However, since the eventual problem is frequently that the upper jaw is too narrow and is virtually never too wide, contraction of the upper arch in infancy is not necessary, even though the most frequent initial deformity is a lateral displacement of the maxillary segment. Control of the maxillary elements therefore resolves itself to either expansion of the upper arch or stabilization of the arch to prevent excessive contraction by the forces used for control of the premaxillary element.

Stabilization of the arch can be achieved by the fitting of a simple upper appliance (Fig. 13.3) which must be used at all times when premaxillary strapping is in place.

Expansion of the upper arch for those few subjects in whom the maxillary segment is displaced medially can be achieved either by the use of a screw

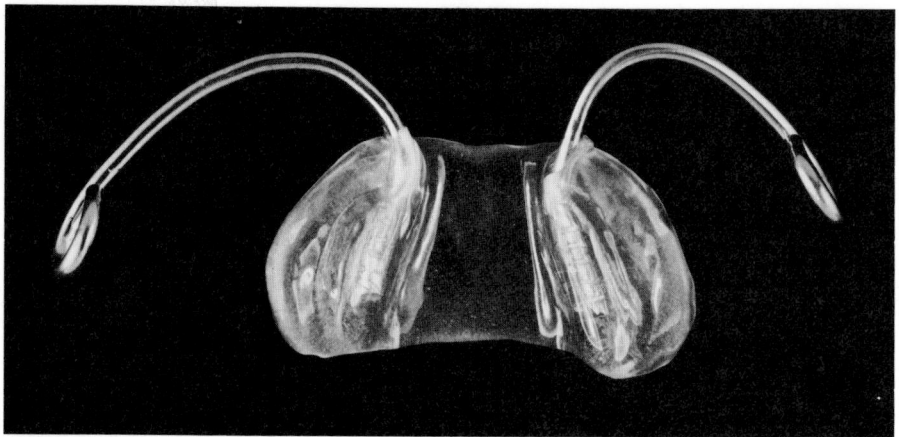

Fig. 13.3 Maxillary appliance used to stabilize the lateral segments of the jaw, and to facilitate feeding by covering the palatal defect. The 'whiskers' are necessary to enable the appliance to be handled from outside the infant's mouth

appliance or by the use of a pre-expanded appliance constructed on a modified model of the jaw.

A simple screw appliance is illustrated in Fig. 13.4. By means of the screw, the appliance can be expanded progessively, and the incorporation of a hinge ensures the appropriate differential expansion of the anterior part of the smaller segment.

Widening of the upper arch by means of a pre-expanded appliance is achieved by first sectioning the model of the upper jaw to separate the segments of the arch. The segments are then repositioned nearer to their correct form, and an appliance made to fit the repositioned model. Forces from the tongue and from the muscles of mastication, acting via the occlusal blocks on the appliance, mould the segments of the arch into a new position. If the initial distortion is severe,

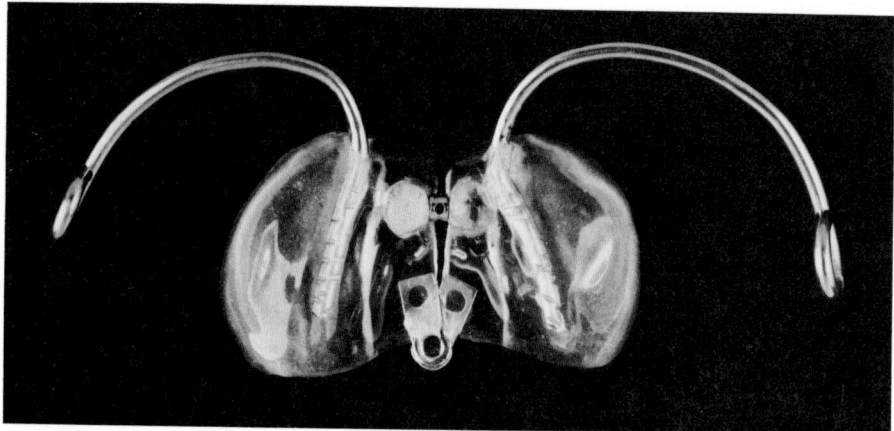

Fig. 13.4 Simple screw appliance to widen the maxillary arch where appropriate, before surgical repair. The hinge enables the anterior part of the maxillary segments to widen more than the posterior part

more than one pre-expanded appliance would be necessary to complete the expansion in stages.

All these appliances are retained in the mouth by the upward force of the tongue and the lower jaw. The extra-oral 'whiskers' are mainly to facilitate the handling of the appliances.

Control of the premaxillary element. In unilateral clefts, slight rotation of the premaxillary element can be corrected with an appliance made on a repositioned model, as described above. However, in most cases, in both unilateral and bilateral clefts, control of the premaxillary element is achieved by means of extra-oral strapping across the premaxilla, attached either directly to the face or to some form of head cap (Fig. 13.5). In unilateral clefts the force of such strapping readily rotates the premaxilla. In bilateral clefts, where the premaxilla is grossly protruded, repositioning is much more difficult. Retrusion of the premaxilla could only be achieved at the expense of distortion of the nasal septum. However, improvement in the premaxillary position can be achieved, and it is felt by some authorities that in bilateral clefts the force of the strapping merely restrains the forward development of the premaxilla while the maxillary segments grow forward to a better relationship (Robertson 1978). As previously mentioned, in complete clefts, premaxillary strapping should never be used without an intra-oral appliance to stabilize the maxillary segments, otherwise the force of the strapping will cause severe contraction of the maxilla.

Infant feeding

In the early stages after birth, the establishment of satisfactory infant feeding in the presence of a wide cleft is sometimes difficult. The hard palate forms part of the suckling mechanism and in its absence good suckling activity may be difficult to achieve. There are also sometimes problems produced by ulceration of the nasal septum. Specially designed feeding-bottle teats are available for use in these conditions, but the problems can also be overcome by the use of an acrylic feeding plate similar to that shown in Fig. 13.3. If it is not employed to stabilize or modify the shape of the upper arch, such an appliance would need to be used only at feeding times. In most cases, feeding aids such as this are needed for only a relatively short time, since most infants rapidly develop the ability to suckle satisfactorily without special aids.

The evidence for and against presurgical treatment

As mentioned previously, presurgical treatment has been the subject of considerable difference of opinion. In arguing in its favour, Maisels (1974) has said that it has major advantages in facilitating lip repair by improving the relationship of the elements of the lip. Huddart (1974) found that the use of an intra-oral appliance restricted further widening of the maxillary arch but allowed normal growth to proceed at the margins of the cleft, thus reducing the width of the cleft. This effect would facilitate operative repair of the palate. There does not seem to have been overt antagonism to the view that lip and palate repair are rendered easier, although many cleft palate centres carry out surgical repair without any presurgical treatment.

Much of the evaluation of the effects of presurgical treatment has been on its

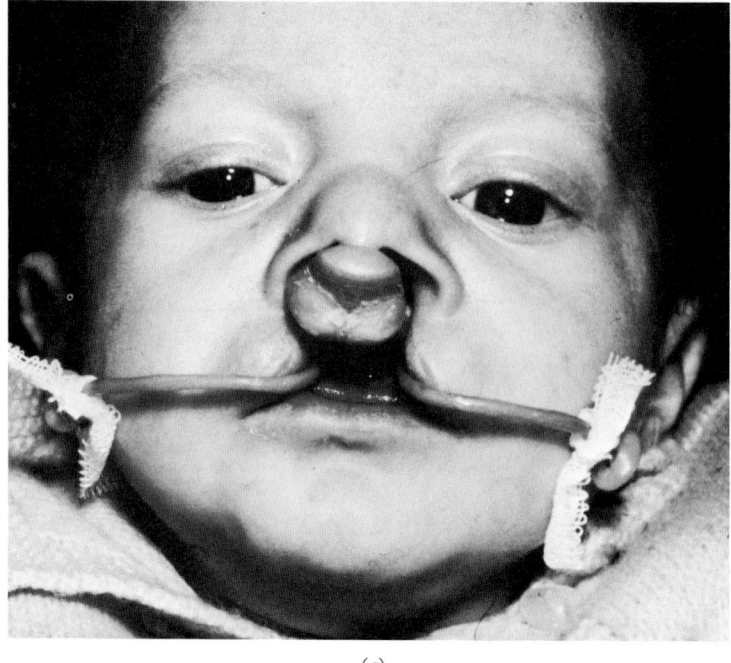

(a)

(b)

Fig. 13.5 Presurgical retraction of premaxillary segment. (a) Infant wearing appliance to stabilize maxillary segments. (b) Protruded premaxilla. (c) Elastic strapping applying gentle continuous force. (d) Premaxilla retruded by strapping

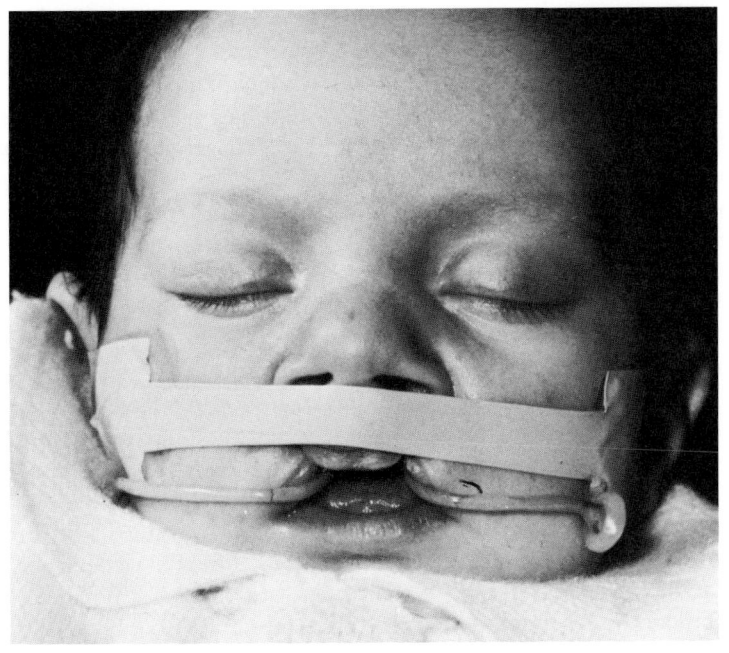

(c)

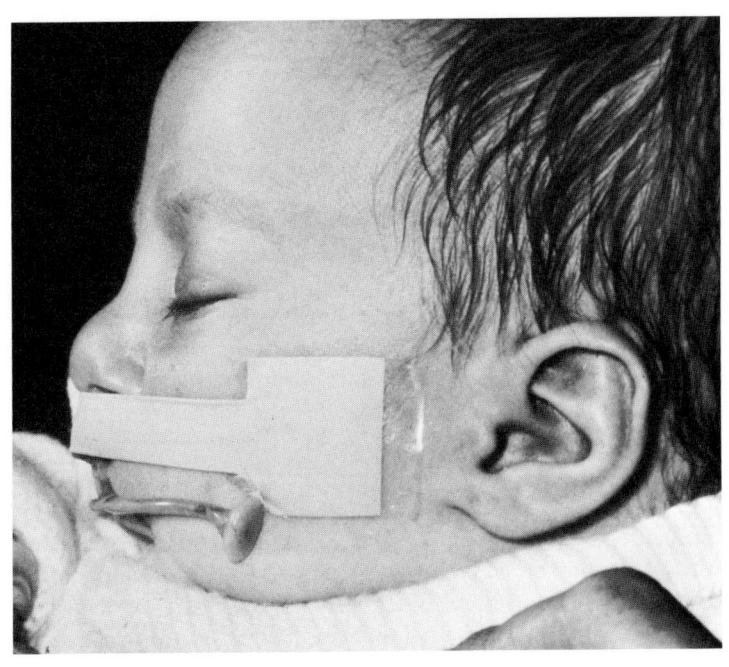

(d)

effects on the occlusion and position of the teeth. Ozerovic & Markovic (1967) claimed that a group of children who had presurgical treatment eventually had less occlusal discrepancies than a group who had no presurgical treatment. Robertson (1973) found that children who had had presurgical treatment had better occlusion in respect of anterior and lateral crossbite and O'Donnel et al (1974) also found significantly less crossbite in children who had had presurgical treatment. However, these studies all compared patients from different treatment centres, and thus variables other than presurgical treatment must have been included. The comparisons are not strictly valid. On the other hand, Huddart (1974) found no differences in arch form and occlusion as a result of presurgical treatment.

Pruzansky & Aduss (1967) have condemned presurgical treatment on the grounds that it is not beneficial to the occlusion. They have claimed that the lip repair always causes coaptation of the segments and narrowing of the palatal cleft, but that the incidence of malocclusion is no greater without than with presurgical treatment.

Thus the controversy over presurgical alignment continues. The protagonists are committed to their differing lines of argument. There have been considerable achievements in the techniques of treatment, but there has not been any controlled clinical trial of them. The value of the method will only be fully assessed by long-term studies in which variables such as surgical skills, technique and timing of operations, degrees of cleft malformation, ethnic and social factors and nursing, nutrition and follow-up care are equalized, and the only residual variable is that of presurgical management. Furthermore, the effects will need to be assessed not only on the dental occlusion but also on the other factors which make up the overall reasons for treatment of children with cleft lip and palate, notably speech, the adequacy of the nasal structures and facial appearance.

Primary bone grafting

When residual problems of the dental occlusion exist in the later stages of development, these problems usually include a deficiency of size of the maxillary arch, both in the sagittal and in the lateral dimensions. Therefore, any presurgical treatment which tends to narrow or to shorten the maxilla will tend to exacerbate such occlusal problems. This applies particularly to treatment aimed at closing gaps in the alveolar process. It is important that such gaps are not closed by moving the segments together, otherwise the total size of the arch will be reduced.

Primary bone grafting into the alveolar defect has been advocated as a method of maintaining the size and form of the arch, often after arch alignment and before surgical repair of the lip and palate. Though at first this seemed a promising innovation (Robinson & Wood 1969; Wood 1970), the longer-term results have been disappointing. Jolleys & Robertson (1972), in a five-year follow-up, found that patients who had had primary bone grafting after presurgical alignment were exhibiting limitation of upper jaw growth with reduced forward development and an increased prevalence of crossbite when compared with patients who had had presurgical alignment but no bone grafting. This finding has been confirmed by other workers. It seems that induced bony union across the alveolar cleft restricts the potential for jaw development. This may have been one of the reasons for poor growth results in some of the cases treated by Brophy's method (Graber 1949). Many centres have now abandoned primary bone grafting as a method of surgical treatment.

THE PRIMARY DENTITION PHASE

The primary dentition begins to appear at about 6 months of age, is completed by about 3 years and begins to be lost at about 6 years of age. Its replacement by the secondary dentition is not completed until approximately 12 years of age. Generally speaking, problems of the dental occlusion and the position of the teeth and jaw segments are less marked in the primary than in the secondary dentition. Defects of growth seem to have a progressive effect, the discrepancies between upper and lower jaws becoming more marked throughout the growth period.

By the time the primary dentition is established it is often possible to see the occlusal problems which will require treatment, either at this stage or later. The common aberrations in segment position are as follows.

1. Medial displacement of the maxillary segments. Medial displacement seems to occur fairly soon after the repair of the lip and palate and would thus appear to be a response to surgical repair. It is often a differential displacement, being more marked at the anterior end of the segment, in the region of the primary canine tooth. The posterior end of the segment is often in the correct relationship with the lower arch (Fig. 13.6).

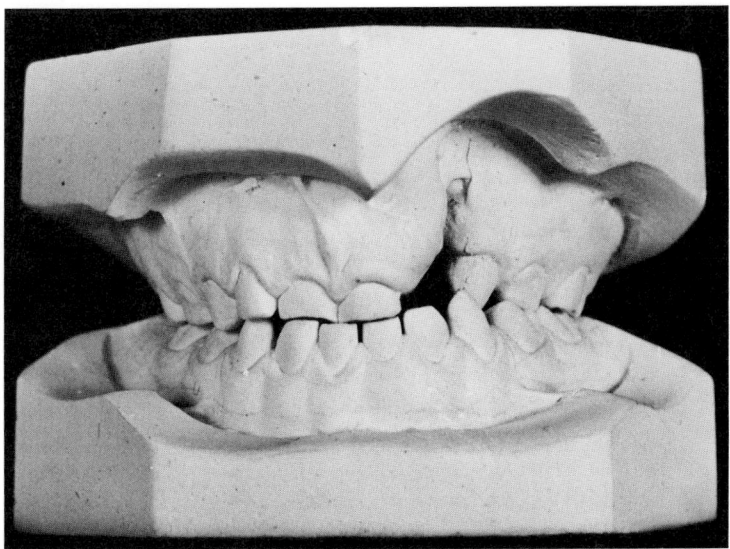

Fig. 13.6 Models of the dental arches in the full primary dentition phase in unilateral cleft lip and palate. There is slight medial displacement of the smaller segment immediately behind the alveolar cleft. The molar regions are in their correct position

2. Displacement of the premaxillary element. In contrast to displacement of the maxillary segment, premaxillary displacement at this early stage seems to be related to the preoperative position of the premaxilla. In unilateral clefts, the force of the repaired lip usually rotates the premaxilla towards its correct position. Maxillary growth deficiency, leading to retrusion of the upper jaw, which is often so marked in the older child, has not usually had much effect at the primary dentition stage, although sometimes the premaxilla is positioned behind the arch of the lower teeth. In bilateral clefts, if protrusion of the premaxilla has not been adequately reduced by strapping before lip repair, the protrusion tends to persist, particularly if it is associated with medial displacement of the maxillary segments. If there has been severe retraction of the premaxilla, either by strapping or from the forces of the repaired lip, there may be a vertical discrepancy between the premaxilla and the maxillary segments, the premaxilla having been rotated backwards and downwards.

3. Alveolar defects. Defects in the alveolar arch are usually limited to aberrations in tooth position, the most common at this stage being palatal eruption of the primary upper lateral incisor. There may be a space in the alveolar arch where an original deficiency of tissue persists (Fig. 13.7).

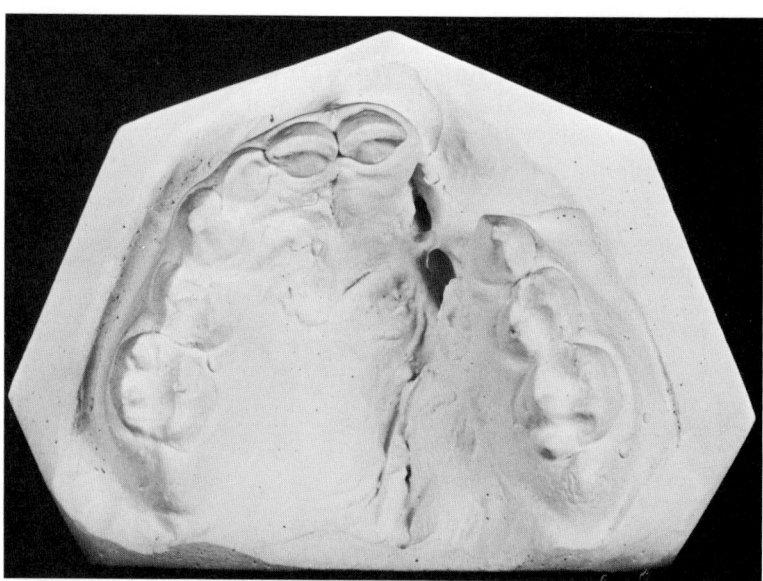

Fig. 13.7 The upper dental arch of a child with repaired unilateral complete cleft, showing a wide defect in the alveolar arch and residual oronasal fistulae

Treatment in the primary dentition

The defects outlined above all have potential for involvement in speech problems. Medial displacement of the maxillary segment causes narrowing of the upper jaw, restricting tongue space. Protrusion or retrusion of the premaxilla, and alveolar defects, may also have a bearing on tongue activity. Since these defects are present at an important time during speech development, it would be reasonable to correct them as early as possible. There are, however, certain barriers to corrective treatment at this early stage. The co-operation of the very young patient in the fitting and long-term management of appliances is often poor. Improvements achieved at this stage have a tendency to progressive relapse with growth, unless mechanically retained. Long-term retention appliances bring their own problems of oral health, especially through the period of natural loss of primary teeth. Furthermore, corrective appliances themselves may interfere with speech, and this can be particularly troublesome at the sensitive stage of starting school.

Nevertheless, improvement can be achieved in the primary dentition if it is considered desirable in relation to speech development or for facial appearance. Since the primary teeth roots are small, and undergoing progressive resorption, it is more reasonable to attempt segment realignment than tooth repositioning. The maxillary segments can be expanded using fixed splints as shown in Fig. 13.12. If there has been sufficient vertical development of the segment to establish a positive locking of the occlusion of the buccal teeth, particularly the primary canine teeth, the expansion of the jaw will be self-retaining. Otherwise, mechanical retention will need to be used until the permanent buccal teeth begin to erupt.

Generally speaking, postalveolar clefts involving only the secondary palate produce few problems in the primary dentition phase. It may be possible to see the early effects on upper jaw growth manifesting as a maxillary retrognathism even at this stage, but most of the problems in the primary dentition arise as a result of clefts which completely separate the two sides of the jaw.

THE MIXED DENTITION PHASE

With the eruption of the first permanent molars and the permanent incisor teeth between the ages of 6 and 8 years, the child enters the mixed dentition phase, which will continue until the eruption of the permanent canine and premolar teeth at about 12 years.

The occlusal problems in cleft lip and palate at this stage can be considered under three headings, these being problems of the dentition, problems of segment alignment and problems of jaw relationship. The first two of these refer particularly to those clefts which involve the alveolar arch, there being little special aberration of tooth and segment position in postalveolar clefts.

The dentition

The most noticeable effects of the cleft malformation on the teeth are often seen with the eruption of the permanent upper incisor teeth. These effects can be foreseen on radiographs before the eruption of these teeth, and it is useful to be able to warn the parent if severe discrepancies of tooth shape and position are likely.

The discrepancies affecting the dentition are as follows.

1. Malformation of the teeth. A high degree of tooth malformation in all areas of the jaws in cleft lip and palate patients has been reported by Jordan et

al (1966), and Foster & Lavelle (1971) have found that the teeth as a whole are significantly smaller in cleft than in non-cleft subjects. Nevertheless, tooth malformation particularly affects the incisor teeth in the immediate vicinity of the cleft, viz. the upper central and lateral incisor on the cleft side of the jaw. As reported in a comprehensive study by Böhn (1963), the lateral incisor is often diminutive and the central incisor is commonly mis-shapen and hypoplastic (Fig. 13.11). There has been some speculation that the repair procedure is to blame for the malformation of the central incisor, but similar malformations can be seen on the teeth in unrepaired clefts (Crabb & Foster 1977).

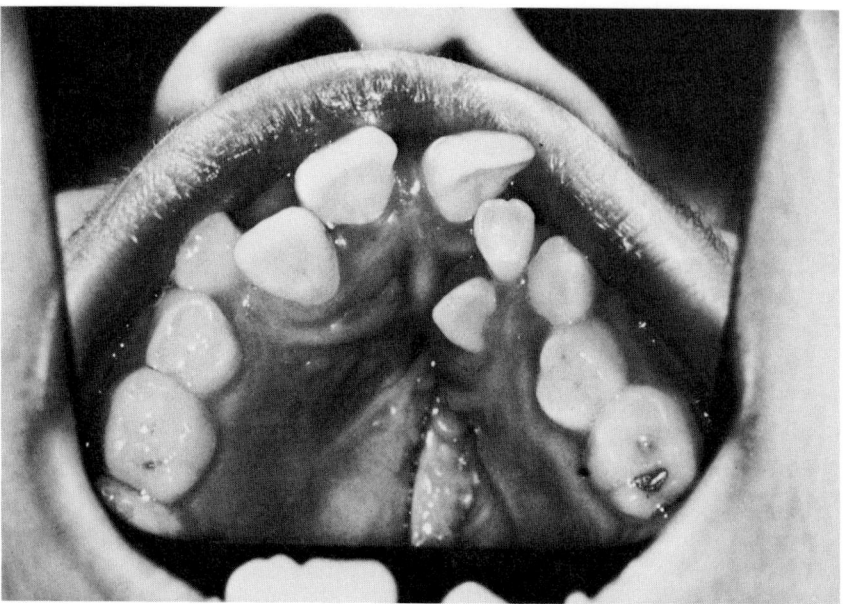

Fig. 13.8 The upper dental arch of a child with repaired unilateral complete cleft in the mixed dentition phase. The permanent lateral incisor on the cleft side has erupted in the palate, and is smaller than its counterpart on the opposite side. Note that both the primary and the permanent lateral incisors on the cleft side are on the maxillary segment

2. Malposition of the teeth. The dental malpositions specific to cleft lip and palate are again peculiar to the upper central and lateral incisor in the vicinity of the alveolar cleft. The central incisor is frequently rotated or tilted, and the lateral incisor is often high in the cleft, sometimes on the premaxilla and sometimes on the maxilla (Fig. 13.8). The eruption of the lateral incisor is often delayed.

3. Anomalies in the number of teeth. Supernumerary teeth and congenitally missing teeth rank high among the dental anomalies in cleft lip and palate. Böhn (1963) found that 75 per cent of 168 subjects with alveolar clefts had either too few or too many teeth, there being 113 supernumerary teeth and 80 missing teeth in the permanent dentitions. The lateral incisor on the cleft side is the tooth most usually affected, and even in subclinical clefts, where

there is evidence from a soft tissue notch or natural scar that a cleft of the primary palate has almost occurred, the upper lateral incisor is not uncommonly defective.

Segment alignment

Segment alignment shows little change in the mixed dentition when compared with the primary dentition. The only change in the teeth in the maxillary segments is the addition of the first permanent molars, which are often in their correct relationship in the lateral dimension. If medial displacement of the maxillary segment has been apparent in the primary dentition, this does not seem to be progressive and is therefore usually no worse in the mixed dentition phase.

Jaw relationship

The relationship between the upper and lower jaws in the sagittal plane provides one of the more noticeable as well as the more variable features in cleft subjects.

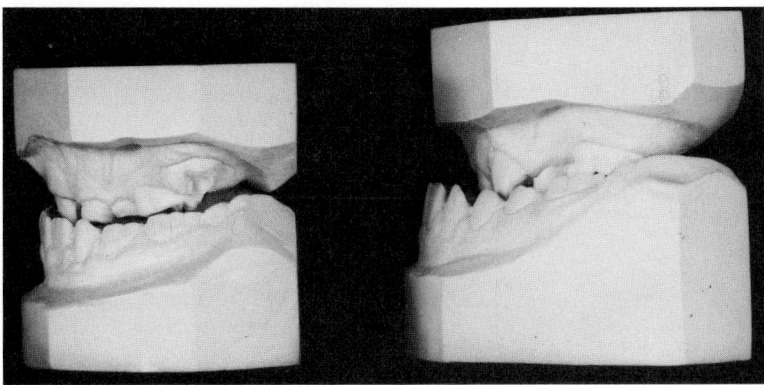

Fig. 13.9 Progressive deficiency of maxillary sagittal growth. Models of the dentition of a child with repaired complete unilateral cleft at age 8 years (left) and 12 years (right). There is a marked increase in the maxillary retrognathism as growth proceeds

In clefts involving only the primary palate, there is usually no fault in jaw relationship other than that produced by normal variation. In clefts of the primary and secondary palate, and in isolated clefts of the secondary palate, the relationship between upper and lower jaws may be correct but is often defective, usually because forward growth of the maxilla is deficient. Relating jaw positions to the cranial base, it has been shown that there is a tendency to mandibular retrognathism but a greater tendency to maxillary retrognathism, so that many cleft subjects show relative mandibular prognathism. If jaw growth is defective, the condition is usually evident at the mixed dentition stage, and may be progressive (Fig. 13.9). The first clinical sign of defective forward growth of the maxilla is often that the permanent upper incisors erupt into a lingual relationship with the lower incisors.

Treatment in the mixed dentition

In the mixed dentition, treatment is usually aimed at correcting the defective positions of the newly erupted permanent incisor teeth. At this stage, the

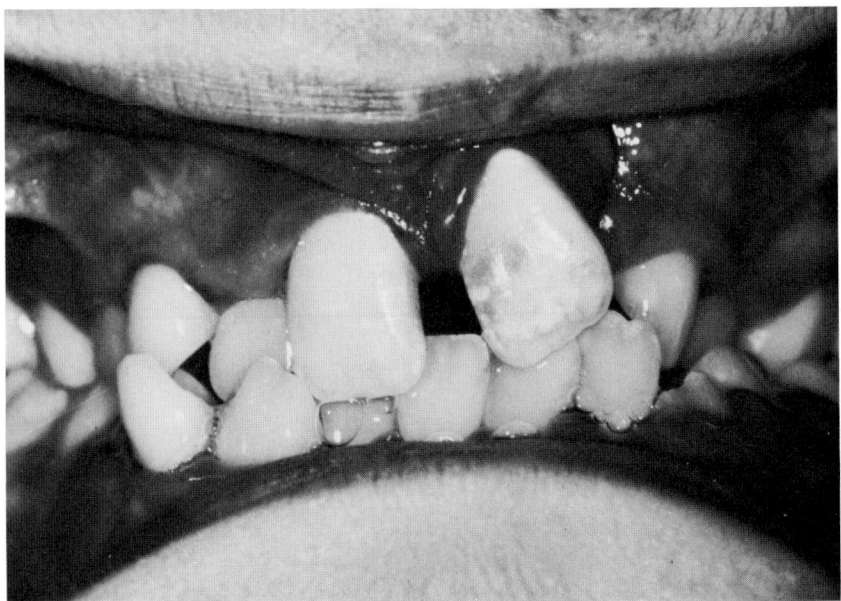

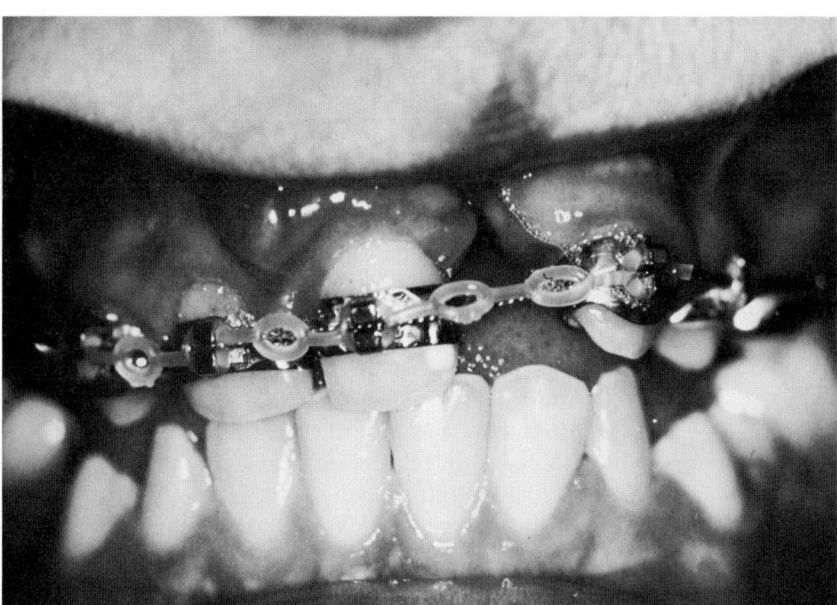

Fig. 13.10 Alignment of upper incisors using a fixed orthodontic appliance

primary canines and molars still present have started to undergo resorption of the roots, and are therefore not suitable for orthodontic movement, nor for the attachment of appliances for segmental movement. On the other hand, the early stage of correction of permanent incisor positions is often possible.

When the upper incisor teeth have erupted inside the arch of the lower teeth it is desirable to correct their position as early as possible so that the maximum space is available for tongue movements. Provided the basal discrepancy in jaw relationship is not too severe, the upper incisors can be moved forward, using fixed or removable orthodontic appliances, into a correct relationship with the lower teeth. Rotation and displacement of the incisor teeth can also be at least partly corrected at this stage, usually with the use of fixed orthodontic appliances (Fig. 13.10). Final alignment of the incisor teeth is usually necessary as the last stage of orthodontic treatment in the permanent dentition.

THE PERMANENT DENTITION PHASE

The permanent dentition, from the age of about 12 years, exhibits just as much variation as any previous phase of dental development. In favourable circumstances there may be little or no malocclusion, particularly if the cleft has not involved the primary palate. More commonly, however, the jaws exhibit growth defects, sometimes in all three planes.

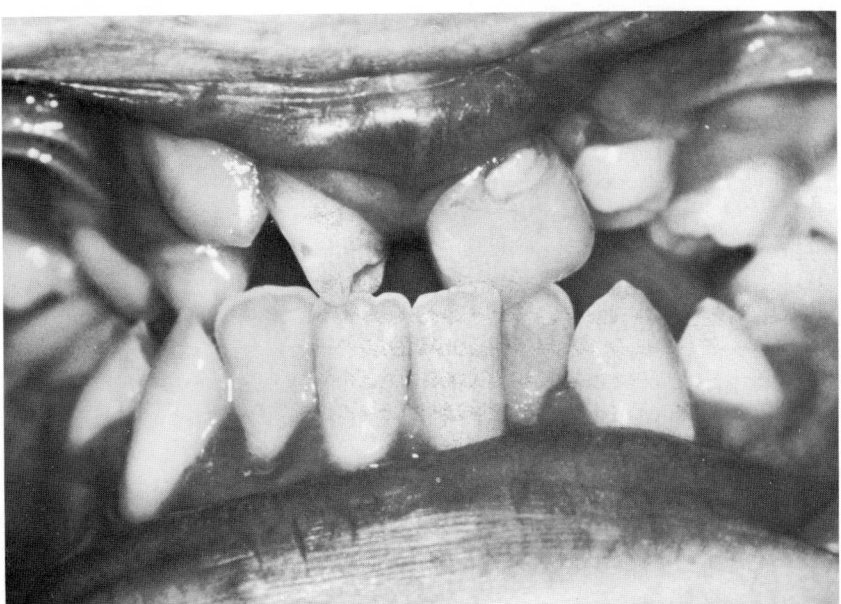

Fig. 13.11 The permanent dentition of a child with repaired complete bilateral cleft. Many characteristic features of the dentition can be seen, including hypoplastic and malpositioned upper incisors, medial displacement of the maxillary segments and deficiency of vertical development in the region of the alveolar cleft

In a complete cleft of primary and secondary palate, where no previous corrective orthodontic treatment has been carried out, the following occlusal defects may be seen in the permanent dentition (Fig. 13.11):

1. Medial displacement of the maxillary segment, giving buccal crossbite, particularly in the canine region. The molars are often correct.
2. Relative maxillary retrognathism, giving reversed incisal overjet.
3. Deficiency of vertical growth of the upper jaw. This may be a generalized deficiency, leading to reduced facial height, or a localized deficiency, which

is particularly common in the region immediately behind the alveolar cleft, leading to a lateral open bite.

4. Dental aberrations, including rotation and malposition of the upper incisor teeth and crowding of the teeth as a result of reduced jaw growth, particularly in the upper jaw. There is also an increased prevalence of hypodontia, the failure of development of upper premolar teeth being more common in cleft subjects than in the normal population (Dixon 1966).

Since the width of the dental arches does not normally undergo a steady increase, but increases with the eruption of new teeth, defects in arch breadth are not progressive, and are no more marked in the permanent dentition phase than in earlier phases. The translative downward and forward growth of the jaws in relation to the skull base is, however, a more steady process, and growth defects in the vertical and sagittal planes are therefore progressive. Thus the relative maxillary retrognathism and reduced vertical height of the face which is so often seen in cleft lip and palate tends to be more severe in the permanent dentition phase than at earlier stages of growth.

Occlusal defects are not so marked in clefts involving only the secondary palate. As the dento-alveolar arch has not been divided there are no specific malpositions of the teeth or segmental malalignments. If the cleft has been severe, there may be a growth defect affecting the forward and downward growth of the upper jaw with residual maxillary retrognathism. In such cases there is usually also crowding of the dentition.

Clefts involving only the primary palate do not usually bring major defects of jaw growth, but may exhibit localized dental malpositions in the region of the lip or alveolar cleft.

Treatment in the permanent dentition

The final stages, and often the major stages, of orthodontic treatment take place in the permanent dentition. The objectives of treatment have been previously outlined—to produce the optimum alignment and relationship of the dental arches for speech, mastication, oral health and facial appearance. It is not always possible to achieve ideal alignment. Orthodontic treatment can move the teeth provided they have adequate bony support, and in cleft lip and palate can produce considerable movement of the segments of the maxilla relative to each other. It cannot, however, overcome the effects of severe disturbance of jaw growth, and some of the more marked defects of sagittal and vertical growth cannot be corrected by orthodontic treatment alone. Furthermore, some of the severe malpositions of the teeth at the margins of the cleft may be difficult to correct and the correction even more difficult to maintain because of the lack of bony support for the teeth unless bone grafts are inserted into the alveolar defect. Thus orthodontic treatment has its limitations and in some of the more severe problems the final alignments may fall short of ideal. At the same time, in most cases much improvement in the occlusion and the shape of the jaw can be achieved, with consequent potential for improvement in oral health and in speech.

The final stages of orthodontic treatment usually begin with the planned extraction of teeth to relieve crowding of the dentition and to make space for alignment of the remaining teeth. At this stage, any supernumerary teeth and grossly malpositioned or malformed teeth may also be removed. Following this, treatment typically consists of correction in the lateral and in the vertical dimensions, and finally alignment of the incisor teeth.

Correction of arch form in the lateral dimension

In the absence of bony union between the two sides of the maxilla, correction of arch form in the lateral dimension is relatively straightforward. Forces applied via the teeth can be made to move the segments of the jaw, often to a considerable degree. The exact method of applying the force will depend on the amount of expansion required and the initial position of the segments. If only a small amount of expansion of the arch is necessary, removable orthodontic appliances may be adequate. Greater amounts of expansion will require the more positive and longer-ranging forces of a fixed appliance (Figs 13.12 and 13.13).

In a few cases equal movement of all parts of the displaced segment is necessary, but in most cases the segment exhibits greater displacement in the immediate vicinity of the alveolar cleft. Frequently there is no displacement of the segment at the molar regions. Therefore some form of differential expansion is often required. This may be difficult to achieve, but appliances such as those shown in Figures 13.12 and 13.13 are capable of producing differential expansion in the lateral dimension (Foster & Chinn 1977).

As there is no mid-palatal suture to be split, expansion of the cleft palate

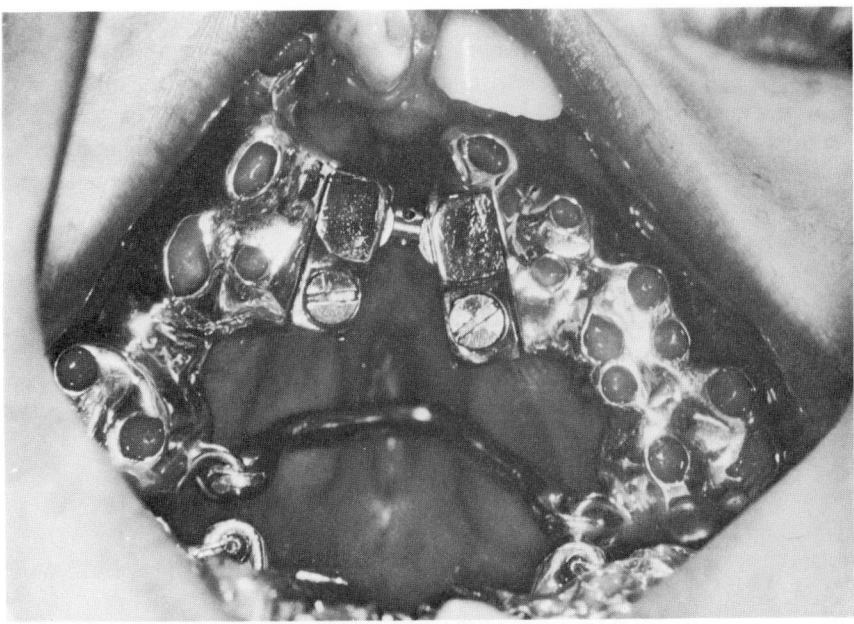

Fig. 13.12 Differential expansion of the maxillary segments in complete bilateral cleft. The appliance consists of a cast metal splint on each segment, with an expansion screw in a rotatory housing, and a bar to prevent expansion of the molar regions

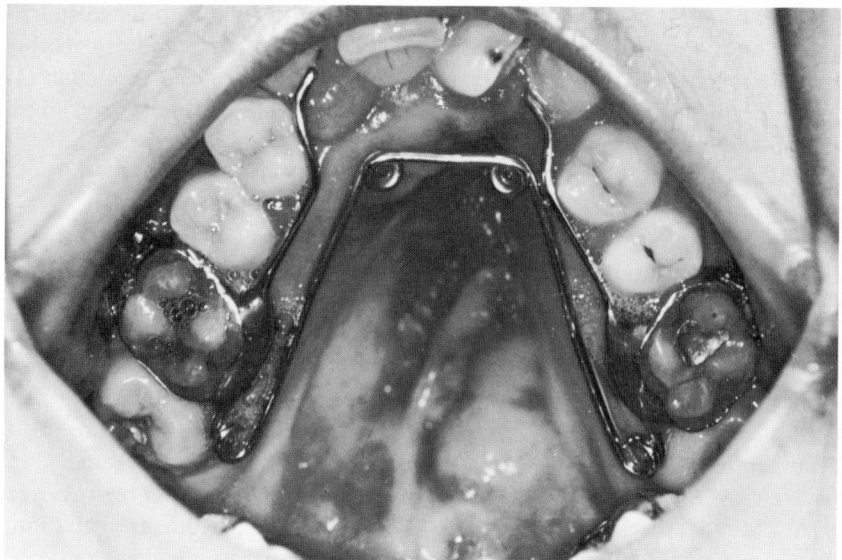

Fig. 13.13 Simple fixed appliance to produce differential expansion of the maxillary arch

does not need to be performed as rapidly as in non-cleft palates, and this slower movement is probably less damaging to the teeth and their supporting structures.

Correction in the vertical dimension
A generalized growth deficiency of the maxilla in the vertical dimension is probably beyond correction by orthodontic treatment alone in the present state of knowledge. Attention has therefore largely been confined to the problems of localized growth deficiency. As previously mentioned, this is most commonly seen in the region immediately behind the alveolar cleft. Unfortunately, this is a problem which is not only very difficult to treat but is also made worse by any expansion of the maxilla in the lateral dimension (Fig. 13.14). Unlike lateral expansion, which is relatively uninhibited by bony attachments, vertical forces on the teeth tend to extrude those teeth rather than produce segmental

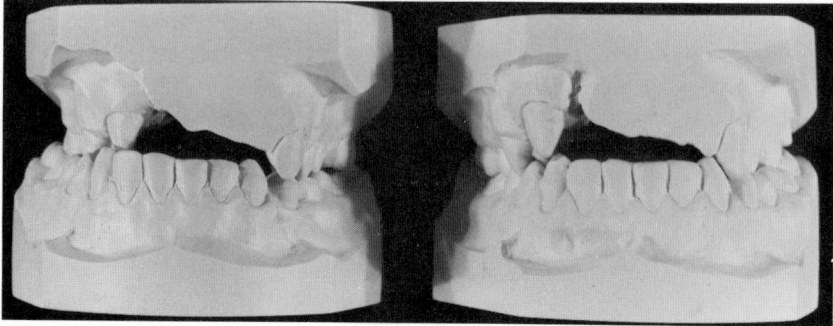

Fig. 13.14 Cutaway models illustrating that expansion of the maxilla tends to accentuate the discrepancy of vertical growth of the lesser segment

movement of the jaw bone. A limited amount of improvement in vertical discrepancies by orthodontic treatment is usually possible, and in some cases may be adequate for complete correction (Fig. 13.15). Generally speaking, however, this is at present one of the less satisfactory aspects of orthodontic treatment in cleft palate.

Alignment of the incisor teeth
If correction of incisor tooth positions in the sagittal dimension has been possible in the mixed dentition phase, final detailed alignment is usually necessary as the last stage of orthodontic treatment. This is best carried out by means of fixed orthodontic appliances, which can produce precise modifications of tooth position. The most difficult correction is usually that on the permanent central incisor nearest the alveolar cleft, which is often grossly malpositioned and malformed and lacks adequate alveolar bone support. If these discrepancies are severe it may be preferable to remove this tooth.

Long-term retention after treatment
Retention of tooth position for a short period after active movement is almost always necessary in orthodontic treatment. Special aspects of the problem in cleft lip and palate make it necessary in most cases to employ long-term retention to prevent relapse of the movements which have been achieved. These special aspects are particularly related to the fact that there is no bony union between the two sides of the jaw and in most cases a bony defect in the alveolar process. The jaw segments and the incisor teeth are thus more mobile than is normal, and though this may make treatment easier, it also makes relapse an ever-present possibility.

Three main methods of retention are commonly employed to maintain stability after active treatment, these being removable prostheses, fixed bridges and bone grafting. All have their advantages and their disadvantages and it seems that up to the present time there is no universal ideal method for ensuring long-term stability.

Removable prostheses
The commonest retention appliance in use is the removable prosthesis. This appliance has the great advantage that it can be fitted quickly and easily after active treatment, and it can be made to replace any missing teeth or to cover a residual palatal fistula. It has the disadvantage that, being removable, it may be lost or broken, with consequent relapse of tooth and segment position. A further considerable disadvantage is the adverse effect of a long-term prosthesis on oral health. This effect is minimized by the use of a carefully designed metal-based prosthesis, utilizing good tooth support and employing minimal soft tissue coverage (Fig. 13.16). Although an immediate acrylic resin prosthesis may usefully be fitted after active treatment, this should normally be replaced by a metal-based prosthesis as soon as possible if optimum oral health is to be maintained.

Fixed bridges
While removable prostheses are of most value in the adolescent years after active treatment and are often used on a lifelong basis, it is possible to use fixed bridges

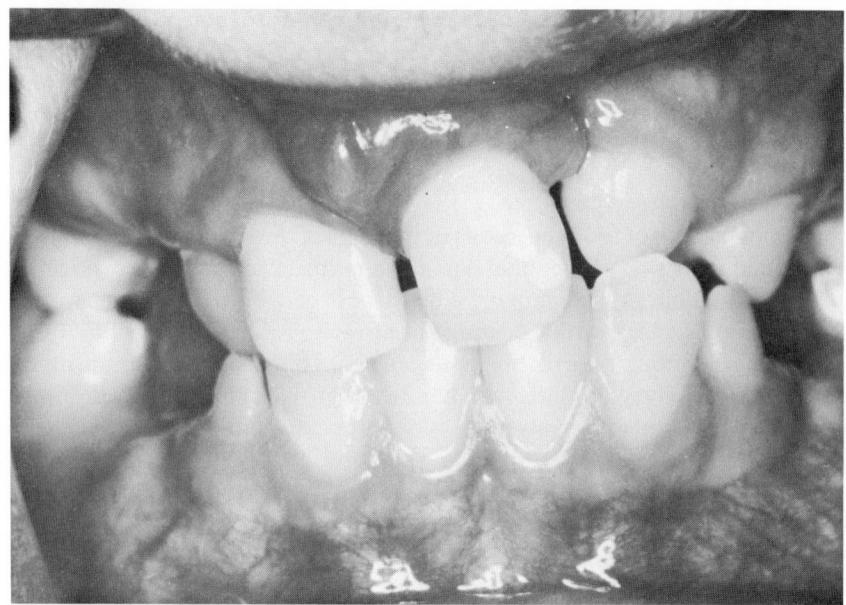

13.15(a)

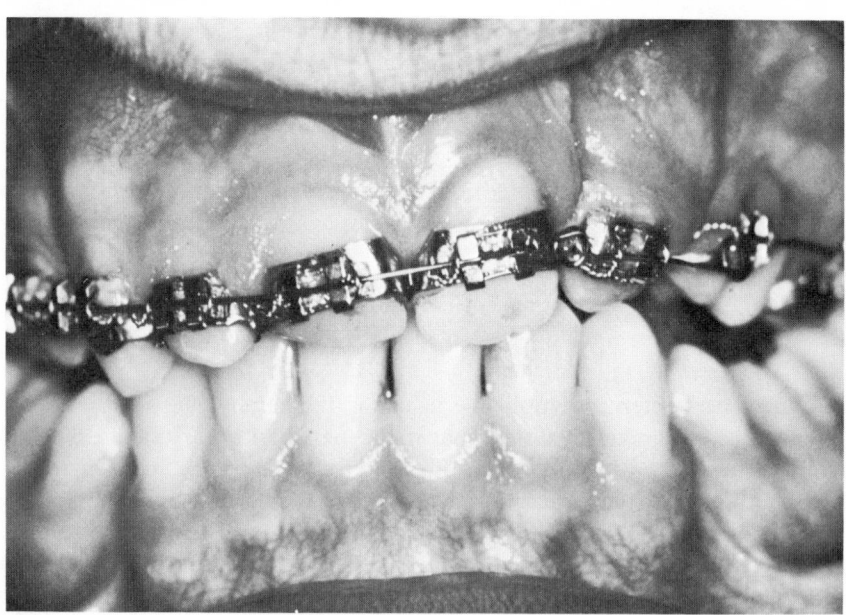

13.15(b)

across the alveolar cleft when growth has ceased (Kantorowicz 1978). The
obvious advantage that a fixed bridge cannot readily be removed and lost is
partly countered by the fact that it does not necessarily provide such stable retention as a removable prosthesis. Furthermore, the construction of a bridge inevitably involves damage to other teeth and in the long-term slow deterioration
usually brings about the need for replacement, which is often more difficult

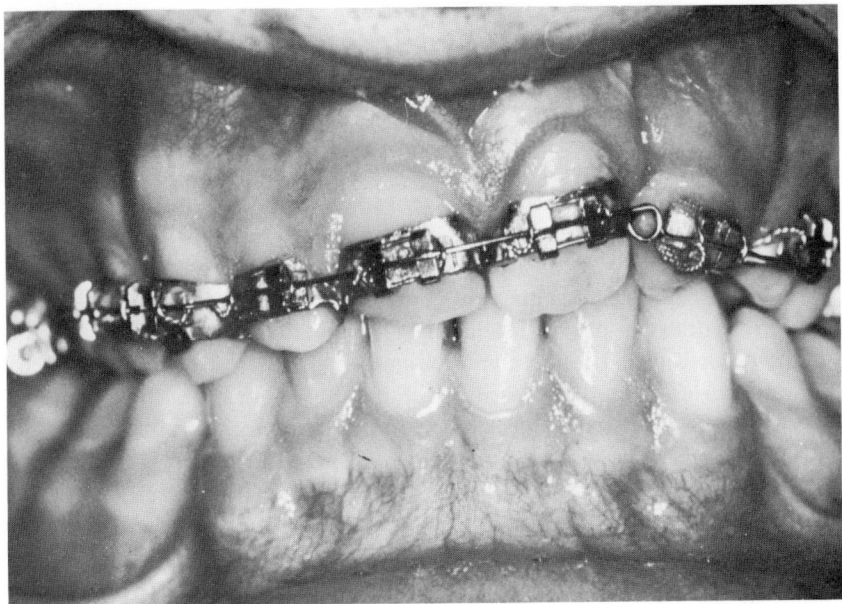

13.15(c)

Fig. 13.15 Improvement of the incisor positions and of minor medial and vertical displacement of the maxillary segment is best achieved with the use of fixed orthodontic appliances

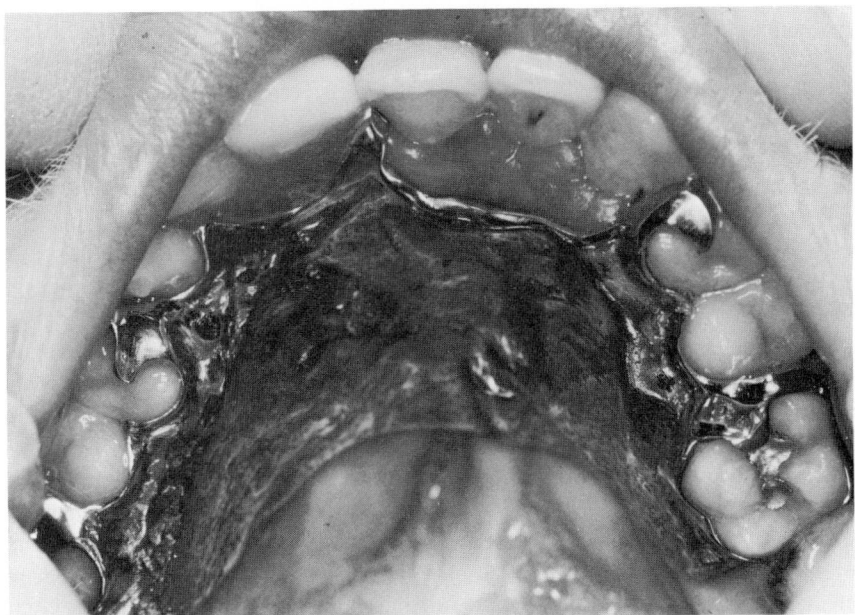

Fig. 13.16 Removable prosthesis on a cobalt–chromium base, replacing missing teeth and stabilizing the maxillary segments after alignment

than the replacement of a removable prosthesis. These factors need to be considered in the decision on what is usually lifelong retention of segment position and replacement of teeth.

Secondary bone grafting

To avoid the need for either a fixed or removable retainer, secondary bone grafting after orthodontic treatment has been advocated. The insertion of a bone graft across the alveolar and part of the palatal cleft seems a logical method of stabilizing the segments. However, early results have suggested that absolute stability is not necessarily achieved. Robertson & Fish (1972) have found that bone grafting does not prevent collapse of the maxillary segment and the recurrence of a crossbite, although the bone grafts appear to remain *in situ* and do not seem to interfere with growth of the maxilla in a sagittal direction.

Thus there does not seem to be an entirely satisfactory method of long-term retention available at present. The method of choice in any individual needs to be determined after consideration of factors such as the condition and shape of the teeth, oral health conditions, the presence of any oronasal fistula and the number of teeth to be replaced. In the adolescent patient, unless there are strong indications to act otherwise, the provision of a carefully designed and constructed removable prosthesis on a metal base gives positive retention and leaves open the option for other types of treatment at a later time.

CONCLUSION

Orthodontic treatment is important for oral health and oral function. In cleft lip and palate, it has particular importance in speech production, and it also has a part to play in the improvement of facial appearance. It is perhaps unfortunate that no single early course of treatment is at present sufficient to correct the developmental anomalies in most children with clefts. It is necessary to apply treatment care throughout the growth period, and because of this orthodontic treatment forms a large proportion of the total treatment for the majority of children. However, orthodontic treatment should not be considered as an isolated treatment regime. If the best results are to be obtained, it is necessary for the orthodontist to work in conjunction with all the other disciplines concerned with cleft lip and palate, and particularly with the plastic surgeon and the speech therapist.

It is important to remember that the dental and occlusal problems associated with cleft lip and palate are likely to be superimposed on those of normal variation, which is very wide-ranging. Even without the cleft malformation many people exhibit discrepancies in jaw growth and tooth position. Although the cleft malformation does not always bring any apparent growth defects, the defects usually associated with cleft lip and palate are those of jaw growth in all three planes. This is most noticeable in the upper jaw, but a tendency towards defective mandibular growth has also been demonstrated. If these growth defects are superimposed on adverse normal variation in any individual, corrective orthodontic treatment is likely to be more difficult and its objectives more limited. Nevertheless, it is usually possible to achieve some improvement, and, in conjunction with surgical treatment and speech therapy, orthodontic treatment can play a very important part in the rehabilitation of the cleft palate patient.

REFERENCES

Böhn A 1963 Dental anomalies in harelip and cleft palate. Acta Odontologica Scandinavica 21: suppl 38

Brophy J W 1927 Cleft lip and cleft palate. Journal of the American Dental Association 14: 1108–1115

Burston W R 1958 The early orthodontic treatment of cleft palate conditions. Dental Practitioner 9: 41–56 (Transactions BSSO)

Crabb J J, Foster T D 1977 Growth defects in unrepaired unilateral cleft lip and palate. Oral Surgery, Oral Medicine and Oral Pathology 44: 329–335

Dixon D A 1966 Anomalies of the teeth and supporting structures in children with cleft of lip and palate. In: Drillien C M, Ingram T S, Wilkinson E M The causes and natural history of cleft lip and palate. Livingstone, Edinburgh

Foster T D, Chinn D 1977 Differential rapid maxillary expansion in cleft palate. British Journal of Orthodontics 4: 139–141

Foster T D, Lavelle C L B 1971 The size of the dentition in complete cleft lip and palate. Cleft Palate Journal 8: 177–184

Graber T M 1949 Craniofacial morphology in cleft palate and cleft lip deformity. Surgery, Gynaecology and Obstetrics 88: 359–369

Huddart A G 1974 An evaluation of presurgical treatment. British Journal of Orthodontics 1: 21–25

Jolleys A, Robertson N R E 1972 A study of the effects of early bone grafting in complete clefts of the lip and palate. British Journal of Plastic Surgery 25: 229–237

Jordan R E, Kraus B S, Neptune C M 1966 Dental abnormalities associated with cleft lip and palate. Cleft Palate Journal 3: 22–55

Kantorowicz G F 1978 Bridge work for cleft palate patients. British Dental Journal 145: 335–336

Kjellgren B 1949 Dental orthopaedic treatment combined with surgery. European Orthodontic Society Transactions p 164–175

Latham R A, Kusy R P, Georgiade N G 1976 An extra-orally activated expansion appliance for cleft palate infants. Cleft Palate Journal 13: 253–261

McNeil C K 1954 Oral and facial deformity. Pitman, London

Maisels D O 1974 The influence of presurgical orthodontic treatment upon the surgery of cleft lip and palate. British Journal of Orthodontics 1: 15–20

O'Donnel J, Krischer J P, Shiere F R 1974 An analysis of presurgical orthopaedics in the treatment of unilateral cleft lip and palate. Cleft Palate Journal 11: 374–393

Ozerovic B, Markovic M 1967 Our experience in early and late presurgical orthopaedic treatment of congenital clefts of the lip and palate. European Orthodontic Society Transactions p 325–336

Pruzansky S, Aduss H 1967 Prevalence of arch collapse and malocclusion in complete unilateral cleft lip and palate. European Orthodontic Society Transactions p 365–382

Robertson N R E 1973 Deciduous occlusion in children with repaired complete clefts of the lip and palate. British Journal of Orthodontics 1: 5–10

Robertson N R E 1978 The orthodontic management of cleft lip and palate patients. British Dental Journal 145: 236–240

Robertson N R E, Fish J 1972 Some observations on rapid expansion followed by bone grafting in cleft lip and palate. Cleft Palate Journal 9: 236–245

Robinson F, Wood B 1969 Primary bone grafting in the treatment of cleft lip and palate, with special reference to alveolar collapse. British Journal of Plastic Surgery 22: 336–342

Wood B 1970 Control of the maxillary arch by primary bone graft in cleft lip and palate cases. Cleft Palate Journal 7: 194–205

14

Assessment and remediation of speech

INTRODUCTION

Assessment, diagnosis and remediation are closely interwoven elements of rehabilitation. Frequent allusion in the literature to 'diagnostic therapy' and to 'therapeutic assessment' lends substance to this view and this chapter will, by its structure, reflect the importance of their interrelationship.

The planning of any therapeutic programme suggests the need for it to be based on certain principles so that appropriate strategies and techniques may be developed. In relation to speech and language disability, these principles could be stated thus:

The need to describe the presenting problem
The identification of information relevant to the problem
The deduction of inferences which may be drawn from this information
Based on these deductions, the pattern of action proposed
The outcome of such action.

This programme represents a logical progress of investigation, diagnosis, remediation and appraisal. It must be emphasized, however, that each stage is closely linked to both its precursor and its successor, and there is therefore a necessity for constant questioning and evaluation on the part of the clinician.

It is not the intehtion here to offer a comprehensive account of assessment and remedial procedures. Instead, an attempt will be made to select aspects which it is hoped will indicate trends and changes which are current in the management of communication disorder associated with cleft palate.

THE ROLE OF THE CLINICIAN

Of primary importance is the need to consider the part played by the speech therapist as a member of the cleft palate team. To some extent this role calls upon different facets of clinical knowledge and skill, at different times and in different environments.

In the first place the multidisciplinary aspect of the treatment programme requires that information about language behaviour shall be available to each member of the team and also that this information shall be presented to that member in a form which has particular relevance to his specialty. The prostho-dontist, for example, may require information about the precise way in which a prosthesis may be influencing speech patterns, while the surgeon will undoubtedly need information regarding the likely effects of any proposed surgery on speech. The orthodontist works closely with the speech therapist and decisions regarding techniques are to some extent the result of mutually shared aims and objectives. A close relationship with audiologist and psychologist may also in certain instances be of benefit in the planning of educational needs, and of speech therapy.

Secondly, there is a requirement from all other members of the team to provide information on structural, physiological, cognitive and social status, so that, taken in conjuction with detailed descriptions of speech and language, an appropriate language programme based on this data may be planned.

These two aspects of the clinician as assessor are not of course mutually exclusive, and indeed the happiest situation is one in which all those concerned with the management of the patient have ready and easy access to each other for ongoing discussion. Alas! save for a few favoured centres, the exigencies of long clinical lists and the constraints of inadequate accommodation inevitably dampen the enthusiasm of even the keenest advocates of consensus management. In many cases, dissemination of information is usually by means of written report and in these conditions the speech therapist must make doubly certain that information contained therein about speech and language is clear, concise, logical and, above all, devoid of incomprehensible streams of professional jargon.

The role of the speech therapist with regard to the patient may vary at different stages between that of advising and that of active intervention.

In the early days, probably around six weeks after birth, parents and baby may for the first time visit the Unit as outpatients. The purpose of this visit is primarily to enable the surgeon to determine his course of action. It also offers an opportunity for discussion of any setbacks which may have arisen; an obvious one is possible feeding difficulty; or if, for example, a feeding plate has been prescribed the orthodontist will wish to ensure that it is satisfactory. Similarly, where appropriate, procedures designed to induce preoperative arch alignment will need checking. This is also an important occasion on which to discuss prognosis and in some cases the advisability of genetic counselling may also be broached at this point.

Discussion and advice about cleft palate may already have taken place following birth, but it must be remembered that at that time the parents may well have been too bewildered and shocked by the impact of the handicap to absorb such information fully. Reiteration at a later stage when they have had time and opportunity to come to terms with the condition may therefore be necessary as well as more effective. At this time too, one of the most commonly voiced anxieties pertains to the likelihood of speech and language disorders. The speech therapist as counsellor must emphasize the probability of satisfactory development. Such a forecast can of course be made with greater confidence if early surgery is anticipated. Pannbacker (1976) reported on the prevalance of incorrect and unrealistic views expressed by parents of cleft palate children in the absence of adequate counselling methods. At this stage a simple description of speech production and of language development can be offered so that if deviations or delays do occur in the future their nature will be better understood.

Arrangements should also be made for a series of regular visits, initially at three-monthly intervals and later perhaps at six-monthly intervals, so that development can be recorded. Most surgeons request tape recordings immediately before operation and then within about three months after surgery. But regular checks during which detailed information about speech and language development can be recorded serve a purpose beyond that of advising the mother. The paucity of recent comprehensive studies on this aspect of development in the cleft palate population has already been noted. Such visits offer a good opportunity to obtain information about early babbling patterns, emergence of the phonological system, development of prosody, early syntactic forms and general communicative ability. Not only can the individual pattern of development be charted, but the collation of such data from a number of subjects over a period of time would ensure more definitive comparative statements in relation to what is known of normal language development.

On these occasions too, the speech therapist must be alert to any signs of possible hearing impairment. Audiological assessment may have already started, but, if not, this should be undertaken as a matter of urgency because of the grave implication of any degree of hearing impairment not only for language development but indeed also for cognitive development.

ASSESSMENT AND DIAGNOSIS

At a level of physical performance the clinician needs to determine the forces which are essential for production of speech.

Respiration
Respiration, for purposes of speech a modified function, needs to be checked. It is important to ensure that structural conditions allow for the rapid inspiratory phase which is followed by controlled and more prolonged expiration. Nasal inspiration may well be impeded by obstruction of the nasal passages, as for example by a deflected septum or enlarged turbinates, or by an overly narrowed pharyngeal isthmus, which is sometimes one result of secondary surgery. Such conditions will commonly also affect resonance and hyponasality may be present. In the case of the unoperated cleft, it must also be remembered that when there is nasal obstruction the normal recourse to mouth breathing may not be as effective since any intra-oral intake will be diffused. Although such impairment may not be sufficiently serious to affect respiration for vital purposes, it may nevertheless have a deleterious effect on the expiratory phase of the cycle and thus, if habitual, ultimately on phonation.

Air wastage resulting in a breathy type of phonation should be checked. This could be a compensatory measure adopted to combat a glottal element in speech by an attempt to introduce a 'soft attack' in phonation. On the other hand, forceful expiration may underlie glottal production and possibly at a later stage lead to the development of vocal nodules.

Phonatory disorders which may occur have been described previously as has their relationship to abnormal positioning of the larynx and/or to increased tension of the vocal cords. Observation of the posture of the patient may give initial

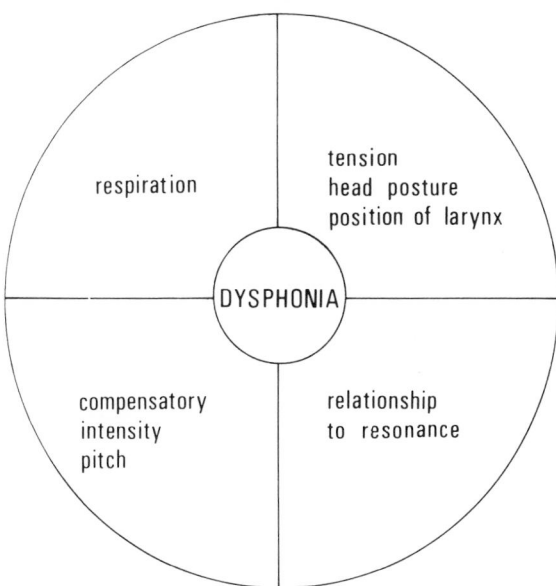

Fig. 14.1 Factors contributing to phonatory disorders in cleft palate

cues, and head and neck position should be particularly noted. Where dysphonia persists or is marked, the opinion of a laryngologist should be sought and laryngoscopy may well reveal the presence of vocal nodules or perhaps inflammation and oedematous changes in the vocal cords (Fig. 14.1).

Hypernasal resonance

Hypernasal resonance is one of the most complex disorders associated with cleft palate. Although there has been a steady decline in numbers of patients presenting with hypernasality over the past years, it is nevertheless a fact that those who do, sometimes constitute almost intractable problems. It is tempting for the speech clinician to regard the alleviation of all such defects of nasal resonance as lying solely within the scope of the surgeon, but the earlier discussion of this condition has indicated that there may be causative factors other than anatomical which can account for this disorder.

Measurement of hypernasality has traditionally centred upon subjective impressions, and until the last ten years or so there has been very little in the way of adequate instrumentation for assessment of ratios of nasal/oral air flows and pressures during ongoing speech. Even so, some of the more recently developed techniques impose some degree of artificiality upon normal modes of speech production, either by the use of facial masks or by other invasive measures such as intra-oral devices, and these may in themselves alter the balance of resonance.

Fletcher & Bishop (1970) first used the term 'nasalance' to define a quantifiable degree of nasality in speech. This measurement represented a ratio of nasal to oral air pressure and was computed by means of an instrument called a Tonar. The term nasalance was used to distinguish this measure from listener-perceived nasality. In order to estimate possible correction between perceived nasality and

Tonar measurements, an extensive study was undertaken. This involved detailed protocols wherein a number of untrained listeners rated degrees of nasality in the recorded speech of a series of cleft palate patients. Although initially there was a wide disparity between judgements, with training this narrowed and at each end of the spectrum, i.e. extreme hypernasality and normality, there was good correlation with Tonar readings. In the middle ranges, where differences were more subtle, predicatably there was less agreement. Fletcher (1978) commented that this study illustrates that it is possible to train listeners to achieve a reasonable level of accuracy in estimating nasality but that this measurement can more easily and reliably be undertaken by use of instrumentation.

At Exeter University a method of measuring nasal air flow has been devised and used clinically. As described by Ellis (1979) this comprises a plastic mask which fits over the nose. This connects with a sensing head mounted in plastic tubing which in turn leads to the anemometer which measures air flow. The instrument also has a facility for recording both air flow and speech on to a stereo tape recorder. This recording can be decoded so that a printout shows associated air flow and speech.

This system is still in relatively early stages of development and Ellis acknowledges the need for further comparative studies before measurement can be adequately quantified. However, in its present stage of development the anemometer does offer a most useful means of visually monitoring speech.

An interesting fact to emerge from the Fletcher (1978) study sheds light on the question of whether evaluation of tape recordings played backwards is more likely to yield accurate results in listener judgement tasks. The findings of this study indicate the converse. Interlistener correlation on this task was significantly lower than when the tapes were played in the normal way. Certainly this seems to be a very reasonable conclusion when one considers the distracting effect of the bizarre sounds coming from backward-played tapes.

Hypernasality can therefore to some extent be quantified. However, these measures simply record the existence and extent of the condition; they reveal no information as to cause. To determine this, the first recourse will again be to instrumental investigation. The objective in this case is to investigate velopharyngeal function. Where as far as can be ascertained this appears to be satisfactory, i.e. where it cannot be established that the physiology of the sphincter is a direct cause of nasal escape, the speech therapist then needs to undertake further assessment. Although the development of new techniques of investigation by means of multiview videofluoroscopy and simultaneous nasendoscopy have greatly enhanced the confidence with which decisions regarding future management can be made, nevertheless there is still a degree of uncertainty present. The use of fibre optics in nasendoscopy, for example, results in some distortion of the picture so that accurate measurements cannot be made (Chapter 15). Again, while it is desirable to obtain multiple views of velopharyngeal function, the basal view entails the subject assuming a position in which there is considerable strain on head and neck (sphinx position) and this in itself may increase nasality.

Causes of nasality have been discussed in the previous chapter. They may be graphically represented as shown in Fig. 14.2.

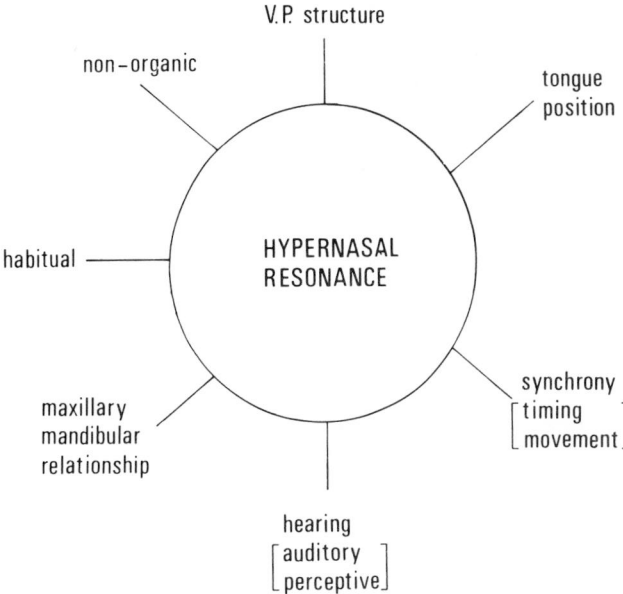

Fig. 14.2 Factors contributing to resonatory disorders in cleft palate

Ascertainment of the more prevalent conditions which may indirectly contribute to nasality are discussed below.

Positioning of tongue
Ongoing rapid tongue movements are probably most satisfactorily measured by means of electropalatography (Hardcastle 1972). The recent inclusion of a printout computer facility has made analysis both easier and more useful. The main problem remains the somewhat lengthy and cumbersome preparations involved in making acrylic palates for each individual and in determining the exact siting for the electrodes.

Subjective observation, both visual and auditory, should give some indication as to whether for example there is abnormal fronting of the tongue particularly on production of the vowel /i/ (Fletcher 1978). This forward position appears to be associated with increased nasal resonance whereas posterior movement is reported to be connected with pharyngeal and glottal articulation.

Diadochokinesis should also be assessed since, as well as its relationship to articulation, Fletcher (1978) noted a correlation between impaired ability for rapid alternating movement and increased nasalance. It is difficult to know whether there is a direct relationship between this impairment and velopharyngeal valving or whether this is an indication of a more generalized oral disability extending beyond the anatomical defect. The latter appears to be a likely, though perhaps at the present time somewhat speculative, hypothesis.

The most usual method of assessing rapid alternative movement is by timing repeated production of /pʌ, tʌ, kʌ/; see Canning & Rose (1974) for norms.

Synchrony of movement

Programming and organization of sequences of movement are essential for the smooth execution of motor activity. Wyke (1969) has described asynchrony of largyngeal muscles with resulting dysphonia. Shelton et al (1964), in a study of cleft palate speakers, observed a considerable variation in the timing and pattern of velopharyngeal closure during ongoing speech. Lateral cineradiography had shown them to be capable of achieving adequate closure. Shprintzen et al (1977) described incongruous movements of lateral pharyngeal walls and the velum in attempts at valving.

These subjects may show considerable variability of response from day to day and the inconsistency of response puts one rather in mind of a verbal dyspraxia. This lack of synchrony could well have its origins in central neurophysiological processes rather than in a peripheral neuromuscular dysfunction. Little investigation of this phenomenon has taken place. EMG studies might be a fruitful source of information, and perhaps more readily the speech therapist could undertake 'a frame by frame' analysis on lateral videography, provided that there was a high-quality simultaneous sound recording.

Maxillary–mandibular relationships

There is evidence that vertical interincisor distance is in inverse relationship to the degree of nasality. The narrower the jaw opening, the greater the degree of hypernasality. Since Class III Angle occlusal pattern is prevalent among the cleft palate population, there is greater likelihood of this occurrence. However, it must be stated that anomalies of occlusion are frequently part of a group of skeletal abnormalities and thus it is difficult to establish a direct correspondence.

Auditory perception

The importance of thorough audiological investigation has already been stressed. It is essential that the subject also be able to differentiate between hypernasal and normal nasal resonance, so that effective monitoring can be encouraged as part of remediation.

Assessment of articulation

On the whole, those children with deviant patterns of articulation are liable to take up more of the speech therapists' time, those presenting with hypernasality forming a smaller proportion of the caseload. O'Riain & Hammond (1972), reporting a study of 249 children aged 5 with cleft palate, stated: 'Articulatory defect was a considerably more frequent characteristic of poor speech than nasality, the ratio being approximately 3:1.'

Calnan (1978), in a review of speech results following primary repair carried out at Oxford between 1950 and 1960, estimated normal speech in 70 to 80 per cent of cases overall. Of a total of 245 cases comprising all groups of cleft palate repaired before the age of 2 years, he gave the following figures: 75.5 per cent with normal articulation; 64.1 per cent with no nasal escape (on 'ee' production). At first sight these figures appear to contradict the findings of the O'Riain & Hammond study, but absence of nasal escape does not necessarily equate with absence of hypernasal resonance, and Calnan does not elaborate on criteria for 'normal articulation'. Within this group there could be those whose deviant articulation was closely related to hypernasal resonance.

Certain types of articulation disorder are closely related to velopharyngeal function. These arise as a result of diminished intra-oral pressure. Failure to impound air within the mouth is likely to have a marked effect particularly on production of fricatives and plosives.

A number of articulatory assessments have been designed to assess this aspect of performance. Among those which are better known are the Iowa pressure test (Morris et al 1961) and the Bzoch error pattern articulation analysis (Bzoch 1964, 1977). Both these tests seek to identify articulatory defects which are associated with cleft palate. Each requires single word elicitation and a traditional type of analysis based on criteria of omission, distortion, etc. Darley (1977), discussing the IPAT, recognizes the limitations of such measures and advocates the necessity of also including a transcription of contextual speech. It is probably most valuable to use them as adjuncts to a routine phonological analysis. In this way a differential description between phonological and physiological patterns can be obtained. Where possible, video recording as an accompaniment to high-quality sound recording is recommended. Where only the latter facility is available, there should be careful notation of visual cues accompanying the sample (Fig. 14.3).

ARTICULATION

Maturational	Physiological
fronting	inappropriate contrasts
deletion of final syllable	backing
weak syllable deletion	nasalization
cluster reduction	pharyngeal realization
	glottal
	inappropriate pauses

---

failure of voiced/voiceless contrasts
failure of stop/continuant contrasts

Fig. 14.3 Differential features of structural and maturational deviance in cleft palate

It is not proposed to describe the physical examination of oral structures since this procedure is well established and has been extensively described in other texts (e.g. Morley 1970). Suffice it to say that the clinician in carrying out such investigations should be alert to the presence of structural irregularities such as palatal fistulae so that their possible significance may be considered in conjunction with other data obtained.

It is also assumed that investigation will not be limited to motor aspects of speech nor to analysis of the phonological system. The vulnerability of cleft palate children to delay in development of many aspects of speech and language has been discussed. It is therefore very important that an assessment of comprehension of verbal language be included and a reasonably detailed description of expressive language in terms of syntax, content and appropriateness of use should form an integral part of investigation. Bloom & Lahey (1978) emphasized the limitations of procedures which regard the analysis of form in language as an end goal, whether this be in relation to comprehension or production (see also Rees & Shulman (1978)); Bloom stated: 'In early language development it seems clear that the child does not learn sounds, words and syntactic structures and then find meanings for these forms; instead it appears that children learn about objects and events and then search for the forms to code various aspects of their experience.'

Categorization of content and use presents, in terms of time, an even more daunting task than does phonetic and syntactic analysis. A detailed discussion of the taxonomies of content and use lies outside the scope of this book and the reader is referred to Bloom & Lahey's (1978) book which includes a comprehensive discussion of the interrelationship between form, content and usage of language. It is important, however, that in relation to cleft palate these aspects of communication should be investigated. Anatomical and physiological abnormalities may well influence many aspects of communication other than those to which they relate directly, and the concern of the speech therapist must be with the totality of language behaviour.

INTERVENTION

Reference back to the principles of intervention cited at the beginning of the chapter has led through from the identification of the problem and the investigations regarding its origins to a consideration of how it may best be resolved. The remainder of the chapter will therefore be concerned with this aspect.

Where hypernasality presents as the outstanding persisting problem a decision has to be made as to whether the first line of intervention should be secondary surgery or whether a satisfactory result can be obtained through a programme of speech therapy designed to re-educate timing and positioning of articulatory organs. Multiview videography should yield information about the potential for achieving velopharyngeal closure and thus enable the surgeon to reach a decision regarding the nature and outcome of any further surgery which may be contemplated. To be of maximal value it is essential that such videography should carry a simultaneous high-quality sound recording so that accurate observations can be made on the relationship between speech and palatopharyngeal movement. The timing of secondary surgical procedures is the subject of some discussion. As with orthodontics, the speech therapist's plea is 'the sooner the better' since the shorter the time in which the child experiences speech in the presence of adverse physical conditions the weaker the habit factor. But conditions relating to growth and natural maturation have to be taken into account, and many surgeons are reluctant to embark upon further pharyngeal surgery before the child is 5 years old. For these reasons, Mazaheri (1977) and his associates do not recommend pharyngoplasty before the age of 6 years.

If the speech difficulties appear to stem directly from an incompetent velo-pharyngeal sphincter it may be hard for the speech therapist to decide on the best course of action. It is unlikely that any direct work aimed at improvement of resonance will be fruitful and at the same time neither will that directed to-wards modifying articulation of plosives or fricative sounds. Furthermore, the poor results may undermine motivation, so that when surgery is eventually carried out subsequent attempts at re-education may well be jeopardized as a consequence of the earlier experience. It is certainly very difficult to go along with Shprintzen's (1978) statement that one of the prerequisites of secondary surgery is that the child should first have achieved articulatory proficiency. All in all, it would appear that when the hypernasality is related to anatomical in-sufficiency requiring further surgery, the speech therapist will be most effective in a supervisory role, by ensuring that aspects of speech and language develop-ment other than those directly related to articulation and resonance are proceed-ing satisfactorily. If secondary surgery is not contemplated before the age of 5 years or so, children will have already started school and it is important that teachers be given full explanation of difficulties likely to be encountered and of the long-term measures proposed.

Many of the techniques used by speech therapists in remedial programmes for other types of disorders are equally applicable to those associated with cleft palate. This discussion is limited to those which may have specific relevance to cleft palate.

Blowing exercises

It appears to be something of a paradox to introduce such a subheading in a book which purports to deal with 'Recent Advances', for surely the origns of 'blow football' and the like are lost in the mists of early speech therapy. Blowing exercises have for many years been regarded as being of doubtful value as a means of improving palatal function, and writers have pointed to the fact that if palatal exercises were effective then the continued experience offered by swallowing would have ensured better results. The only concession made was that they might play some part in improving oral breath direction. Calnan & Renfrew (1961), Moll (1965) are among many authors disputing the efficacy of blowing. Their arguments were based on the contention that closure mechanisms for blowing differ from those necessary for the rapid ongoing movements involved in speech. In a paper written by Shprintzen et al (1974), based on multiview videofluoroscopic recordings, compelling evidence is offered to show that there are striking similarities between the closure pattern for blowing, whistling and speech, but that this pattern differs markedly from that of swallowing and gag-ging. The main differences reported are in the much more specific movement of the lateral pharyngeal walls and in the point of contact of the velum with the posterior pharyngeal wall in the first group of activities where air-stream mechanisms are involved. These authors suggested that previous work showing differences between movements for blowing for speech might be due to the fact that the blowing tasks involved considerable force (a carnival blower and a man-ometer in the two studies cited above). What was not revealed in the Shprintzen et al study, however, is whether there is a difference in the rate of movement for blowing and speech. Fritzell's (1969) EMG study refers to the need to investigate timing mechanisms. Blowing activity appears to be an 'all or none' phenomenon, whereas during speech there is a much more refined and changing degree of muscular control commensurate with the changing demands of context.

Conflicting reports have been given about the ability to modify blowing exercises to meet speech requirements. Powers & Starr (1974) undertook a therapy programme based on muscle training in non-speech tasks with four subjects with repaired clefts of the palate. These exercises were undertaken on an intensive basis over a period of six weeks; no attempt was made to carry them over to speaking tasks. The results were disappointing. At the end of the experiment there was no significant change in velopharyngeal gap nor in the degree of perceived nasality. In the case of one patient, some reduction in V–P gap was observed which appeared to be associated with *increased* nasality.

In their study, Shprintzen et al (1974) did not advocate whistling and blowing exercises as a method of improving closure. What they did suggest was that these activities which shared a similar pattern of velopharyngeal action as speech could be carried over to speech production. This was demonstrated in a study which was based on techniques of behaviour modification (Shprintzen et al 1975): four patients with repaired cleft palate who had normal closure for whistling and blowing, but not for speech, participated in a programme during which they were shown how to introduce phonation simultaneously with blowing. Once this pattern was established, the non-speech element was gradually extinguished and the phonatory activity was reinforced. A visual feedback device called a scape-scope was used to monitor nasal escape. This is a small, clear, plastic cylinder containing a piston. At one end a flexible plastic tube connects with a rubber end-piece which fits into and occludes the nostril. The other end of the cylinder has a small opening which allows air to escape. A qualitative estimate of nasal escape is provided by the piston moving up and down the cylinder during speech. This programme also was based on intensive therapy and schedules of reinforcement were rigidly maintained. Initially visual feedback was the determinant of success (no nasal escape of air = no movement of the piston), but subjects were encouraged to monitor speech through auditory and kinaesthetic pathways as treatment proceeded. Three out of four subjects, including one who had recently undergone pharyngeal flap surgery, achieved normal V–P closure during ongoing speech. The fourth had an accompanying hearing loss and although capable of closure did not manage this consistently. In the absence of auditory feedback, reliance had to be placed on kinaesthetic feedback and in the scheduled time of the programme this was not firmly established. Follow-up of the other subject for periods up to eight months indicated maintenance of acceptable levels of oral resonance. The authors contend that faulty mechanisms can be the result of learned behaviour. If surgery is not undertaken before the age of about 12 months, then deviant habits will have become established. Blowing and whistling are unlikely to be affected since these activities do not form a significant part of infant behaviour! The argument in favour of habit strength is the fact that in this study the oldest subject required the greatest amount of therapy to extinguish incorrect patterns. The study is, it must be said, very conservative in the claims it makes and strict criteria are laid down regarding the suitable type of subject and the regime to be followed. The improvement in resonance appears to be based on subjective evaluation since no quantifiable measures were used. Videofluoroscopy after treatment in each case showed approximation to normal closure of the velopharyngeal valve during speech.

Feedback
A number of therapy techniques are based on strategies of feedback. Among the earlier ones to be used clinically in this country are the visual speech aid and later the palatal training device (Tudor & Selly 1974). The palatal training appliance consists of an acrylic palate, the posterior edge of which has a loop of orthotic wire attached to it. This touches the soft palate at rest. The patient is encouraged by this sensation to lift the soft palate. To facilitate training a further aid has been developed as a supplement. This also consists of an acrylic base plate into which are embedded two electrodes at the point of contact with the soft plate. When the palate is at rest the current passes through and a light shows in the control box. When the palate is elevated the circuit is broken and the light is extinguished. No full study of the technique's effectiveness has yet been reported. Curle (1979) has outlined a programme based on its use in clinical practice which demonstrates a measure of success. Nevertheless there is evidence that some subjects achieve the correct response, i.e. the light is extinguished, while still retaining marked nasal resonance on speaking. Perhaps the placing of the electrodes allows for monitoring of contact in an anteroposterior relationship but not for dysfunction of lateral pharyngeal walls.

The nasal anemometer can also be used as a feedback device.

Fletcher (1978) described in some detail a therapy programme based on learning theory principles and employing Tonar to compute nasal oral air pressure ratios. Subjects were given a series of short sentences which were graded in order of difficulty with regard to nasality. Base-lines were established for each subject and a token system operated relating to success on each subgoal. This was a comparatively short programme (13 sessions of 20 to 30 min duration) so that definitive results are not claimed. From the 19 subjects who received treatment it was possible to grade response into four separate groups. These ranged from those (42 per cent) who were readily able to meet and maintain criteria for reduced nasality through to one subject who was unable to sustain any reduction whatsoever in nasality.

For those subjects who are anatomically potentially capable of achieving closure such biometric programmes may prove very useful. Postoperatively too, they may be effective since it by no means follows that new patterns of oral behaviour will automatically be adopted after surgery.

Another point which emerges from these studies is the demonstration that although the desired response may be achieved initially through visual feedback, underlying all the training is the necessity of establishing auditory and kinaesmenting the work of the speech pathologist in carrying out specific training programmes. Such self help groups are also now being set up in the UK.

Auditory perceptual dysfunction, particularly in relation to discrimination, has been demonstrated as a frequent mutually occurring condition with cleft palate. An interesting study based on the effect of feedback filtering on nasalization has been described by Garber & Moller (1977). It was observed that under conditions of low pass filtering where subjects heard their own speech with cut-off frequencies of 100, 500 and 300 Hz there was a marked decrease in nasality. This fact might have relevance to a training programme if linked to visual and kinaesthetic monitoring. There is also some evidence which indicates that there may be a corresponding impairment in tactile kinaesthetic awareness.

If assessment reveals deficiencies, then training to improve these skills should certainly form a part of any treatment programme. Most clinicians will be familiar with techniques of auditory training, but because the relevance of tactile kinaesthesia has been less extensively documented a brief description of some techniques which may be appropriate is given.

One of the patterns of articulatory dysfunction has been shown to be related to an apparent diminished awareness of tongue tip activity. Programmes based on principles of proprioceptive neuromuscular facilitation (PNF) have, in this writer's experience, met with some degree of success. Such a programme relies on increasing oral awareness by the use of contrasts in temperature and texture. A cold agent, such as iced mousse for example, is placed on the tip of the tongue, and is conveyed to various parts of the oral cavity with the subject reporting on the location of the cold sensation. This is contrasted with a sensation of heat induced by a heated metal tongue depressor being placed on the tip of the tongue. In particular, movement between tongue tip and alveolus is emphasized. Two-point discrimination tasks with toothpicks are also used, although a device called an esthesiometer has been developed (Ringel & Ewanowski 1965) which permits more exact study.

Transfer to production of alveolar plosives /t/ and /d/ in neutral vowel context follows (/tʌ, dʌ/). Modification of other deviant realizations [ç] [ʝ] and [ɬ] meets with success once new patterns of tongue movement become established. Again, an intensive programme of therapy to facilitate generalization is advocated, and some form of visual feedback would undoubtedly help as an initial reinforcer of newly learned patterns.

TYPES OF INTERVENTION

In the foregoing discussion repeated reference has been made to the advantages of intensive therapy programmes. The educational pattern in North America, where children attend summer school camps during the long vacation, has provided the opportunity for such courses. Schendel & Bzoch (1971) described a representative six-week summer programme which has been carried out over a period of ten years in the University of Florida. The practical advantage of such a programme is that it brings together children from widely scattered rural areas where little opportunity exists for regular individual therapy. This was one of the determining factors in the decision to run such courses at the Canniesburn Hospital in Glasgow (Huskie 1979). An intensive therapy project is now under way at Frenchay Hospital, Bristol, following a successful six-week pilot study (Albery et al 1979). This project seeks to compare the effectiveness of intensive therapy with conventional patterns of once-weekly treatment. During their time at the Unit, children have three sessions of therapy daily, two of these being individual and one in a group. Additionally, there is reinforcement provided by lay helpers who go through the programmes written up each day in each child's notebook. Following the six-week block, periodic reviews take place over the next two years. Initial investigation includes assessment of articulation, vocabulary, and linguistic ability based on the ITPA. Additionally a screening test has been developed which differentiates the children with palatal incompetence and these are excluded from the study. The assessment also includes subjective evaluation of nasality and intelligibility and hearing tests are also carried out. This study should yield interesting and important information though there may be certain reservations about the feasibility of making a straight comparison with the control group because of the multiplicity of variables involved and the fact that the overall sample is unlikely to be very large. Nevertheless the measurement of progress of each child undergoing the intensive programme should prove valuable and, if the results are encouraging, it is hoped that this experience may act as a catalyst for the setting-up of other intensive programmes elsewhere.

Group therapy also has much to commend itself although it should be seen as an adjunct of individual based treatment. Andrä & Diekmann (1976) reported successful results from a series of such programmes. These covered a wide age range (0–18 years) and at the lower end of the scale it was the parents who received the training. Advantages of such concentrated programmes are that motivation is likely to be much better, the realization that the child shares his disability with a number of others, and above all a much better opportunity for stabilization of newly learned skills. Against these advantages must be set the question of desirability of removing children from their homes for periods of around six weeks, which imposes a limit on the lower age range of children who can be seen. This is difficult in so far as it is the younger children who are likely to be in most need of help.

For these younger age groups a programme of parental counselling has been suggested. Undoubtedly one of the best ways of overcoming parents' anxiety is by involving them actively in the rehabilitation progress. Involvement requires more than a five-minute talk at the end of the session. It means that the parent should be present throughout the treatment, that the therapist should demonstrate the manner in which the desired response can be obtained, and that the parent in turn should have the opportunity to practise the technique in the clinic. In this way difficulties or queries can be resolved at the time and there is less danger of wrong methods being used which may have unfortunate results. Hansen et al (1977) reported on the development in the United States of self-help programmes for parents of cleft palate children. With experience, parents of older children have assumed the role of 'lay counsellors', supplementing the work of the speech pathologist in carrying out specific training programmes. Such self help groups are also now being set up in the UK.

There is little to commend the pattern of once-weekly therapy unless this session is used mainly for planning a daily home programme during the ensuing week. Many therapists seek to achieve progress through the exercise of some form of behaviour modification programme. This type of therapy has little value unless it includes regular reinforcement to stabilize the desired behaviour.

Clinical experience, the development of new techniques and the considerable advances made in the different specialties concerned with cleft palate have produced a change in the emphasis of treatment for speech and language disability. While the clinician is now less frequently faced with the gross unintelligibility formerly associated with this condition, the difficulties which do occur place considerable demand upon skill in analysing the problem and in finding the appropriate pattern of remediation.

REFERENCES

Albery E 1979 Intensive speech therapy with cleft palate children. In: Ellis R, Flack F C (eds) Palatoglossal malfunction. College of Speech Therapists, London

Andrä A, Diekmann O 1976 Group treatment of children with speech disorders. Stomatology DDR 26–6: 390–395

Bloom L, Lahey M 1978 Language development and language disorders. Wiley, New York

Bzoch K 1964, 1977 Bzoch error pattern articulation analysis

Calnan J 1978 Recent advances in plastic surgery. Churchill Livingstone, Edinburgh

Calnan J, Renfrew C E 1961 Blowing tests and speech. British Journal of Plastic Surgery 13: 4

Canning B A, Rose M F 1974 Clinical measurement of the speed of tongue and lip movements in British children with normal speech. British Journal of Disorders of Communication 9 (1): 45–50

Curle J 1979 Therapeutic methods. An introduction. In: Ellis R, Flack F C (eds) Palatoglossal malfunction. College of Speech Therapists, London

Darley F L 1977 Appraisal of articulation. In: Darley F L, Spriestersbach D C (eds) Diagnostic methods in speech pathology. Harper and Row, New York

Ellis R 1979 The Exeter nasal anemometer. In: Ellis R, Flack F C (eds) Palatoglossal malfunction. College of Speech Therapists, London

Fletcher S G 1978 Diagnosing speech disorders from cleft palate. Grune and Stratton, New York

Fletcher S G, Bishop M E 1970 Measurements of nasality with tonar. Cleft Palate Journal 7: 500

Fritzell B 1969 The velopharyngeal muscles in speech. Acta otolaryngologica supplement 250

Garber S R, Moller K T 1977 The effect of feedback filtering on nasalization in hypernasal speakers. In: Proceedings of the third international congress on cleft palate and related craniofacial anomalies. Toronto, Canada

Hansen S, Hansen P, Schmidt J, Schmidt J 1977 A role for parents assisting the cleft habilitation process. In: Proceedings of the third international congress on cleft palate and related craniofacial anomalies, Toronto, Canada

Hardcastle W J 1972 The use of electropalatography in phonetic research. Phonetica 25: 197–215

Huskie C 1979 The Glasgow experience. In: Ellis R, Flack F C (eds) Palatoglossal malfunction. College of Speech Therapists, London

Mazaheri M, Harding R L, Krogman W M, Riski J E (1977) Pattern of velopharyngeal growth in cleft palate patients with or without pharyngeal flaps. Proc. 3rd Int. Congress cleft palate, Toronto, Canada

Moll K L 1965 A cinefluorographic study of velopharyngeal function in normals during various functions. Cleft Palate Journal 2: 112–122

Morley M E 1970 Cleft palate and speech, 7th edn. Churchill Livingstone, Edinburgh

Morris H L, Spriestersbach D C, Darley F L 1961 An articulation test for assessing competency of velopharyngeal closure. Journal of Speech and Hearing Research 4: 48–55

O'Riain S, Hammond B N 1972 Speech results in cleft palate surgery. British Journal of Plastic Surgery 25 (4): 380–387

Pannbacker M 1976 Survey of publications for parents of cleft palate children. Cleft Palate Journal 13: 57–60

Powers G L, Starr C D 1974 The effect of muscle exercises on velopharyngeal gap and nasality. Cleft Palate Journal 11: 28–35

Rees N, Shulman A 1978 I don't understand what you mean by comprehension. Journal of Speech and Hearing Disorders 43 (2): 208–219

Ringel R L, Ewanowski S J 1965 Oral perception 1. Two-point discrimination. Journal of Speech and Hearing Research 8: 389–398

Schendel L L, Bzoch K R 1971 In: Grabb W C, Rosenstein S W, Bzoch K R (eds) Advantages of intensive summer training programmes in cleft lip and palate. Little Brown, Boston

Shelton R L, Brooks A R, Youngstrom K A 1964 Articulation and patterns of velopharyngeal closure. Journal of Speech and Hearing Disorders 29: 390–408

Shprintzen R J, McCall G N, Skolnick M L, Lencione R M 1974 Selective movement of the lateral aspects of the pharyngeal walls during velopharyngeal closure for speech, blowing and whistling in normals. Cleft Palate Journal 12:

Shprintzen R J, McCall G N, Skolnick M L 1975 A new therapeutic technique for the treatment of velopharyngeal incompetence. Journal of Speech and Hearing Disorders 40: 69–83

Shrpintzen R J, Rakof S J, Skolnick M L, Lavarato S 1977 Incongruous movements of the velum and lateral pharyngeal walls. Cleft Palate Journal 14: 148–157

Tudor C, Selley W G 1974 Palatal training appliance and visual speech aid for use in hypernasal speech. British Journal of Disorders of Communication 9: 117–122

Wyke B 1967 Recent advances in the neurology of phonation. British Journal of Disorders of Communication 4: 1–14

Assessment of velopharyngeal function

THE FUNCTION OF THE VELOPHARYNGEAL ISTHMUS

The velopharyngeal isthmus acts as a device to conserve the vibrating air stream from the lungs for modulation by the tongue and to a lesser extent the lips into what we recognize as intelligible speech. Failure to conserve the air stream results in shortened utterances and increased effort till a point is reached where only two or three syllables per breath can be produced.

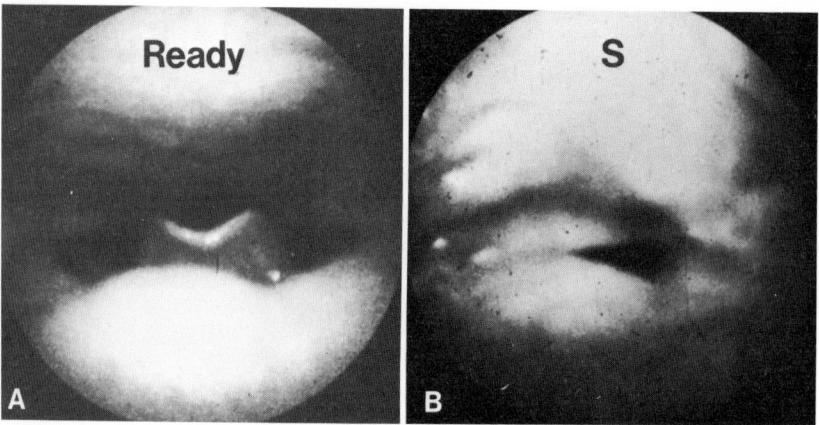

Fig. 15.1 Frames taken from 16 mm cine film of the endoscopic assessment of a normal volunteer during counting to 20 show incomplete closure of the pharyngeal isthmus on the 's' of sixteen. (a) Ready position; (b) on 's'

Total obstruction of flow is not necessary. That is to say, a few English people with speech perceived as normal who have volunteered for assessment of velopharyngeal function can be seen endoscopically to be failing to close the isthmus completely (Fig. 15.1). But a correctly timed rapid reduction of nasal flow is essential.

Speech may be fully intelligible, but not normal, where articulation is perfect but nasal escape is detectable. In such people resonance qualities of the voice are usually also affected. This will be found in the child who had normal speech until his adenoids were removed disclosing a previously undiagnosed submucous cleft palate or pharyngeal disproportion. The same situation may be found after surgical removal of portions of the soft palate. It does also occasionally

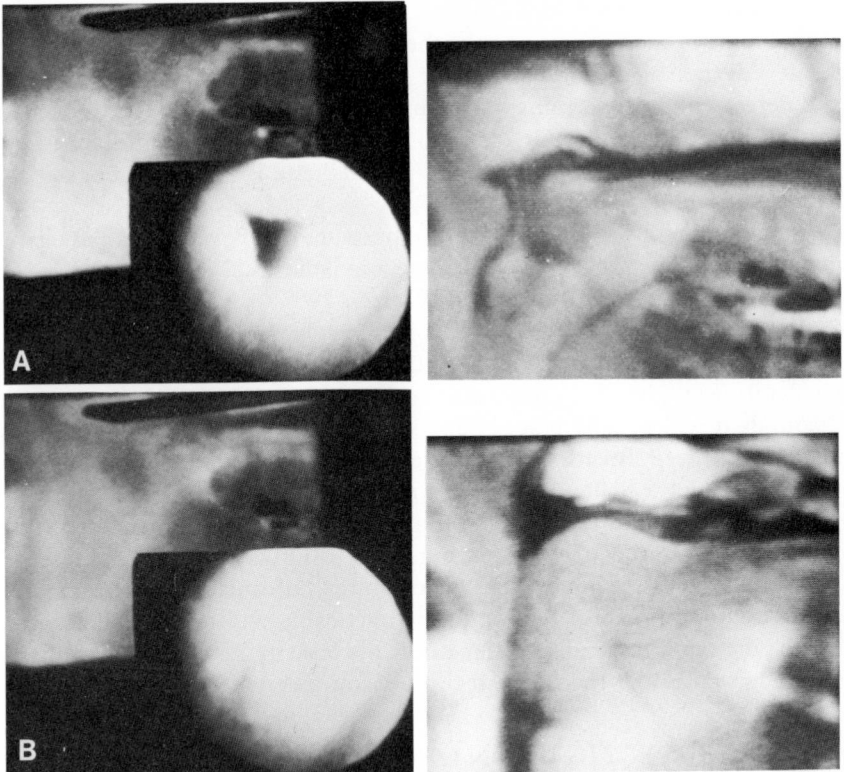

Fig. 15.2 Frames taken from a videotape recording of an adult with an unrepaired submucous cleft whose intelligibility was perfect, nasal escape moderate and who complained of aching in the throat when lecturing or dictating. This was cured by repair of the submucous cleft.
(a) Preoperative frames of split-screen and lateral radiograph of barium-coated pharynx on 's'. Note Passavant's ridge. (b) Postoperative frames on 's'. Palate lengthened by the Veau–Wardill–Kilner technique. Passavant's ridge not formed.

occur in adults whose cleft palate has broken down after surgery or who have never had a palate repair. They will, however, exhibit a variable degree of nasal escape and they will tend to speak in short phrases. They may become breathless and even notice a degree of aching in the throat if they attempt to speak for prolonged periods (Fig. 15.2).

In assessing the function of the velopharyngeal isthmus, two levels of attainment have to be considered. The ideal is a virtually complete, rapid, correctly timed reduction of isthmus area, providing optimal rationing of the available air. Or, a lesser degree of reduction, which may not abolish nasal escape, provides less than optimal rationing, but nevertheless raises the oral breath pressure to a level where correct use of the tongue will result in intelligible sounds of a reasonable volume, which can be joined together into words and sentences of an acceptable length. Because of the multiplicity of factors which determine what is an adequate breath pressure in any individual, absolute figures are not used.

Assessment of velopharyngeal function should therefore be primarily an attempt to assess whether adequate oral breath pressure can be achieved all of the time, some of the time, or none of the time. If adequate oral pressure cannot be achieved, then an attempt should be made to define the site, size and shape of the defect and to determine which muscles may be utilized to produce an adequate, or preferably total, reduction of nasal air flow at the appropriate moments in speech, while still leaving an adequate isthmus for normal nasal resonance on open sounds.

Although very sophisticated nasal/oral pressure and flow studies can be made from which the functional area of the defect in isthmus closure may be deduced and the flow of escaped air measured (Warren 1967) (see Chapter 16), primary assessment tends to be subjective. It often resolves itself into a classification of the degree of audible nasal escape. If this is more than + on a four-point scale (0, nil; +, slight; + +, moderate; + + +, severe) during plosive and fricative sounds it will usually be advisable to assess by what methods the escape could be minimized. Breath direction exercises and aids such as the Selley visual speech aid (Tudor & Selley 1974) or the progressive reduction of size of isthmus obturators (speech bulbs) have been found helpful. Quite often, resort to some form of surgery to the structures around the isthmus will be considered. To monitor the success of any of these procedures, information from as many of the known modes of investigation as is practicable will help to eliminate the fallacies inherent in any individual method, not least in the subjective assessment of the result of any of the above techniques on perceived nasal escape.

MODES OF INVESTIGATION OF THE ISTHMUS

Information on the resting structure and muscular function may be obtained by: (i) ear (Chapter 8); (ii) eye; (iii) electromyography (Chapter 6); (iv) studies of air flow and pressure (Chapter 16); (v) ultrasound.

At the present time the role of ultrasound is not well defined. It has the theoretical advantage of being non-invasive and without radiation hazard. However, the information obtained so far is not precise although eventually ultrasound may become a valuable routine mode. This chapter is therefore principally concerned with assessing the relative value of information obtained by the eye, directly or indirectly.

Visual assessment of the function of the isthmus may be considered under the following headings:

1. Direct examination of the oral cavity
2. Endoscopic examination
   a. Oral pharyngoscopy
   b. Nasopharyngoscopy
3. Radiological assessment

Direct examination of the oral cavity

In assessment of velopharyngeal function the apparent length and mobility of the soft palate is notoriously misleading since one cannot know the configuration of the posterior nasopharyngeal wall. Thus an apparently short palate with a poor lift may produce closure in the horizontally disposed isthmus of a child

(Calnan 1958) while a long mobile palate may not reach the vertical wall of a cavernous box pharynx (Neiman et al 1975).

The stigmata of submucous cleft should be sought. Of these, the most reliable is the absence of a well-defined bony eminence in the middle of the back of the hard palate, due to the divided posterior nasal spine, or even a definite notch. A broad diffuse (Roman arch) lift of the palate or two definite points of lift more than 2 cm apart ('square' arch) are frequently associated with the condition while the bifid uvula and the so-called 'classical' translucent zone are certainly not necessary to make the diagnosis.

The horizontal ridge of mucosa which develops on the posterior pharyngeal wall described by Passavant in 1863 may sometimes be noted immediately below the palate as the patient says 'ah' and adduction of the lateral walls of the pharynx which contain the salpingopharyngeus muscle may sometimes be noted. If they are not seen, it cannot be assumed that these movements could not occur in the forced speech sounds since 'ah' and 'eeh' may not evoke a maximal effort of the muscles around the isthmus. Unfortunately they are the only sounds available for this test.

A fistula of the palate may result in audible nasal escape on certain sounds. It can sometimes be obturated by chewing gum or wax to simplify the diagnosis of the competence of the isthmus as well as by selecting test sounds where the tongue would naturally obturate the fistula.

As already stated, a capacious oropharynx is no guide to the size of the isthmus.

Endoscopy

Endoscopes have a number of physical characteristics which are illustrated in Fig. 15.3. A satisfactory view of the velopharyngeal isthmus depends on achieving a view precisely through that section of the isthmus at which closure does or could be presumed to be most likely to take place. For the purpose of this presentation it is defined as a tangent to the posterior wall at the upper limit

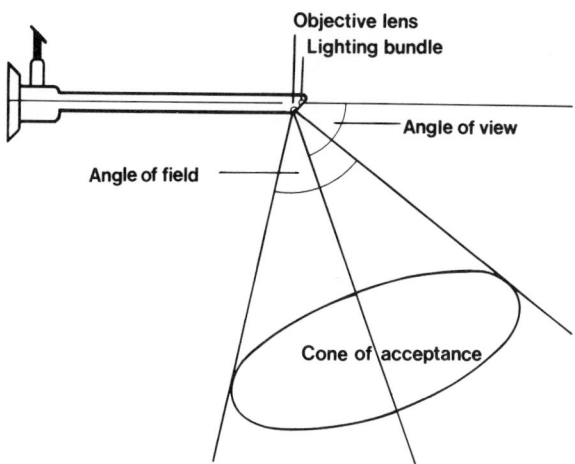

Fig. 15.3 Endoscope terminology

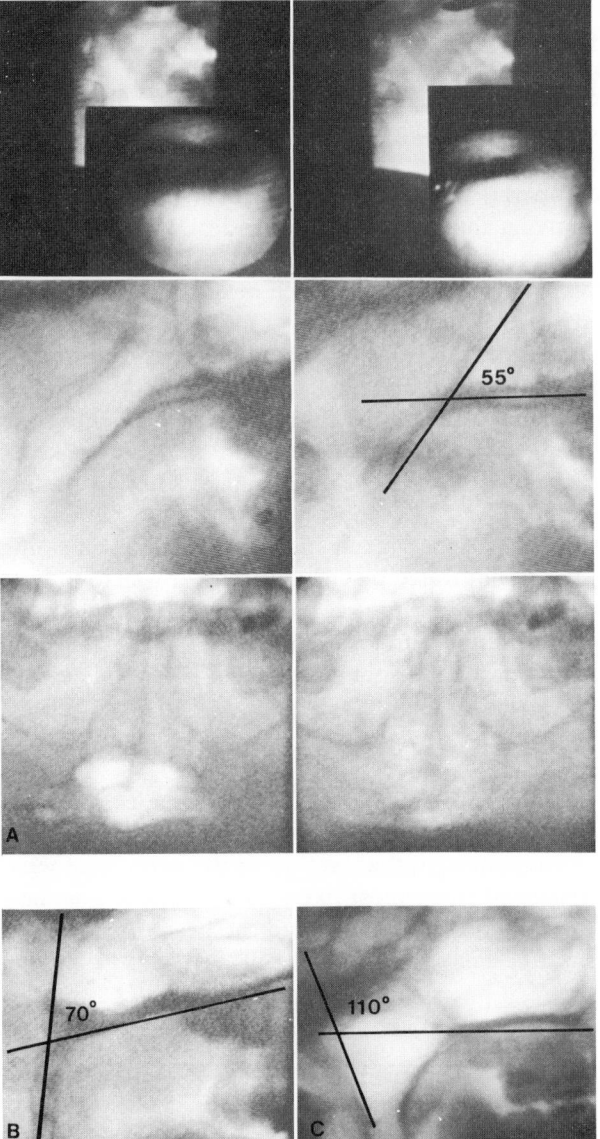

Fig. 15.4 The ideal angle of view (i.a.v.). (a) Seven-year-old; infantile pharynx; i.a.v. 55 degrees. Upper pair of photographs were taken from the split-screen videotape recording in the open and attempted closure position and show no closure achieved; middle pair show lateral X-ray film of barium-coated pharynx, which could be accepted as closure of the pharyngeal isthmus; lower pair of basal view radiographs confirm no closure. (b) Fourteen-year-old; normal pharynx; i.a.v. 70 degrees. (c) Twenty-three-year-old; 'box' pharynx; i.a.v. 110 degrees

of the presumed point of contact of the levator eminence if movement had continued in the manner observed on lateral videofluoroscopy (Fig. 15.4). It will be referred to as the presumptive closure plane (p.c.p.) and an angle which may be measured between it and the projection of a line along the hard palate will be referred to as the ideal angle of view (i.a.v.). An endoscope having a viewing angle close to this will have an ideal, central and therefore minimally distorted view. When the local anatomy makes it impossible to place the tip of the endoscope on this line a compromise view has to be accepted and unfortunately the viewer can be totally unaware of this unless a simultaneous lateral radiograph is being obtained.

Oral pharyngoscopy

Mme Susanne Borel-Maisonny (1937), working with a laryngopharyngoscope with a retrograde angle of view of 11 degrees, and a nasopharyngoscope with a retrograde angle of view of 33 degrees, introduced over the tongue, was able to observe the isthmus in isolated sounds. She showed, for example, how an inadequate palate might achieve closure against a Passavant's ridge (which could be diagnosed by lateral pharyngeal radiography) or with the help of lateral walls adducting to meet in the sagittal plane (which could not).

The technique does not appear to have gained popularity, perhaps because lateral pharyngeal radiography was coming into vogue. But in 1966 Taub published the findings obtainable with an oral panendoscope. This right angle viewing instrument has a 50-degree cone of acceptance, incorporates a bulb requiring a heat shield but has sufficient illumination for colour cine and video recording. After topical anaesthesia patient tolerance is reported to be good and information on the approximate range of movement of each wall of the isthmus and residual orifice size on testing with 'ah–pah' sequences can be recorded. Unfortunately conversational levels of speech muscle activity cannot be assessed. In particular, s and s blends, which are of all sounds the most likely to exhibit a lack of activity in cleft patients, cannot be tested.

Because of the optical characteristics of the panendoscope the maximum retrograde angle of view to a tangent to the posterior edge of the lower border of the soft palate is 25 degrees. This may result in failure of observation of the levator eminence in small children with a horizontally disposed isthmus. With the Storz nasopharyngoscope this ability to view 'retrograde' i.e. anterior to the right angle view, is 35 degrees owing to its exceptional cone of acceptance (Fig. 15.7). Consequently, the author usually attempts an oropharyngeal view prior to nasopharyngoscopy. Even when unsuccessful, it appears to give the child some confidence in tolerating the instrument and is of course sometimes the only endoscopic view obtained.

Nasopharyngoscopy

Instrumentation. It was not until the advent of the fibre-lighted endoscope that attempts to see the site of closure of the isthmus via the nasal passage were successful (Pigott, 1969) as the distal bulb kept the objective lens too far anteriorly and the view tended to be obscured by the levator eminence at the moment of attempted closure.

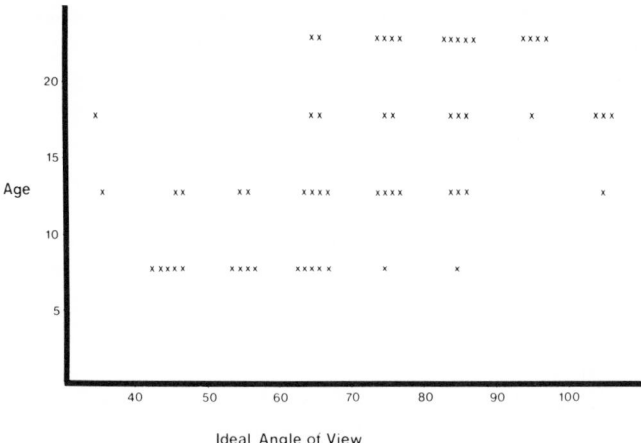

Fig. 15.5 The ideal angle of view plotted against age, taken from a random sample of 60 consecutive patients

Nasopharyngoscopy permits observation of the isthmus in unhindered speech, and with patience a satisfactory view of the isthmus and the muscles surrounding it can be achieved. It is, of course, an invasive technique, cannot be performed under general anaesthesia and even sedation has proved to be counterproductive. Preliminary practice on volunteers is absolutely essential both to learn the normal appearances and to become accustomed to the technique.

Several instruments have been assessed in the author's clinic and these may be grouped into rigid and flexible types.

a. Rigid endoscopes. (i) Storz-Hopkins 70-degree nasopharyngoscope. The most commonly used instrument, because of its superb optical characteristics, has been the 70-degree Storz-Hopkins nasopharyngoscope. This angle of view most nearly approximates the presumptive closure plane (p.c.p.) of the isthmus in the average examination (Fig. 15.5). However, if the closure plane is considerably less than 40 degrees from forward view, examination at the extreme periphery of the field of view is somewhat distorted from the wide angle effect (Fig. 15.6). The wide angle effect will be discussed more fully later. The Storz instru-

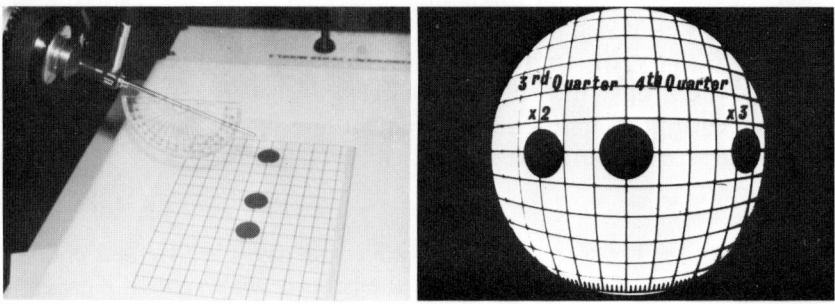

Fig. 15.6 The endoscopic view of a grid with three pennies placed upon it compared with the experimental set-up. The correction factor for the apparent size of the penny in each quarter radius is shown as a simplified multiple

ment is oval in section, measures 4.2×3.5 mm in cross-section and has a convenient working length. It uses the Hopkins rod lens system (Fig. 15.7), which permits greater light transmission for a given overall diameter and better optical resolution than conventional lens systems. Its exceptional cone of acceptance of over 110 degrees in air permits the entire isthmus to be visualized in one field. This makes orientation unequivocal, and the inexperienced examiner will have much less difficulty in siting the endoscope. The rigid stem also makes it possible to lift the tip of the endoscope up away from the isthmus (in many cases) to increase the field of view without losing the essential view along the p.c.p. On other occasions the endoscope will be trapped by the anatomical relations of the inferior turbinate and septum and can be advanced in only a limited axis. It is in these patients that a wide angle view is particularly valuable. The oval section of the endoscope makes rotation beyond about 30 degrees uncomfortable, especially in children and adults with a markedly deflected septum,

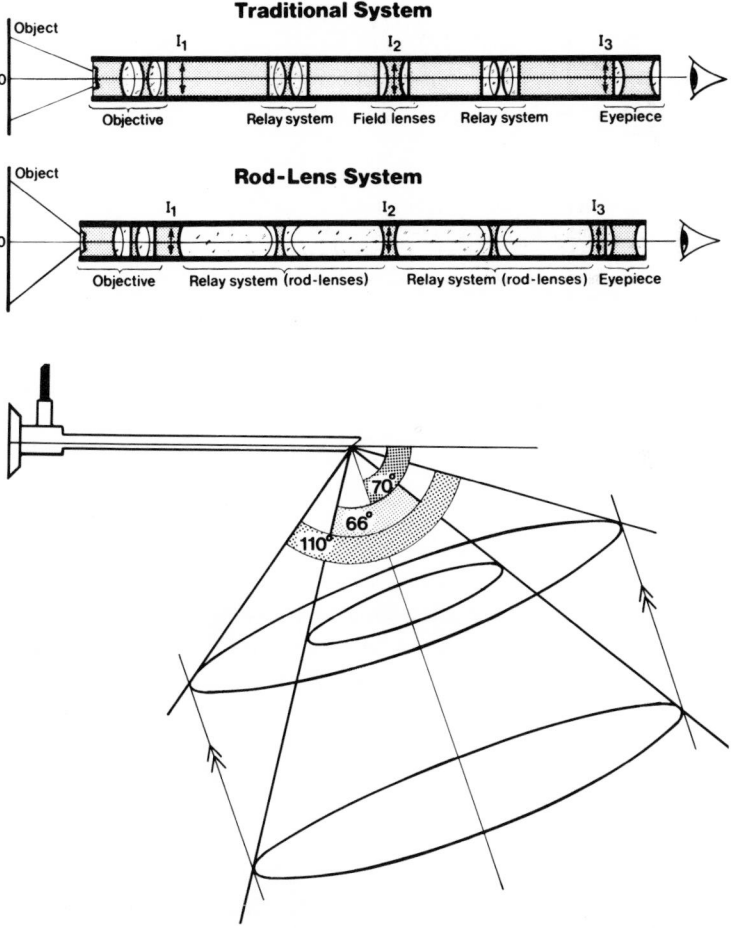

Fig. 15.7 The rod-lens system (field angle 110 degrees) compared with the conventional system (field angle 60 degrees) (by courtesy of Professor H. Hopkins, FRS). The effect on the field of view at a given distance is shown

and may make visualization of the Eustachian tubes' orifices impossible. These are notably slit-like in patients with cleft palates, and of reduced mobility on swallowing compared with the normal. The integral lighting cable from light source to instrument tip avoids the 30 per cent light loss at each air/glass interface. The success rate is shown in Fig. 15.8 and the inferences from this are discussed later in the section on the impact of endoscopic assessment on management.

(ii) The American Cystoscope Company's infant cystoscope telescope is also oval and has overall dimensions of 3.5×3.2 mm and a cone of acceptance of 40 degrees. Although 0.3 mm does not sound a big difference, the smaller instrument was found to pass on four out of seven occasions when mechanical obstruction to the Storz instrument had been encountered. The relatively smaller light

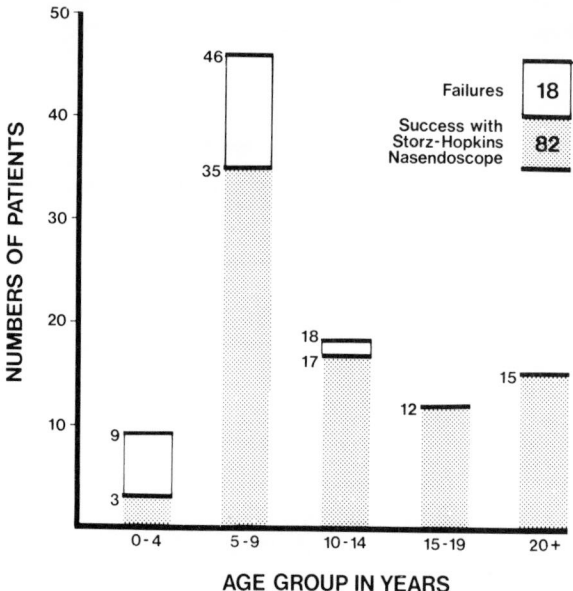

Fig. 15.8 Success rate in passing the Storz-Hopkins nasopharyngoscope in 100 randomly selected patients

bundle, non-integral cable, smaller cone of acceptance with greater difficulty in orientation make this instrument a long way inferior for this purpose. Nevertheless, the availability of a smaller instrument is clearly advantageous.

(iii) The West German firm of Richard Wolff market excellent endoscopes of circular cross-section, with both 30-degree and 70-degree viewing, and 4.2, 3.8 and 3.2 mm diameter. These have been used extensively in the Unit of Professor A. C. Huffstadt in Gröningen (Mulder 1976) and in conjunction with a directly coupled 35 mm reflex camera excellent still pictures of the isthmus may be obtained. Mulder has found the 30-degree oblique instrument generally more satisfactory, and it is obviously an advantage to be equipped to view at both angles. However, it can be seen that if one takes the undistorted field of view of 30 degrees each side of the central viewing angle (i.e. for the Storz-Hopkins 70-degree scope 40–100 degrees and for the Wolff 30-degree scope

0–60 degrees) the relative proportions of the random sample in Fig. 15.5 would be approximately nine-tenths of the sample for the 70-degree scope and one-third for the 30-degree scope. This makes no allowance for the tilt which can be imparted to the Storz instrument in some cases. It can be seen that if a 20-degree tilt up of the tip were possible in order to simulate a smaller angle of view, the Storz figures would rise close to 100 per cent. Conversely, downward tilting of the tip of the 30-degree instrument to simulate a greater viewing angle is not possible because of restriction of movement at the nostril. Preliminary assessment of the p.c.p. from examination of the lateral radiograph could well be the deciding factor in selection of the telescope for that individual.

b. Flexible endoscopes. The 4 mm overall diameter Machida fibre optic naso-pharyngo-laryngoscope has an overall length of 30 cm with markings at 10 cm. The angle of view is 0 degrees, i.e. forward, and the field of view has been measured by us as 66 degrees. The tip is controlled to flex over 90 degrees from its main axis. At this curvature the tip is 3 cm away from the main axis (Fig. 15.9a) which, in practice, means that the endoscope main axis would have to

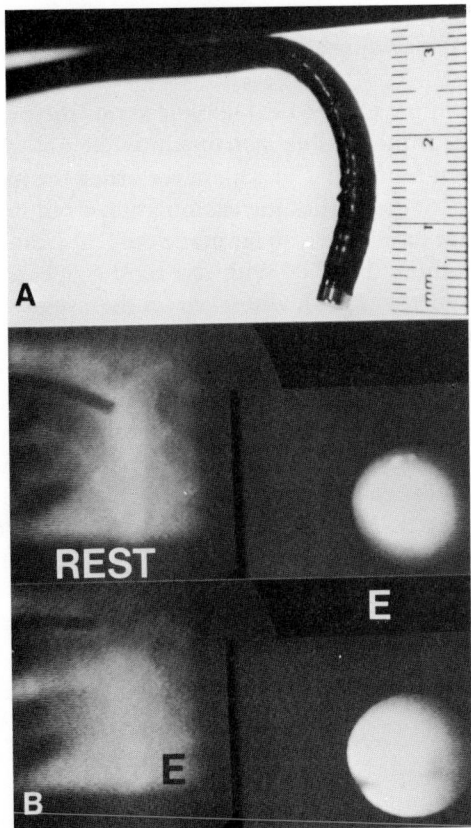

Fig. 15.9 (a) The Machida endoscope tip lies 3 cm from the main axis at 90-degree flexion. (b) Two frames taken from a videotape recording show the endoscope being moved by the palate and the tangential view of the isthmus

be about 3 cm above the level of minimum isthmus circumference to be able to look down the mean presumptive plane of closure. Because the endoscope cannot usually be passed above the inferior turbinate and will therefore tend to lie along the floor of the nose, it is not infrequently too close to the isthmus to make use of the tip flexion facility. The observer frequently finds himself with a tangential view across the p.c.p. Unfortunately, this can give the observer the impression of a smaller orifice than is the case, or even a false appearance of closure. This phenomenon will not be appreciated by the examiner unless the endoscope is simultaneously monitored by lateral videofluorography (Fig. 15.9b). If the level of minimal isthmus circumference is well below the plane of the hard palate, or where the endoscope passes above the inferior turbinate, a true view is obtained, as it obviously is where the p.c.p. approaches the horizontal.

Despite these criticisms there are many patients whose diagnosis can be made with the flexible endoscope prior to pharyngeal flap pharyngoplasty. Ironically, the higher the base and the less restrictive the pharyngeal flap or the longer the palate, the more liable a minor degree of incompetence is to be out of sight. It is undoubtedly easier to pass the flexible endoscope although its flat tip and slightly greater diameter (than the width of the Storz-Hopkins instrument) has resulted in occasional failure to pass it where the rigid instrument subsequently succeeded.

It has proved impossible to be dogmatic about the proportion of small children who will accept the flexible instrument while not tolerating the rigid endoscope. It has been found that in whichever order the instruments are used, the child's tolerance for the continuing examination is reduced for the second instrument. The author has, in fact, so far made only 50 examination with the flexible scope as against more than 500 with the rigid scope, so that the experience of Croft (Shprintzen et al 1977), who gave up the use of the Storz instrument for the Machida fibrescope, must be borne in mind. Success rates of over 90 per cent are being achieved in samples including reasonable numbers of children under five (R Shprintzen 1978, personal communication).

The 4 mm Olympus fibre bronchoscope requires its own light source and does not appear to have any other advantages over the Machida laryngoscope. Both fibrescopes are between five and ten times more expensive than the rigid endoscopes. The shorter Machida laryngoscope can be coupled to a teaching attachment to permit suitable patients to obtain visual feedback of their palate in action, as recommended by Matsuya et al (1973).

A summary of the advantages of these endoscopes is shown in Table 15.1.

Table 15.1 Summary of endoscope characteristics

Characteristic	Type of instrument		
	Storz-Hopkins	Conventional	Fibre optic
Ease of introduction	+	+	+++
Clarity	+++	++	+
Field of view	+++	++	+
Manœuvrability	++	++	+

(a)   (b)

The technique of endoscopy

Whichever endoscope or preferably combination of endoscopes is selected, the technique will have a number of points in common.

Patient selection. The writer has found it very difficult to anticipate which child will tolerate endoscopy well. Personality plays a big part so that children between the ages of 3 and 6 years have occasionally responded without apparent fear. The age of 6 has been taken as a dividing line in that most English children will have had at least one term at their primary school. Generally, the statistics listed in Fig. 15.8 may influence the decision as to whether to attempt an endoscopy, particularly in a child where the diagnosis is already known (such as submucous cleft) or can be obtained from radiological investigation (such as pharyngeal disproportion). Children in this age group are of course in most need of help to rectify anatomical faults prior to being in a position to benefit from the explosive need to communicate that comes from going off to school.

Ideally, all children would have had adequate corrective surgery for velopharyngeal incompetence (v.p.i.) before school age, and although such surgery can obviously be undertaken with little or no preliminary investigation the surgeon will learn little or nothing about the cause of his failures. Thus the pressure to investigate as fully as possible as young as possible seems inescapable. It has occasionally been helpful to see a shy child several times in the outpatient clinic at fortnightly intervals until he will sit on one's knee and name objects or count. A child who will not talk in the clinic almost never talks 'on the day'. It is our practice to ask children's parents to wait outside in the first instance in order for the examiner to make the most direct contact with the child. Occasionally if this is a failure a few children can be cajoled by their parent into submitting. This is exceptional and the parents usually find themselves unable to exert their normal authority over the child for fear of seeming to bully the child in front of strangers.

The examination room and equipment. Although any room with a couch or dental or ENT examination chair will do, we now prefer a semi-upright seated position for the patient. Most control of the patient's head is achieved with the examiner standing looking over from behind the patient with the heel of his hand on the forehead (Fig. 15.10a). Sudden movement by the patient then automatically moves the hand with it and the endoscope is unlikely to hurt the child or indeed to be bent. In practice, we have the child sitting in a dental chair* and examine from in front due to the constraints imposed by simultaneous X-ray recording (Fig. 15.10b).

A light airy room is preferable to a theatre or dental-surgery type of environment. A sink, towels and tissues will be needed, in addition to a small trolley for the fibre light source and to rest the endoscope on. Suction tubes and catheters may be required if tenacious mucus cannot be removed by sniffing and blowing the nose (which should always precede endoscopy). A worksurface for notes is useful, and a book for recording date of examination and, if videotape recordings are to be obtained, tape foot-counter and reel numbers. Previous investigation reel and footage can usefully be noted here. Our current documentation form is illustrated in Fig. 15.11. We have found that several replays

---

* Many hospitals have old-pattern dental chairs in their storerooms for the asking.

of the videotape recordings may be required to be certain of the findings, and a panel assessment is ideal.

Anaesthesia. While cocaine is undoubtedly the most effective agent it is a dangerous drug. Facilities for resuscitation must be available. However, a number of colleagues do use it and have also found adrenaline and phenylephrine a help.

In practice, 4 per cent lignocaine hydrochloride is used. Not more than 1 ml is drawn up into a syringe through a No. 10 Portex intravenous cannula, to the end of which a wisp of cotton wool has been attached to form a bud and

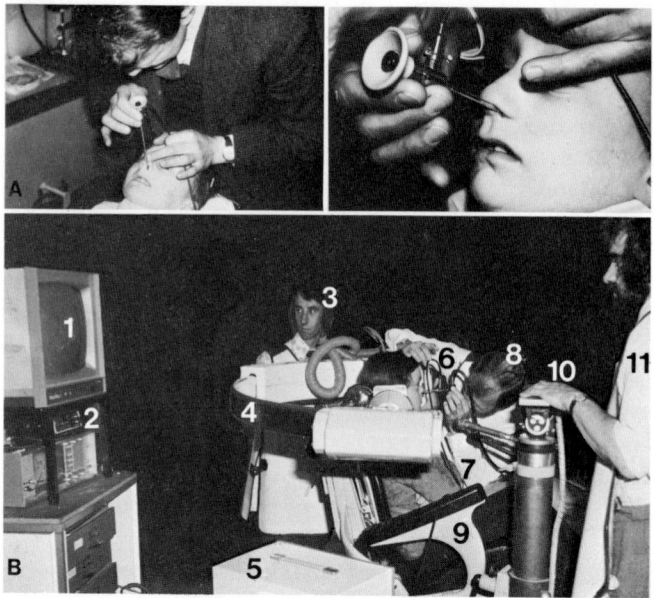

Fig. 15.10 (a) Examination of a 9-year-old boy shows that tension relaxes once the endoscope is in place. (b) Examination of a 12-year-old boy during split-screen recording. 1, Monitor; 2, split-screen unit; 3, radiographer; 4, 'C' arm image intensifier; 5, light sources; 6, endoscope with light source and fibre optic teaching attachment leads; 7, microphone; 8, endoscopist; 9, dental chair; 10, TV camera; 11, audiovisual controller

held in place with a twist of Micropore (Fig. 15.12). The bud should be tested for security before being introduced and it should be of such a size that when soaked with lignocaine it has a comparable size to the endoscope. This provides useful information on the relative ease with which the endoscope can subsequently be inserted on one side of the nose or the other. The lignocaine stings and tastes bitter. Several ploys are worth attempting to get over this, in many ways the most difficult, phase of the whole procedure in that the majority of children who have submitted to it will also tolerate endoscopy.

Prior to anaesthetizing the nose the patient is asked to blow his nose and sniff repeatedly until no wet sounds can be heard. Each nostril is inspected and each is blocked while the patient sniffs to determine the most promising side for the endoscopy to be performed. In older patients it is best performed bilaterally

FRENCHAY HOSPITAL	Hospital No.	D.O.B.
PALATOGLOSSAL MALFUNCTION	Name	G.P.
	Address	
INVESTIGATION		Cons
Referred by Unit No.		Date

KEY. Nil = 0 Slight = I Moderate = 2 Gross = 3 Not applicable = 8 Not assessed = 9

HISTORY   Grade

Feeding difficulty
Deprived home
Temperamental
Low I.Q.
Hearing loss
U.R.T.I

SPEECH ASSESSMENT   Additional Grade   Variable = 6   Manner

Previous speech therapy   Resonance hyper   Plosive faults
Impaired intelligibility   hypo   Fricative
Impaired articulation   mixed   Affricate
Nasal escape overall   Stimulability   Continuant

Area: Labio-dental [] Alveolar [] Palatal [] Velar [] Pharyngeal [] Glottal [] Sub GI []

PREVIOUS OPERATION

EXAMINATION

Reduced lip mobility [] Gothic lift [] Hard palate notch [] Passavant ridge []
Alveolar collapse []   Norman lift [] Translucent zone []   Lateral wall []
Fistula []   Box lift []   Bifid uvula []   movement

ENDOSCOPY   Tape No.   Minutes   Obliquity
Scope   I 2   Obscurity
Not attempted
Nostril R [] L
Easy
Difficult
Tearful
Obstructed
I.
2.
Estimated minimum area
R   x   mms   Observed   Corrected
L   x   mms   Observed image to be drawn in appropriate angular field
Take R for total in non flap cases

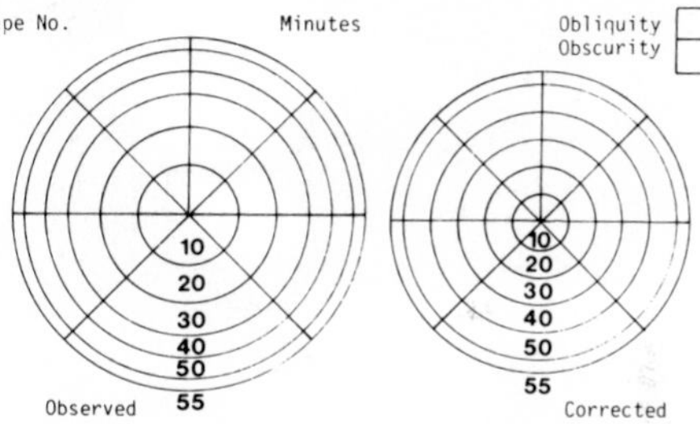

RADIOLOGY   Basal []   Fronto-occipital []

Coating   Complete []   Obscurity []
           Incomplete []

Lateral   Ant. [][][][][][]   Post

Frontal   Right [][][][][][]   Left

        Closure Angle [][]

DIAGNOSIS

a) Principal Diagnosis
b) Underlying Cause
c) Other relevant condition
d) Principal Investigation   Assessment of Palatoglossal malfunction

OPINION

Fig. 15.11 Velopharyngeal function assessment form

to minimize optical errors, but in small children it may only be practicable to inspect one side.

The tip of the nose is elevated, the cotton bud on the tip of the catheter is placed in the vestibule. The child may tend to put his hand up to pull it out but will probably leave it if the examiner at that moment takes his hand away and distracts the child by offering him a small sweet. When the child starts to suck the sweet the catheter is gently but firmly advanced about an inch, taking great care to keep it along the floor of the nose, while telling the child to suck hard to take the taste away. At the same time, the examiner's other hand holding the syringe out of sight behind the child's head dribbles in the lignocaine. After

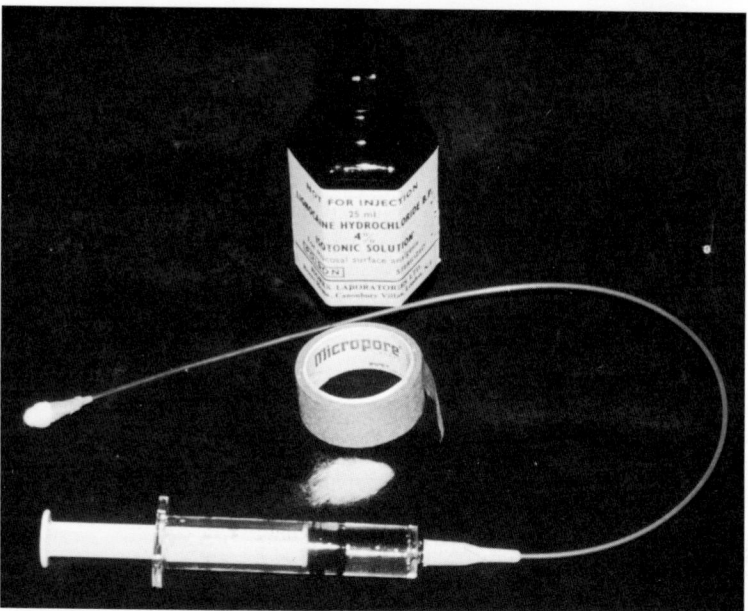

Fig. 15.12 One ml of lignocaine hydrochloride (4 per cent) drawn up through the cottonbud-tipped Portex No. 10 catheter

another repeat of this manœuvre the child may be getting distressed. The examiner then tells the child he is going to take it out but in fact advances it steadily forward till it passes the posterior choana, when resistance suddenly drops and again the child tends to relax. The catheter can then be easily advanced to touch the posterior wall. Sometimes this can be felt as resistance and a little more lignacaine is instilled and the child asked to swallow to anaesthetize the posterior wall. If the catheter descends into the oropharynx a gag reflex will be evoked, and the catheter is immediately and steadily withdrawn, the child being told that this is being done—which he can, of course, see. Ideally both nostrils are prepared. If the catheter hits a tight obstruction on the first nostril—usually at the anterior end of the turbinate—it is withdrawn and the other side tried.

Endoscopy. The endoscope is laid against the child's nose tip and the child asked if that is all right. Usually the answer is yes. (Occasionally the child bursts into inconsolable tears and as the view would be totally obscured by tears and mucus in the nasopharynx, the investigation has to be abandoned.) The nose tip is firmly elevated and the endoscope is very slowly and steadily advanced along the floor of the nose, feeling for resistance and watching the angle of the endoscope and head. Gentle angulation is tried and slight pressure can be applied. Quite often the tip must be angled laterally after about two inches of the scope have been inserted to get round the posterior border of the vomer. This is most common if the normal nostril of a unilateral cleft is examined because of the convexity in the cleft nostril in the mid zone and corresponding deflection of front and back borders into the normal nostril.

Once the endoscope passes this resistance the examiner's eye is applied to the eyepiece and the final advance made looking down onto the upper surface of the palate. The final advance is made slowly so as not to bury the tip in the adenoids. Although more than two or three drops of blood have never yet been caused, even one spot of blood on the light emission pupil or the objective lens ruins the examination, requiring withdrawal of the endoscope. Pressing on the posterior wall also causes quite a severe ache felt in the ears.

Once a clear view down the posterior pharyngeal wall to the back of tongue and epiglottis is obtained, the patient is asked to swallow. Speech closure will be above and, in the endoscopic sense, beyond this level. The tip of the endoscope is then made to 'hunt' for the optimal position by being raised gently or advanced a little or both and the patient asked to say a group of sounds. The following sequence is used and tests the closure effort in different positions of the tongue. Pah, pah, pah, sah, sah, sah, tah, tah, tah, dah, dah, dah, cha, cha, cha, kah, kah, kah, and gah, gah, gah. The patient is then asked to count to 20 slowly and then as fast as he can. Any suggestions of a deterioration of function between 10 and 20 can be followed by a request to count to 40, though the numbers 15 to 20 are in practice a very good guide.

Flexible endoscopy technique is the same in all essentials except manipulation of the tip with the rotation knob into very slight flexion at the very start of the examination to ensure insertion along the nasal floor. Direct viewing throughout the insertion is, of course, valuable in this forward viewing instrument.

Finally a scan of the Eustachian tubal eminences is attempted while swallowing and the opposite nostril examination performed if indicated.

The passive configuration and movement of each wall of the isthmus is noted and an attempt is made to gauge the size of the isthmus. Shprintzen et al (1977) have used a catheter of known diameter, introduced through the opposite nostril and fed down the isthmus as a reference for approximate magnification, while the author has used data from a simultaneous lateral radiograph as a split-screen image recorded on video tape, the width of the endoscope being the absolute measurement giving the anteroposterior depth of the isthmus from the lateral radiograph. This can then be related to the lateral extent of the isthmus on the endoscopic view and also gives an approximation of the area. However, the technique becomes cumbersome if really accurate results are needed and is only of research interest.

Fallacies of endoscopic (monocular) assessment. It is essential for the observer to be aware of the fallacies inherent in monocular viewing.

1. Underestimation of the area of failure to close. This may occur because it is further from the eyepiece than the examiner imagines and obeys the inverse square law. More insidious than this is the precise relationship of the field of view to the cone of structures above the approximately cylindrical isthmus. If one is not looking directly through the plane of the isthmus it is possible to fail to appreciate its area regardless of magnification. This can be seen in Fig. 15.13. Moving the endoscope slightly back and forth, will allow the examiner to find the correct point of view, provided that the angle is appropriate to that particular patient. If the viewing angle is grossly incorrect, no matter where he places the tip of the instrument the examiner will not be able to get his angle

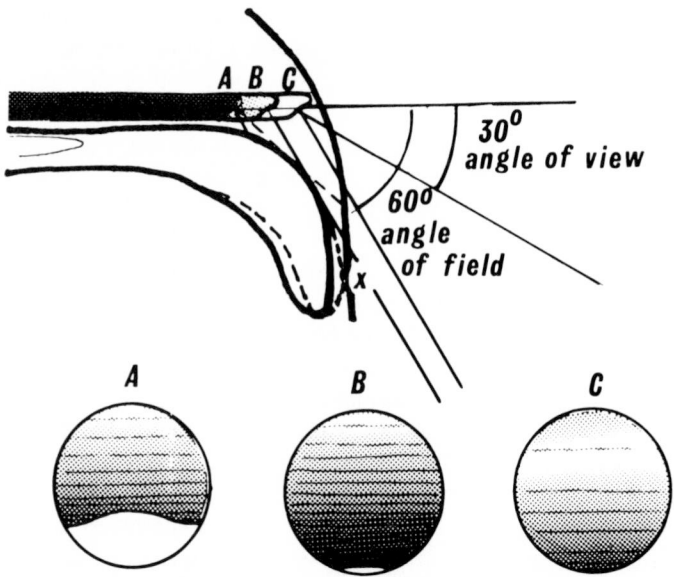

Fig. 15.13 With a small telescopic viewing angle and a 60-degree field of view, a critical situation can occur where the examiner cannot know if closure is occurring at X. Position A, no shadow—impression of closure; B, moderate shadow—impressions inconclusive; C, palate out of view—impressions inconclusive

of view to correspond to the plane of closure and a false impression of closure is likely to be deduced.

2. Underestimation of movement of structures around the isthmus. Objects that move towards the eyepiece become more brightly illuminated and yellower. One is aware of movement occurring but not of how much. Movement across the field of view is appreciated as genuine although movement at the periphery will seem reduced (Fig. 15.14). Because of the frequent siting of the endoscope tip very close to the centre of what may often be a spherical contraction of the isthmus, much of the movement may occur almost directly towards the eyepiece. Again panning of the tip allows the mind to build up a concept of what is really happening provided that the endoscope can be manœuvred sufficiently to view all movements angularly. Unfortunately, this is not always possible, especially in the very horizontal isthmus with a low basi sphenoid.

3. The wide angle effect. The very strength of the wide angle system which allows one to view the entire circumference of the isthmus from very close, commits the observer to making conscious corrections for the compression of objects at the periphery. This is most easily appreciated from a study of Fig. 15.6. The problem is less important with the fibrescope since objects at the periphery will only need to be enlarged by a factor in the region of 1.0 to 1.5, but in the outer two quarters of the radius of the field of view of the Storz instrument the multiplication would need to be twice and three times respectively, assuming that the isthmus plane is at right angles to the central angle of view of the telescope. This becomes very critical when one attempts to assess the extent of

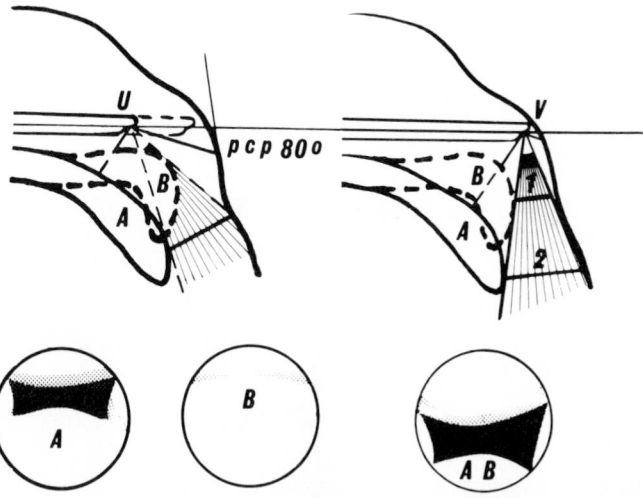

Fig. 15.14 Failure to view along the p.c.p. from position U gives impression of excellent palate movement from A–B and closure occurring (endoscope with 110-degree angle of field). From position V there is no appreciable palate movement, and the examiner will be unaware that the orifice has reduced to half the diameter. Scanning from U to V allows the examiner to conclude that there is fairly good palate movement with substantial failure to close

failure to close of the further port of a failed pharyngeal flap operation. This will be (a) further away and therefore perceived as smaller, (b) more obliquely seen and therefore perceived as smaller, and (c) not infrequently at the periphery of the field of view and therefore perceived as smaller.

Recording endoscopy
The simplest recording system has been described by Sommerlad et al (1975). (This is manageable by the endoscopist on his own.) Essential points in video and cine recording have been described by Pigott & Makepeace (1975) whose system is designed to permit simultaneous biplane examination and requires a minimum team of three people, even when the system has been simplified by the use of a teaching attachment. A custom-built split-screen unit is also required as commercially available units will not displace the X-ray image from the centre of the screen or synchronize the X-ray pulses with the endoscope television camera.

Radiology

Lateral pharyngeal radiography

The literature on the radiological aspects of VPI is immense. Scheier (1897) has been given credit for the first application of single-exposure lateral radiographs in speech. Lateral and frontal tomograms have produced useful information. The disadvantage of single frame exposures is that the film may be mistimed and that sustained test sounds are not representative of conversational speech. Cineradiography of velopharyngeal function was developed in the 1950s with the use of image intensification (Carrell 1952) and synchronization of the X-ray generator with the film frame.

The dimensions of the bony and soft tissue isthmus, the range and timing of movements of the soft palate related to speech, the presence of Passavant's ridge movement and the presumptive closure plane of the isthmus can be analysed. The p.c.p. is of the greatest importance in selection of the most suitable endoscopic or *en face* radiographic viewing angle.

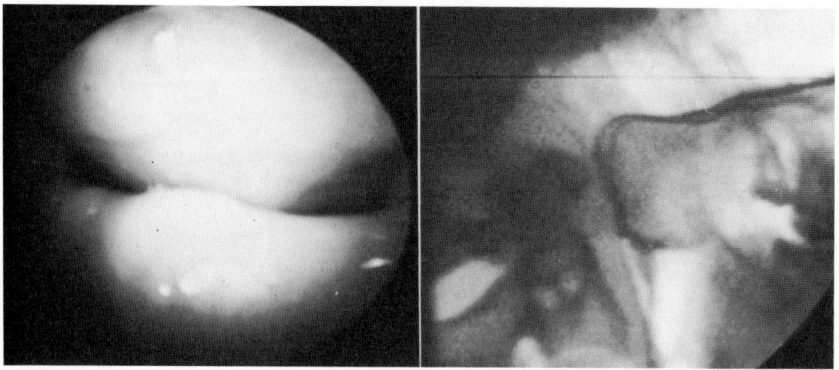

Fig. 15.15 Patient with 'firm closure' on lateral pharyngeal videofluorography who has bilateral patent gutters endoscopically

An X-ray picture is two-dimensional and because of the confusion of shadows the lateral view has always been the most simple to interpret. However, both the tongue dorsum and the walls of the pharyngeal isthmus have complex curves and it is only those structures which form a reasonable thickness of tissue or surface (in the case of tissue/air interfaces) which register. It is therefore perfectly possible to have a lateral radiograph showing apparent firm closure when it is the listener's opinion that the isthmus is incompetent (Fig. 15.15). Barium contrast will be squeezed out of firmly closed orifices as a rat's tail, but a sufficient coating of barium-impregnated mucus may persist on each side of the salpingopharyngeus muscle, for example, to give the impression of two walls failing to close by several millimetres in a patient whose endoscopic view gives indisputable evidence of firm closure across the full width of the isthmus. Measurement of soft tissue dimensions even from a cephalometric lateral radiograph must therefore also be interpreted with caution.

Because of X-ray dosages there are limits to the safe exposure time of cinefluorography which are cut down by a factor of 1000 by image intensifier (Cooper & Hoffmann 1955) and reduce the radiation factor of the three minutes of an average X-ray assessment multiplane examination to less than that of one chest film.

Basal view (hyperextended submentovertical)
The need for examination of the isthmus *en face* was realized by Skolnick (1969), who found that if the patient is placed in what he describes as the Sphinx position, with the neck hyperextended, the X-ray beam could be made to pass at right angles to a line from the corner of the mouth to the external auditory meatus avoiding the cervical spine shadows and in this position the pharyngeal isthmus of many patients would be seen *en face* (Fig. 15.16a). He used primarily a video recording system. The technique has the great advantage of being non-invasive (apart from the instillation of barium contrast) and of keeping the radiation dosage very low because of image intensification. The technique also overcomes one of the major objections to endoscopic interpretation in that the effective beam is more nearly parallel and at right angles to the critical plane of

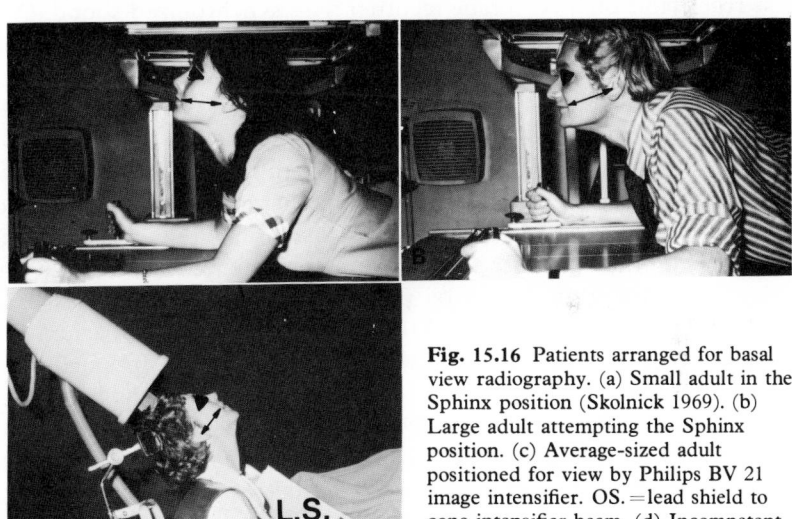

Fig. 15.16 Patients arranged for basal view radiography. (a) Small adult in the Sphinx position (Skolnick 1969). (b) Large adult attempting the Sphinx position. (c) Average-sized adult positioned for view by Philips BV 21 image intensifier. OS. =lead shield to cone intensifier beam. (d) Incompetent isthmus at rest and on 'E'

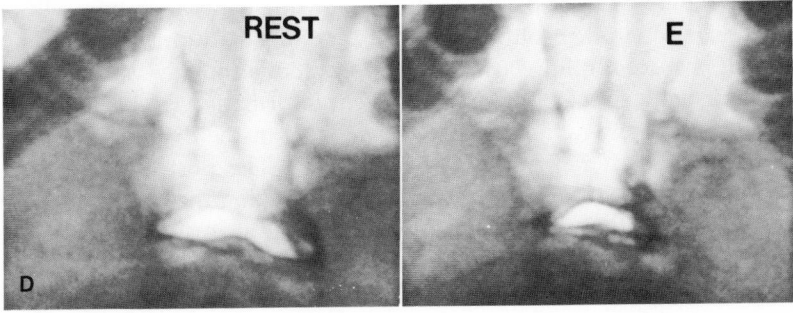

movement. This applies particularly to the invaluable investigation of lateral wall movement. (Such movement is required for superior and inferior based pharyngeal flap surgery to create the conditions for allowing a fully closed and an open state). Skolnick combines the basal view with lateral, oblique and frontal views (Skolnick & McCall 1972) to get the most complete information possible from this mode of investigation.

Coated lateral and basal view radiographs have been used in this clinic routinely since 1974, so that a comparison of information obtainable from each mode could be made. Disadvantages of basal view radiography may be summarized as follows.

A problem may arise in positioning a large adult (Fig. 15.16b) in sufficient hyperextension beneath the buckey of a horizontal screening table. The Philips 'C' arm BV 22 or 21 image intensifier gets round this problem (Fig. 15.16c). It will be found to be available in many hospital orthopaedic theatres and is normally only in use for relatively short periods of the week. It does not require a consultant radiologist to use it provided that a competent radiographer is available and the examiner knows what he is looking for. Gibson & Pigott (1976) have found that factors of the order of 100 kV and 1–2 mA will be needed. The image is recordable on a videotape recorder with synchronized sound. (Videotape recorders are also available in many hospitals and also tend to be used for short periods of the week.) Even with this equipment, some adults with a short neck cannot extend sufficiently to get the isthmus *en face* and in some children the isthmus is so horizontal that an *en face* view cannot be obtained.

There are a number of other problems with this technique which need to be appreciated. Firstly, in patients whose velopharyngeal closure is just competent in normal postures of the head, hyperextension (Fig. 15.17) may make them incompetent (or increase the area of incompetence in those that are not competent, with the head in neutral position). However, this is not likely to invalidate observations on mobility of the lateral wall. Secondly, barium coating may produce several 'rings' at any level down the isthmus. In small children with a rather horizontal p.c.p. who should be closing against the basi sphenoid rather than the true posterior pharyngeal wall (Calnan 1958), an apparent and incompetent isthmus will be seen which has nothing to do with the level of closure. This became apparent when previous endoscopy had shown the isthmus well and the basal view could not be made to 'fit'. In such patients a fronto-occipital view may occasionally be more representative but does, of course, depend on a good coating. This is only rarely achieved as the posterosuperior wall is not brushed by the soft palate in the swallowing act, which one relies on to coat the posterior wall in older patients. Instilling barium in the head-down recumbent posture should get round this problem although we have not done so, having usually already obtained sufficient information from the endoscopic view. The basal view radiograph is least reliable in the diagnosis of the small incompetent port after pharyngeal flap surgery. The port often blocks completely with barium although bubbles of mucus leaking through it are a helpful pointer. The axis of the port is not infrequently at a considerable angle to the vertical plane and several rings of barium may be noted. Without previous endoscopic information to help the interpretation it is impossible to say which is

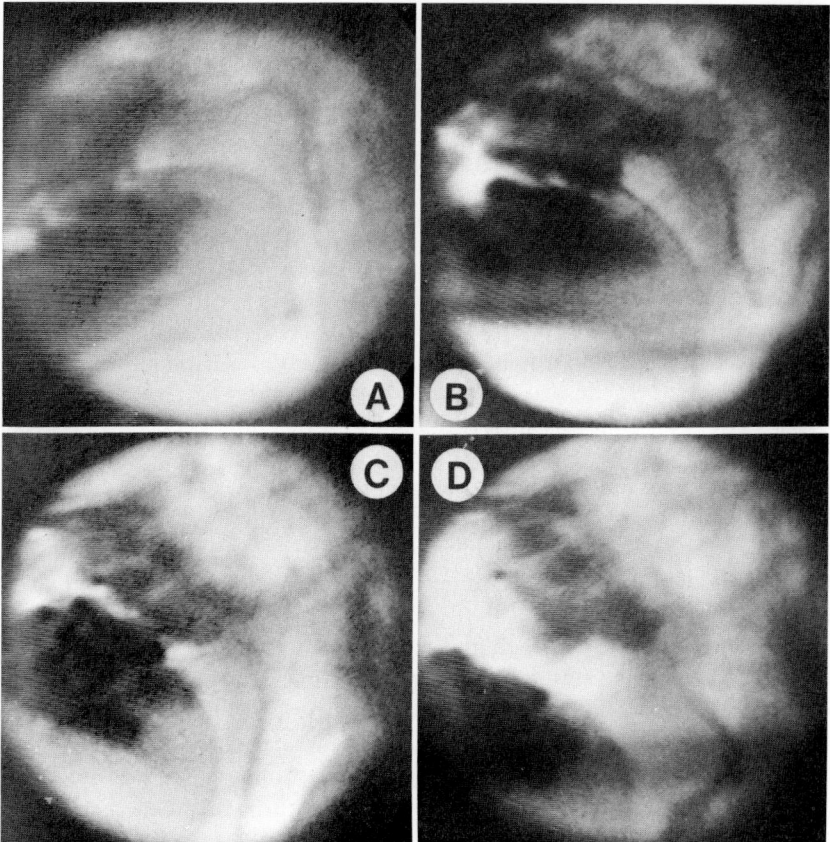

Fig. 15.17 A series of frames taken from the lateral videofluorographs of a young child progressively hyperextending the head into the basal view position

the relevant shadow. Indeed, with foreknowledge from the endoscopic view, specific manipulation of the head to align the port to the X-ray beam may eventually allow a correct image to be obtained.

From the foregoing it can be seen that no single mode of investigation is entirely reliable, and the more modes which can be used either simultaneously or in series, the more accurate the interpretation is likely to become. These methods permit the observation of unhindered speech and allow considerable progress to be made in the understanding of palatopharyngeal and tongue movements.

Simultaneous lateral pharyngeal videofluoroscopy with video nasopharyngoscopy
The advantages of simultaneously recording the lateral radiograph with the endoscopic view have been summarized by Pigott (1977) and, apart from a number of observations already made, include facilitation in placement of the endoscope tip for optimal viewing of the isthmus, i.e. the greatest distance above the isthmus consistent with viewing along the presumptive closure plane. Apart

from this, there is no good reason for making simultaneous recordings routinely. But in that case radiological investigation should be done first to define the p.c.p. and sufficient time must elapse for barium coating to disperse before the endoscopy is undertaken.

Really accurate assessment of the orifice area by simultaneous recording proved to be enormously complex and seems unlikely to become a clinical tool.

ORGANIZATION OF THE ASSESSMENT CLINIC

Clinics are held by the author with the cleft palate speech therapist. Because of the complexity of equipment being used it has been of the greatest value to have present a specialist in audiovisual techniques. Originally a consultant radiologist developed the use of the BV 21 image intensifier for this purpose and made the radiographic examinations, but it has now been found adequate for the endoscopist and a skilled radiographer to produce the X-ray recordings. It should be emphasized that this rather large team is only necessary if it is decided to undertake simultaneous multiview recordings. Sommerlad et al (1975) have shown how simply one person can obtain videotape recordings of the endoscopy. Speech assessment and radiological examination can then be obtained at other times.

The patient will have a speech and nasal air flow recording made first. Then endoscopy is performed simultaneously with radiography of the uncoated lateral pharynx. The pharynx is then coated with barium sulphate by instilling 2 ml into each nostril and asking the patient to swallow repeatedly. The lateral frontal and finally the basal view radiographs are then obtained.

The members of the clinic see patients from a number of sources, including speech therapists, general practitioners, community physicians, ENT surgeons, paediatricians and plastic surgeons, but may not be responsible for subsequent treatment. A summary of the findings is made including, on occasion, copies of the videotapes from which the treatment plan may be decided by the referring physician.

THE IMPACT OF ASSESSMENT OF THE VELOPHARYNGEAL ISTHMUS ON THE SELECTION OF TREATMENT

At the present time in this clinic the following options are considered after analysis of a speech recording, lateral and basal radiography, and rigid and/or flexible endoscope videotapes.

No treatment
No nasal escape. Misdiagnosis of speech immaturities. Some neurological patients.

Speech therapy
Minimal nasal escape, or nasal escape on some sounds with good effortless closure on others. This is taken as an indication that, with therapy, the patient should be given an opportunity to correct the incompetence.

Surgery

Sufficient lack of oral breath pressure in the opinion of the therapist to be inhibiting the development of normal articulation patterns. Palatal incompetence
which has not responded to speech therapy.

Over the last five years two principal pharyngoplasty operations have been
practised on the majority of cases. Detailed analysis of the results will be
published, but the clinical impression is as follows.

Posterior wall advancement. The indication has been a mobile palate coming
to within five millimetres of the posterior pharyngeal wall. Silastic sponge implants and latterly custom-built Silastic sheath, gel-filled, Dacron-backed pillows
with volumes up to 2.5 ml are being assessed. On the whole, the results have
not been very satisfactory due to early extrusion in a few cases and the persistence of the patient's habit of forcing the air stream up the nose in some others.
The level of audible nasal escape should probably not be more than moderate
for this method to have a chance of effecting a cure and 5 mm is probably an
optimistic distance to advance the pharyngeal wall.

Palate lengthening with simultaneous pharyngeal flap. This technique, first
published by Hönig in 1963, has been used on the majority of other patients
who have symmetrical defects as seen on endoscopy or basal radiographs. The
impression is that although the operation is technically difficult sometimes and
fairly time-consuming, it has a high success rate in abolishing nasal escape.
(Because of the subjective nature of grading nasal escape, the terms 'reduction
of nasal escape' and 'improvement of speech' should probably be avoided.) In
really successful cases the re-repaired lengthened palate produces the natural
closure pattern against the pharyngeal wall. In less successful cases the pedicle
acts as an obturator and one relies on lateral wall adduction for closure as in
the classical superiorly based flap. Hönig* points out that if necessary the pedicle
can be divided if hyponasality or catarrh prove to be a problem, without loss
of competence. If the palate appears to be well united, the aponeurosis is merely
stripped back off the nasal layer for about 0.5 to 1.0 cm before the transverse
division of the nasal layer is made. In some cases a really worthwhile pushback
will not be achieved unless this incision is continued up the mucosa over the
medial pterygoid plates, and a flap the full width of the posterior pharyngeal
wall let in a 'U' shape.

Offset and bilateral pharyngeal flaps. In cases where mid-line closure has been
found with bilateral gutters, bilateral pharyngeal flaps have been let into the
palate from above or a Skoog or Orticochea type of operation from below. For
asymmetrical cases an offset Honig procedure has been used. A number of these
cases have had a previous pharyngoplasty and it is in these that endoscopic and/
or basal view radiography has been most helpful, resulting in an encouragingly
high conversion to the 'no nasal escape' group. Apart from patients whose incompetence resulted from adenoidectomy exposing velopharyngeal disproportion, postoperative speech therapy is almost invariably required.

Innumerable other pharyngoplasties exist and maybe some are better than

---

* Hönig states that he saw Professor Sanvenero Rosselli use this technique to get himself out of
a difficulty in a demonstration case in Hamburg in 1954. However, Sanvenero-Rosselli did not appear
to consider it a fundamentally essential manœuvre, did not use it routinely or publish it subsequently.

those mentioned. But the biggest lesson to be learned from increasingly sophisticated assessment of velopharyngeal function is that intelligibility is almost entirely a function of the tongue not the palate. The corollary of this is that parents should be warned that the success of a pharyngoplasty may not be appreciated by them and that their child will not become intelligible as a result of the operation.

If real progress is to be made towards achieving the eventual goal of improved intelligibility it seems essential that thought must be directed to modifying the faulty habits of the tongue rather than by devising yet more pharyngoplasties.

ACKNOWLEDGEMENTS

The investigation of velopharyngeal function at Frenchay Hospital is a team activity and I would like to express my very grateful thanks to all the team members over the past 10 years who have helped to build up the present system. Their expertise and enthusiasm have been invaluable, as has been the support of the Regional Health Authority for an equipment research grant and the district and sector management teams for other facilities and accommodation.

The members of the present team immediately responsible for the investigation are: Mrs E. Albery, BSc, Cleft Palate Speech Therapist, Department of Speech Therapy, Frenchay Hospital, Bristol; Dr M. J. Gibson, BSc, MB, ChB, FFR, DMRD, who developed the use of the Philips BV 21 image intensifier in this field and who trained radiographers of the Department of Radiology, Frenchay Hospital, to operate the system; Mr A. P. W. Makepeace, Specialist in Audiovisual Communication Techniques, Department of Medicine, University of Bristol, developed and operates the complex recording system.

REFERENCES

Borel-Maisonny S 1937 Resultats photétiques obtenus dans les fissures palatines. Revue de Stomatologie 39: 733–754
Calnan J 1958 Modern views on Passavant's ridge. British Journal of Plastic Surgery 10: 89–113
Carrell J 1952 A cinefluorographic technique for the study of velopharyngeal closure. Journal of Speech and Hearing Disorders 17: 224–228
Cooper H K, Hoffmann F A 1955 The application of cinefluorography with image intensification in the field of plastic surgery, dentistry and speech. Plastic and Reconstructive Surgery 16: 135–137
Gibson M J, Pigott R W 1976 Combined radiographic and endoscopic assessment of the nasopharynx. Medica Mundi 21: 43–46
Hönig C A 1963 Over pharyngoplastick. Acad. Diss., Bosch, Utrecht.
Hönig C A 1967 The treatment of velopharyngeal insufficiency after palatal repair. Archivum Chirurigicum Neerlandicum 19: 71–81
Matsuya T, Yamaoka M, Miyazaki T 1973 Assessment of velopharyngeal closure by use of fibrescope. Abstracts of second international congress on cleft palate, Copenhagen
Mulder J S 1976 Velopharyngeal function and speech. Doctoral thesis, University of Gröningen. Van Gorcum, Assen/Amsterdam
Neiman G S, Peterson S J, Pruzansky S 1975 Delayed pharyngeal flap success: Report of a case. Cleft Palate Journal 12: 244–246
Passavant G 1863 Cited by Calnan 1957 Modern views on Passavant's ridge. British Journal of Plastic Surgery 10: 89–99
Pigott R W 1969 The nasendoscopic appearance of the normal palatopharyngeal valve. Plastic and Reconstructive Surgery 43: 19–24
Pigott R W 1977 The development of endoscopy of the palatopharyngeal isthmus. Proceedings of the Royal Society B195: 269–275
Pigott R W, Makepeace A P W 1975 The technique of recording nasal pharyngoscopy. British Journal of Plastic Surgery 28: 26–33
Scheier M 1897 Über die Verwerthung der Röntgenstrahlen in der Rhino- und Laryngologie. Archiv für Laryngology 6: 57–66

Shprintzen R, Croft C, Lewin M 1977 The relationship of perceived hypernasality to velopharyngeal gap size during speech. Third international congress on cleft palate, Toronto

Skolnick M L 1969 Video velopharyngography in patients with hypernasal speech, with emphasis on lateral pharyngeal motion in velopharyngeal closure. Radiology 93: 747–755

Skolnick M L, McCall 1972 Velopharyngeal competence and incompetence following pharyngeal flap surgery: video fluoroscopic study in multiple projections. Cleft Palate Journal 9: 1–12

Sommerlad B C, Hackett M E J, Watson J 1975 A simplified method of recording in nasal pharyngoscopy. British Journal of Plastic Surgery 28: 34–36

Taub S 1966 The Taub oral panendoscope: a new technique. Cleft Palate Journal 3: 328–346

Tudor C, Selley W G 1974 Palatal training appliance and visual speech aid for use in hypernasal speech. British Journal of Disorders of Communication 9: 117–122

Warren D 1967 Nasal emission of air and velopharyngeal function. Cleft Palate Journal 4: 148–156

16

Aerodynamic and phonetic analysis

The primary purpose of most secondary surgery in cleft palate treatment is to help the patient to achieve normal speech production. The speech of such a patient is abnormal because it has a distinctive nasal quality and this is considered to be due to nasal escape or hypernasality, or a combination of both. The reasons for this have been discussed in previous chapters. In most cases it is velopharyngeal incompetence—to use the American term—which is the problem, and the task of the surgeon is to reduce the size of the orifice at the nasal port and to try to provide a functioning soft palate. Without adequate closure of the nasal port by the soft palate there will be airflow through the nose at inappropriate times during speaking, and there will be a more constant acoustic coupling of the nose and nasopharynx to the vocal tract. In spite of successful surgery the speech may remain poor because the patient has mild deafness, poor dentition or lack of sensation in tongue and lips. The intelligence level of the child and the amount of parental encouragement must also be taken into account. Moreover, these patients are children who are at, or have just passed through, that important period in their lives when their articulation and phonation are changing rapidly to give them the adult form of speech. It is not surprising to find that they devise many forms of compensation for their disability and that the quality of their speech can range from being just perceptibly different to almost impossible to understand.

The surgeon may find himself in the unenviable position of trying to decide on the most appropriate course of treatment without having the necessary background knowledge of phonetics and speech production, and having to assess on his own the results of that treatment. He will more usually have the assistance of a speech therapist whose assessment will be based on a wide experience of speech defects, but must depend largely on subjective judgement of the quality of the patient's speech. Objective methods have been devised to estimate the ability to prevent nasal escape and these methods have been described in previous chapters. However, it is questionable how much the results tell us about what is happening in the production of normal continuous speech.

We can look on our speech mechanism as a kind of wind instrument that we play to produce a changing stream of sound that is recognized by the listener as a signal carrying a message. Our thoracic system acts as the bellows to provide the aerodynamic requirements of the reed, the larynx, and we modify the acoustic spectrum of this voicing source by altering the cavity sizes of the vocal tract by movements of our articulators. The soft palate is an articulator with a special function, in that it allows an extra cavity, that of the nose, to be joined to the oral cavity. This adds sound from the nose to that of the mouth but the main effect is to change the spectrum of the acoustic output of the mouth. The changes can be quite complex and depend not just on the size of the nasal port, but on the articulatory configuration at the time (House & Stevens 1956). When the soft palate is lowered to open the nasal port and the lips are opened, the air from the lungs will divide between the two branches. A knowledge of the dynamic pattern of air-flow division, derived from measurement, is therefore essential if abnormal is to be distinguished from normal. This chapter considers speech production from this qualitative viewpoint, trying to unravel the rapid and precise changes that must occur in phonation and articulation for intelligible speech.

We might start by looking at the kind of variation one might expect in the air flow through the two channels of nose and mouth. The glottal stop, for instance, which occurs more frequently during speech than most people would like to acknowledge, is really a complete closure of the airway through the larynx. During the closure there can be no air flow through nose or mouth and so, strictly speaking, there can be no sound. A stop consonant such as [t] in the word 'tea', [ti], on the other hand, is made by raising the tongue behind the upper teeth to close off the mouth passage and the soft palate against the back wall of the pharynx to close off the nasal passage. Although the method of closure is different from that of the glottal stop, again there can be no air flow during the occlusion phase and no noise, the actual [t] sound being heard as the pressure behind the mouth closure is released and there is a short period of turbulent air (called aspiration) which occurs just before the vowel begins. If we are considering normal relaxed speech at conversational loudness, that is, at the acoustic intensity level that would be used by adults in a reasonably quiet room, the oral flow during vowels will be about 150 ml/s (millilitres per second), but in aspiration, depending on context, it might reach a peak of over 1 litre/s. The flow through the nose, on the other hand, is in general much smaller and during vowels would be expected to be very small indeed, perhaps only 15 ml/s; this will be variable, depending on the individual, the context and the vowel itself. If the word were 'team', [tim], then we would expect the nasal flow to increase throughout the vowel in anticipation of the nasal sound, and when the actual occlusion is made at the lips for the nasal [m] the flow rate will be about 40 ml/s.

These figures give an idea of the range of rates involved and show that the flow through nose and mouth is an everchanging function. Speech is normally produced on expiratory air flow from lung volumes above the level of functional reserve capacity, with inspirations being taken between phrases and words depending on context, mood and respiratory requirements. During these egressive flow periods there is, as we have tried to show, a great variation in flow rate from instant to instant, but the regulatory structure of speech ensures that the mean flow from speech group to speech group will be fairly constant and in the adult this will be only a little more than that for vowels. Relaxed respiration involves volume changes of about 500 ml of air and so speech makes no great extra demands on the ventilatory system. Over an extended period of speaking, then, the Average Lung Volume Level (Anthony & Farquharson 1975) would be expected to be only slightly greater than that for quiet breathing. This is for the adult, however, and as yet we have little information on flow rates and lung volume changes in children's speech.

Initial consideration of the cleft palate problem raises a number of quite fundamental questions, the main two concerning the measurement of nasality and the definition of nasal voice quality. It would appear that no universally agreed scale of quality has been established from physical data, and one would wonder if this is due to the difficulty of reaching consensus on the subjective judgement or the complexity of the measurement record, or both. Should age, sex and accent be taken into account? One would wonder how far the judgement of nasality is influenced by nasal escape and whether listening to tape-recorded samples is ever completely satisfactory. What other, or extra, articulatory, acoustic and aerodynamic constraints are imposed by velopharyngeal incompetence? Is it possible to predict the compensatory forms of articulation and phonation that the patient will develop?

Figure 16.1 shows the kind of record being developed to look at some of these questions. It is designed to allow easy comparison of one physical quantity with another and to give satisfactory phonetic segmentation. The paper speed is 25 cm/s as shown by the 50 Hz signal of trace 1; this scale of 40 ms/cm appears to be almost optimum for showing the fine detail of articulatory change in nasal and oral air flow. Two traces are used for each air stream; the lower trace of each pair is the 'true' waveform and the upper is its low-pass filtered (smoothed) version. Traces 3 and 4 show nasal flow, and traces 6 and 7 oral flow. It should be noted that these traces are calibrated and that at any instant the flow rate is known to an accuracy of better than 10 per cent. Traces 2 and 5 are the outputs of integrators connected to the flow signals of nose and mouth respectively; scales are not shown here for lack of space, but the saw-tooth waveform resets after a change of volume of 70 ml. Trace 8 is the voicing signal (Lx) derived from a laryngograph (Fourcin 1974, Anthony 1978). Trace 9, labelled Fx, shows the frequency of the vocal cord vibration, that is, the fundamental frequency or the 'pitch'. Air-flow measurement is made by means of a pneumotachographic flow head (Fleish 1925), which is basically a small diameter tube in which is set a fine wire gauze to act as a resistance. The pressure drop across this resistance will be proportional to the flow through it, and a small sensitive semiconductor transducer connected to the pneumotach has an output voltage proportional to the pressure difference. The chain of calibration used in this study is standardized in that a pressure difference of 1 cm H_2O gives an output of 1 V from the transducer and its amplifier and this, when applied to the high-speed oscillograph, gives a deflection of 2 cm. The calibration (static) of a pneumotach gauze requires, then, the measurement of the flow through the head necessary to give a pressure drop of 1 cm H_2O.

The resistance of the flow-measuring system should be low compared with the internal resistance of the speech mechanism to ensure that it has as little effect as possible on production. For the pneumotach arrangement used here, a compromise must be made between the gauze resistance and the electrical

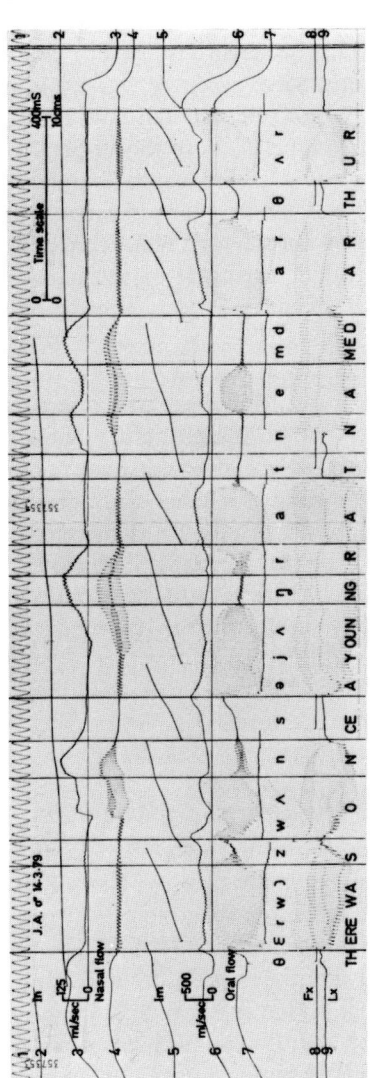

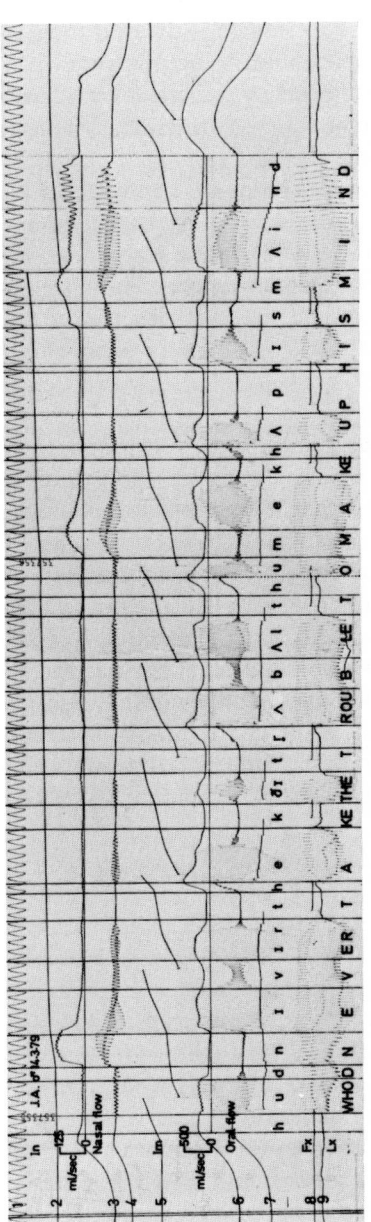

Fig. 16.1(a) and (b) Oscillogram showing air-flow rate and volume, vocal cord vibration waveform and frequency for the standard test spoken by a normal adult

amplification necessary to provide adequate amplitude of the traces on the record. With the low flow rates involved in this work, the limiting factor is the signal-to-noise ratio and at the present time the gauze resistance is close to the average resistance of the oral tract. To give traces of comparable amplitude for nose and mouth normally requires that the amplification in the nasal channel be increased by a factor of 4. Occasionally, for the very small child, the gain has to be raised by as much as a factor of 10, so that the sensitivity is very great indeed, and it is difficult to establish and maintain zero.

Anaesthetic masks can be modified to hold separate pneumotach flow heads above and below a rubber divider piece that fits tightly across the upper lip (Comroe 1950). Good repeatable records of nasal and oral flow can be obtained but articulatory movement is restricted (Lubker & Moll 1965) because the human face does not lend itself to a simple shape of mask which will be flexible and airtight. The effect on respiration of the added resistance of the gauzes should be small (Milic-Emili & Pengelly 1970) but this has not been investigated formally.

Many children are a little apprehensive when they see the mask and its associated equipment for the first time. If it is pointed out, however, that one can see through the gauzes quite easily, and if a mask is then placed lightly against the face to allow the child to check that breathing is not affected, he accepts it quite readily. A head harness is necessary to ensure a good fit, but the child is always asked for his co-operation in supporting with his hands some of the weight of the combined mask and heads. The most intractable problem is the acoustic effect of the mask on speech. Although there is little loss of intelligibility, the voice is muffled and it is almost impossible to hear the detail of sounds with high frequency content such as stops and fricatives. For this reason, the analysis of the utterance must be done from the first recording made without the mask; this is clearly a less than satisfactory procedure.

THE ANALYSIS OF THE RECORD

The excerpt from the aerodynamic oscillographic recording spoken by an adult male (Fig. 16.1) is the first sentence of the standard text, 'Arthur the Rat'. This is a phonetically balanced text long enough as a task when read aloud to bring out voice and ventilation problems. From the traces a wealth of data can be extracted such as average flow rates for nose and mouth, peak values and long-term ratios. It is only when the waveforms are analysed in terms of phonetic elements, however, that we can begin to describe the dynamic organization of phonation and articulation and understand the constraints imposed on speech by the mechanical system. It can clearly be seen from the record that speech is not composed of separate discrete sounds or syllables, and so the division into segments or 'sounds' must necessarily be artificial and arbitrary to some degree. But we must have units and conventions that will establish their boundaries in terms of what we know of the mechanics and aerodynamics of speech production. The zero flow lines play an important part in this respect, and they are drawn here for the filtered air-flow traces. Some parts of the record can never satisfactorily be segmented: diphthongs for instance, where one vowel blends imperceptibly into the other in air-flow pattern and in sound. There may be an overlap of one factor on another in a sequence which makes it difficult to choose a beginning point or an end point, but however difficult this is, consistency must be maintained. Segmentation depends on the interpretation of all the information that is available and one must guard against reading more into the record than is justified. This is particularly a danger where children's speech is concerned, because we know so little about their production of speech. Along with the segmentation there must be a phonetic transcription but the amount of detail or 'narrowness' (Abercrombie 1967) of the transcription will depend on the context and the particular problems being investigated. Here a phonetic transcription of a fairly simple type is given along with the text in normal orthography fitted, as far as possible, to the segmentation.*

Nasal sounds are easily recognized in the pattern of nasal flow, and the word 'named' [nemd] gives a good starting point for the analysis. At the beginning of the [n] air flow through the mouth is decreasing almost to zero because the tip or blade of the tongue is rising towards the teeth ridge while at the same time there is increasing flow through the nose as the nasal port is opened by the soft palate. The laryngographic oscillation (Lx) does not start until about halfway through this segment, showing that the sound [n] was devoiced initially. This is not, however, unusual for this subject, and it has been found in the records of normal children. The whole question of the devoicing of nasals (Barry & Kunzel 1978) requires investigation in view of its possible influence on the judgement of nasal quality. As the tongue moves towards the position for the vowel, the nasal flow decreases (but not to zero) as the oral flow increases. Then as the bilabial closure for [m] is being established the oral flow decreases, but not immediately, to zero as the nasal flow increases. This is the characteristic pattern for this word in this context, with the duration of the second nasal being greater than that of the initial nasal and having a greater amplitude of air flow. This seems to be the case in English whether the initial or final nasal consonant is [m] or [n] (Jespersen 1909). The voiced stop [d] following requires a high intra-oral pressure for its production and hence a good velopharyngeal closure. Here we see the nasal air flow decreasing almost to zero as the mouth closure is maintained until the point of plosion. Voicing continues until the fricative [θ] of 'Arthur' but it can be seen that the waveform of vocal cord movement distorts and falters just before the release of [d]. This is because over the short period of total occlusion the intra-oral pressure is rapidly rising to equal the subglottal pressure; without a transglottal difference of pressure there can be no air flow and no vocal cord vibration. The oral air flow increases during the [ɑ] and the approximant [r] preceding the unvoiced fricative [θ] and there is a small nasal flow also. This reduces to zero for the fricative and remains zero until the end of the phrase. The fricative is produced by forcing air into turbulence between tongue and teeth and this segment has a characteristic downward and upward curving shape. In this sequence 'named Arthur' we may distinguish the main two functions of the soft palate in speech: first, in 'named', to change the acoustic coupling and hence the flow through the nose in a smoothly varying way and secondly, at the end of the first syllable of 'Arthur', and more particu-

* This transcription indicates the Scottish pronunciation of the speakers

larly in the [d] preceding it, to act as a two-position switch closing and opening the nasal port. In the first, it is the degree of nasality that is being controlled, whereas in the second it is the intra-oral pressure that is being maintained or released. In 'named' the vowel is nasalized under the influence of the initial and final nasals and nasalization can also be seen in the sequence 'young rat' in the segments preceding and following the velar nasal. The sequence 'once' is interesting in that the nasalization occurs abruptly after the approximant [w], and in the fact that the nasal flow reduces smoothly as the oral flow for [s] increases. Note also that the oral flow during the nasal is not zero. The [s] flow reaches its maximum as voicing begins again for [ɑ] and so one could consider that in the spoken form the [s] 'belongs' to the following syllable rather than to the preceding one, which raises awkward questions of syllable division. If the nasal air flow can be equated directly with soft palate movement, then it would appear from the record so far that there are considerable constraints on the speed of movement, particularly on closing. At the beginning of Fig. 16.1b, however, there is an example of the nasal air flow being 'switched' on. The sequence 'who'd never' has the vowel [u] followed by a voiced stop [d] which is released as the nasal [n] commences, giving nasal plosion. One should note that there is little nasal flow throughout the second phrase apart from that for [m] in 'make' and 'mind'. The combination of [s] and [m] in 'his mind' is of interest in that there is an unexpected nasal flow during the fricative [s]. This flow increases as the lip closure is made for the [m] and like the first segment of 'named' this nasal is initially devoiced.

The air-flow record of Fig. 16.2a and b presents the contrasting pattern of a typical cleft patient. This boy, who was 9 years old when the record was made, had primary surgery for cleft lip and palate in infancy. At 5 years of age his speech was considered to be largely unintelligible, but at 6 he had a dental plate made and he was given intensive speech therapy. Further surgery for a palatal fistula was carried out at 8 years. At the time of the recording he had a voice quality typical of cleft palate, and although his speech was intelligible his production of dental fricatives, sibilants and aspirated plosives was not acceptable.

The calibrations for air flow for Fig. 16.2a and b are only slightly different from Fig. 16.1a and b (354 as against 333 ml/s/cm) and so they can be compared by eye more or less directly. Integrators were not used for this oscillogram. Traces 2 and 3 are now nasal flow, and traces 4 and 5 oral flow. Trace 6 is Lx, trace 7 is Fx and trace 8 (Ao) is the acoustic pressure waveform of the microphone placed in front of the mouth but a little to the side of the pneumotach head. It will be noticed that there is less detail in the oral flow trace for the cleft palate child, and this is generally the case. The speech is produced a little more slowly than that recorded in Fig. 16.1, and this excerpt starts with the second last segment of 'once' where the nasal flow rate is 40 ml/s, compared with 130 ml/s for the adult, followed by a long period of nasal flow during the [s], with a peak value of 150 ml/s compared with zero for the adult. An estimate of the volume escaping through the nose during the [s] would be about 30 ml—not a large amount of air, but it may produce an audible noise. In normal circumstances, this noise would be masked by the characteristic high frequency acoustic spectrum of the orally produced [s] sound, but here

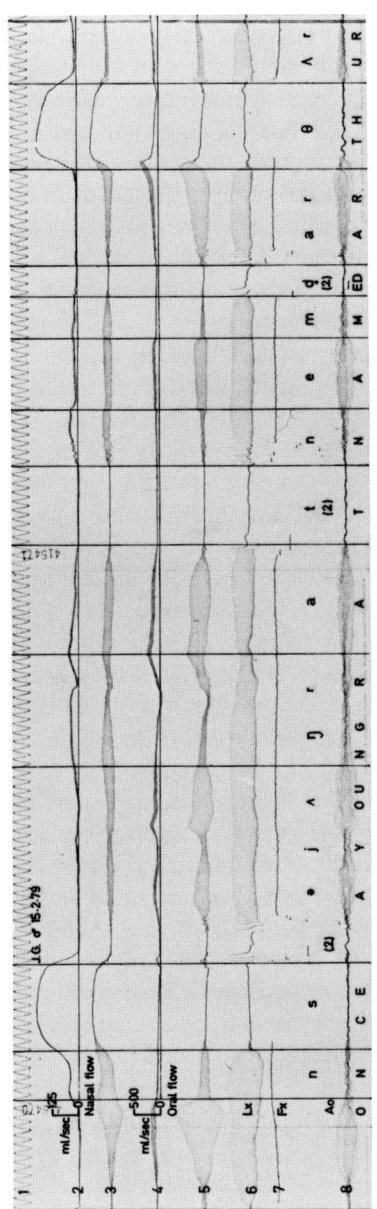

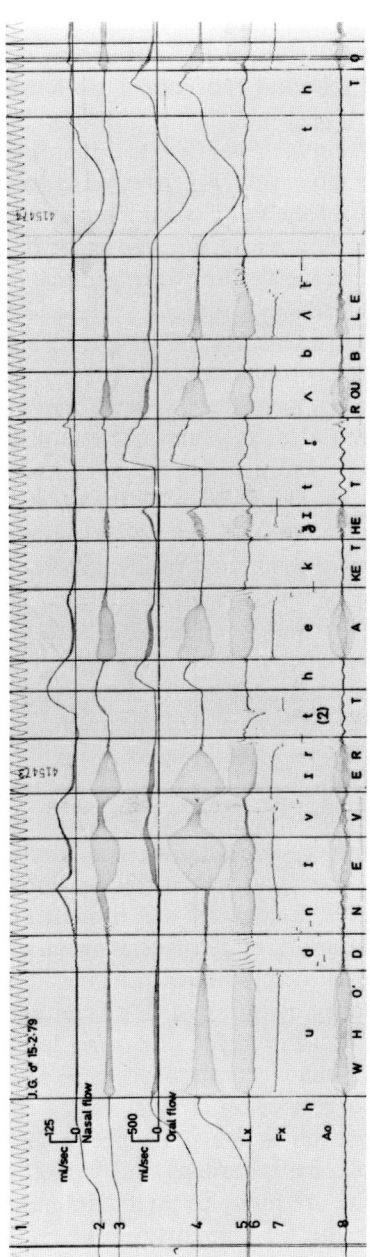

Fig. 16.2(a) and (b) Air-flow record for a typical cleft palate in a child aged 9 years. For details see text

the acoustic intensity of the [s] must be very low as the oral flow at its maximum is only 15 ml/s, and this may, in fact, be below the critical rate for turbulence. The same considerations apply to the dental fricative [θ] in 'Arthur' where again the oral flow shape is different from that of the adult. In the second phrase (Fig. 16.2a) there are inconsistencies in nasal flow; [ɾ] (devoiced) of 'trouble', [h] of 'to' and [k] of 'make' do not have high nasal flow, but [h] of 'take' and [h] and [z] of 'his' (not shown) do. The initial sequence of 'take' deserves closer inspection in view of the fact that the nasal escape is large and starts some 50 ms before the oral flow. If this were due to early relaxation of the soft palate then it would have to be considered as what might be called nasal pre-plosion. The answer, however, lies in the shape of the laryngographic waveform (Lx), which shows a glottal stop preventing all flow through the larynx while the tongue is in the closure position. At the end of the glottal stop there is no flow through the mouth because the tongue closure is still made, but there is flow through the nose because the soft palate is not closing the nasal port. This is a well-known compensatory articulation, although it may also be part of the child's sound system. It is almost certainly used at the end of 'named', after the [s] of 'once', and possibly at the end of 'rat'. Actual nasals have a fairly small flow never exceeding 50 ml/s. In 'named' we have the opposite nasal flow pattern to that found, and expected, in the adult, the [n] being longer and of higher amplitude than the [m]. Finally the high nasal flow during the [v] of 'never' should be noted. This is a speech sound formed by the lower lip against the upper teeth and requiring a high intra-oral pressure for its production. The difference between it and the other fricatives discussed already is that it is voiced. The internal resistance of the air-supply system is increased by that of the larynx and therefore greater difficulty in preventing nasal escape should be expected for this type of sound.

This kind of analysis gives an insight into dynamic organization of speech production and draws attention to the problems that arise when some part of the anatomy and/or muscular function is abnormal. Palatal deficiency or lack of movement creates extreme difficulty in building up adequate intra-oral pressures to generate a turbulent air stream for fricative sounds or to signal the release of stop plosives. Normal nasal flow in nasal contexts appears to follow fairly well-defined rules and gives the possibility of describing the voice quality of nasality in terms of flow, context and acoustic spectrum. The record and the transcription describe many facets of the patient's speech at one particular time and allow comparison to be made between samples of speech before and after surgery or therapy. It has an equally important function in concentrating attention on the specific speech problems that must be investigated by, for example, nasendoscopy and videofluoroscopy.

There are many problems in endoscopy of the soft palate, with both rigid and flexible instruments, but given that the nasendoscope can be brought into a position slightly beyond the hard palate, then the whole of the superior surface can be seen when it is rising. With the rigid endoscope, if the palate is relaxed the open port area and shape can be checked and through the orifice the back of the tongue is often visible with the epiglottis and vocal cords further away. The action of the soft palate can be compared in speech and swallowing, but the view is a distorted one (see Chapter 15). It is also difficult to judge the size of the nasopharynx above and the shape of the posterior wall below the level of the hard palate. With the normal palate, one often has the impression of the soft palate moving up the back wall vertically, and in such cases the nasal port is obscured as the raising muscles contract and a 'knuckle' is formed against the back wall. From several points of view, then, the best observations are obtained with the most abnormal palates. However, direct observation by nasendoscopy is always worth striving for, no matter how serious the practical difficulties are, because so much can be learned of the palate's capability of movement and the organization of control in specific phonetic contexts. It is possible to make a reasonable judgement of the size of the orifice caused by some deficiency in length or shape, and one can see if the gap is unilateral or bilateral. The seriousness of the lack of closure can be judged by the strength of the jet-stream of mucus through the gap in fricative and plosive production.

The movements of the soft palate in speech are much too fast to be captured by eye and related to changes in the air-flow record. With the video recorders available at present, stopping the machine is not satisfactory because human reaction time is so variable (particularly with speech), and there are no facilities for numbering consecutive frames or for shuttling the tape back and forth, listening and looking, until the exact instant is found. One approach which has proved useful and effective, though open to some objection, is to have the word or phrase spoken 'very slowly', 'drawn out' or made 'much longer'—all these instructions are understood by the smallest child, though an actual spoken example is always given at the time. Some patients will extend the consonants by holding the closure for a stop, for instance, while some will continue the vowels but the word will be lengthened by a slower articulation in one form or another. It will be said that this is not normal speech and this, of course, is quite true but it becomes a valid method of studying the movement of the soft palate if we know how 'drawn-out' speech differs from normal rate speech. When the air-flow pattern of 'named' (which is well defined in normal speech) is compared with the same word said lengthened, a similar waveform is found. There may be slight differences in amplitude but it differs, as expected, primarily as a new function of time. The pattern of movement from the video recording of 'named', said slowly, corresponds closely to the 'slow' air-flow pattern but it is the mirror image of it; as the palate rises, the air flow decreases and vice versa. Obviously, detailed studies must be done to confirm how closely air flow and observed movement do match, but this method appears to provide a practical answer to the problem at the moment.

The general pattern of normal palatal action as described from the lateral radiograph seems fairly clear (Calnan 1956). The palate at rest is seen to slope downwards and backwards from the posterior margin of the hard palate at an angle of about 40 degrees, and closure consists of a pulling backwards and upwards, bending the soft palate into a near-horizontal part and a vertical part which is brought in close to the back wall of the pharynx. If the closure is a firm one then the upper part against the back wall will be squeezed into a 'knuckle', but however firm or tight the closure is, the vertical part will not necessarily lie against the back wall. But the anatomy of this region and the mechanics of movement of the soft palate of the cleft palate patient seldom fit this simple description, and in many cases it is only the study of the videotape, particularly using 'drawn-out' speech, which shows the immense problems which have been imposed on the patient. Tentatively, palates might be divided into three types: type 1 is the normal already described; type 2 bends backwards and downwards in a long unbroken curve, giving the impression that the lower end is tethered; type 3 hangs limply, almost vertically, from the hard palate. Type 2 closure movement preserves its curved shape and so even if contact is made with the back wall it is seldom extensive and never seems to be firm. The level of contact will be somewhat below the level of the upper surface of the hard palate. In types 1 and 2 it is seldom that the tongue comes in contact with the underside of the soft palate, but type 3 requires the tongue to push it up into position. In many cases this is only accomplished by a kind of fast ballistic movement of the tongue from an anterior articulatory position and the point of contact is therefore very variable, not firm, and occurs only momentarily. The shape of the back wall is important; in one patient it sloped downwards and backwards so quickly that, although she had a type 1 palate, contact was made over only a small area and the air-flow record confirmed that closure was not complete. The soft palate of the patient of Fig. 16.2a and b could be classed as type 2, and it moves as a curve to make contact at a level well below that of the hard palate. Good closure should be possible, though, because the curve of the palate when raised fits a curved portion of the back wall. This is confirmed by the air-flow record, but closure is not consistently made. It is good on [t] of 'two' on [f] of 'four', but the [θ] of 'Arthur' shows a large gap. There is relaxation of the palate on aspiration, and [s] never shows movement even in the sequence [st] of 'stamps' (one of the standard words used in the speech assessment) (Ingram et al 1971) where the [t] has closure.

Progress in research depends on the unexpected. Up to this point, the airflow analysis and the nasendoscopic and fluoroscopic observations have been shown to support a close relationship between velopharyngeal incompetence and the quality of the speech produced. Perhaps this is too simple a view. If we take the tape recording of the patient of Fig. 16.2a and b referred to above, and use a speech microscope to allow very careful listening to small portions of it, we find that the [s] fricative is never acceptable but the other fricatives are not judged to be abnormal whether or not the air-flow record shows nasal escape. The record of the next patient to be discussed (Fig. 16.3a and b) shows airflow rates through the nose which are quite enormous (perhaps the highest that are likely to be found in records of this kind) but the oral airflow pattern is preserved and his speech is quite intelligible. There is certainly a nasal quality to it, but serious nasal escape is not heard in his reading and it is only the consonants [s] in 'was', [d] in 'day', [b] in 'blade' and 'but' and [v] in 'given' and 'ever' in the whole of the 'Arthur the Rat' text that are not acceptable.

This boy, who was 15 years old at the time of recording, suffered severe craniofacial injuries when he was aged 7 as the result of a car accident. He lost one eye and little remains of his soft palate. When he says [a] only a little movement is seen at the top of the arch when looking into his mouth. Nasendoscopy showed no traces of palatal movement, and when the nasendoscope was used

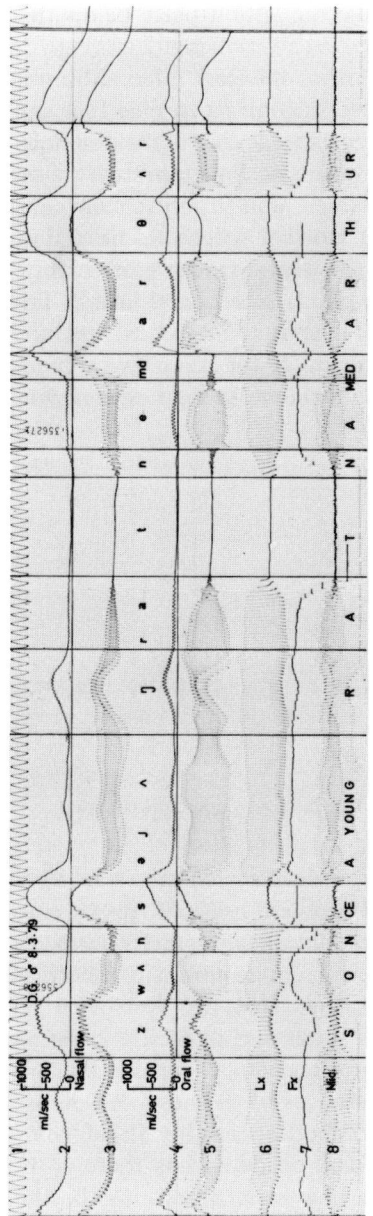

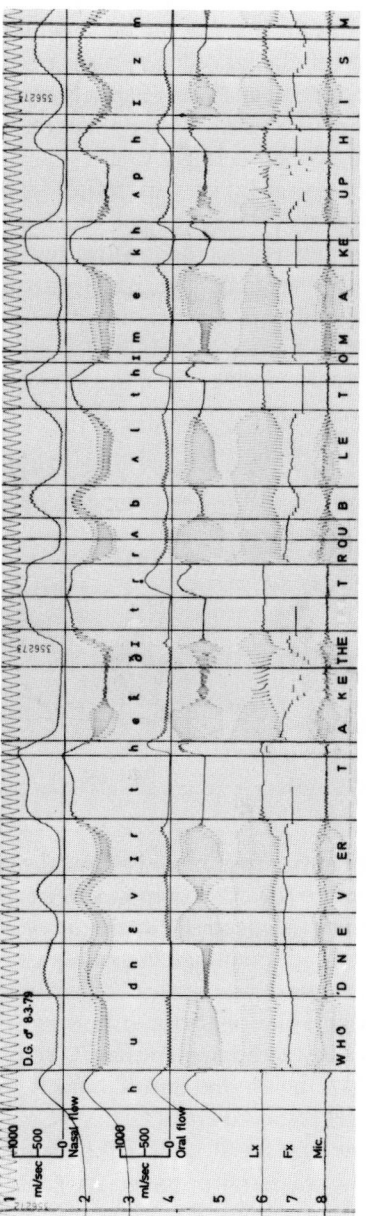

Fig. 16.3(a) and (b) Air-flow record for a patient (aged 15 years) with acquired velopharyngeal deficiency. For details see text

intra-orally to look up the nasopharynx a large polyp was seen in the left naris with a large vertical cleft extending above it. Videofluoroscopy shows that the upper part of what remains of the soft palate moves slightly in speaking and appears to attempt the normal movements, while the lateral parts below that bend upwards or are pushed against the back wall in swallowing. Figure 16.3a starts with the [z] of 'was' in the first phrase of 'Arthur the Rat'. The calibration for both nasal and oral channels in this oscillogram, in contrast to Figs 16.1 and 16.2, are the same but even then the nasal flow often exceeds that of the oral flow. Nasal escape is clearly seen at all the expected points in both phrases; in the first phrase at [z] of 'was', [s] of 'once', [d] of 'named' and [θ] of 'Arthur', and the peak value reached is 945 ml/s. The ratio, in normal speech, of nasal flow to oral flow is less than unity, but here during the dental fricative of 'Arthur' it is 4.5, the total flow, nasal plus oral, at that point exceeding 1 litre/s. The actual volume of air escaping during the segment itself is about 100 ml and over the whole phrase it is about 300 ml, which would suffice for about two seconds of normal speech production at conversational level. How, then, is near normal speech produced by this subject?

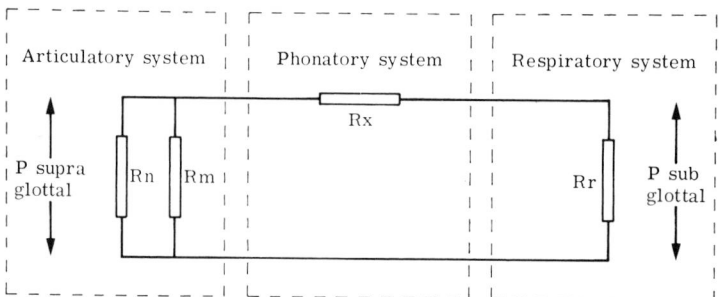

Fig. 16.4 Simple electrical analogue of the aerodynamic system in human speech production

The answer seems to be that the patient's respiratory system has learned to respond to the extra demand. We can look at the problem best perhaps by constructing the electrical analogue of a much-simplified aerodynamic system. In such a model, voltage is analogous to pressure, current to flow and electrical resistance to mechanical (flow) resistance. In Fig. 16.4 the resistance R_r represents the distributed flow resistance of the lungs and bronchial passages (here considered negligible), R_x represents the flow resistance (considered constant) of the larynx, and R_n and R_m are the resistances of the nose and mouth passages respectively. The first segment of Fig. 16.3b, the aspiration [h] of 'who', has oral and nasal flows of the same shape and amplitude and as there is the same supraglottal pressure for each channel the flow resistances must be the same, that is, $R_n = R_m$. There is confirmation for this in other, voiced, parts of the record where oral and nasal flows have the same amplitudes. We can consider three static cases. During vowels a reasonable supraglottal pressure would be 0.5 cm H_2O giving 2.5 Ω (ohms) (aerodynamic) for both nose and mouth resistances, a laryngeal resistance of 2 Ω and a subglottal pressure of 1.3 cm H_2O. For the voiced fricatives with a nasal flow of 800 ml/s and an oral flow of 200 ml/s the supraglottal pressure would then be 2 cm H_2O and the subglottal pressure 4 cm H_2O. For the occlusion periods of stops when the resistance of the mouth is considered infinite the nasal flow is again 800 ml/s, the supraglottal pressure is again 2 cm H_2O but the subglottal pressure is then 3.6 cm H_2O. It should be stressed that this is a grossly oversimplified model, but these figures suggest that the increase in subglottal pressure which is necessary to produce these high nasal flows is not as great as might be expected. More important is the requirement that the ventilatory system must provide, very rapidly, high flow rates to build up the supraglottal pressures that are essential for plosive and fricative production. The nasal air-flow trace for [md] of 'named' (and of the first segment of 'there') rises proportionately with time, and, assuming that this is the result of a corresponding linear rise in pressure below the larynx, the time constant is about 70 ms. A more probable figure would be about 100 ms, which corresponds to the minimum figure that has been found (Rothenberg 1968). It cannot be much longer, one would think, if the phonetic requirements of plosives and other speech sounds are to be satisfied. One would wonder, too, whether this time constant plays a decisive role in determining the maximum speed of speaking for this patient. Confirmation of these estimates and the conclusions drawn from them will require other tests and measurements. There is a great dearth of data on the pressures developed above and below the larynx in speech and this is almost certainly because the insertion of pressure-sensitive devices through the nose into the nasopharynx is considered invasive. But modern transducers are only 2 to 3 mm in diameter (Anthony & MacLachlan 1969) and if the correct technique is used there is little discomfort.

If we accept that we can describe how this boy has overcome his disability, we must ask why most children with congenital cleft palates do not have such good speech. But are they comparable? The child with the congenital cleft palate has both to learn to speak and then to develop the accepted adult form with a deficient mechanism; this boy, on the other hand, had already acquired mature speech (and a facility in controlling it) before his sudden loss of velopharyngeal function. After the accident he did not change his established pattern of articulation or phonation (perhaps it would have been difficult for him to do so even at 7 years of age) and he adapted his ventilatory organization instead. From an understanding of the means by which he retained his adult form of speech we may learn how to help children with congenital cleft palates to improve their speech and achieve equally good results.

REFERENCES

Abercrombie D 1967 Elements of general phonetics. Edinburgh University Press, Edinburgh

Anthony J, MacLachlan D 1969 A small transducer for subglottal pressure measurement. Work in Progress no. 3, 56–59. Department of Phonetics, University of Edinburgh

Anthony J, Farquharson I M 1975 Clinical research in speech pathology. Journal of Laryngology and Otology 89: 1169–1183

Anthony J 1978 The Voiscope. Health Services Bulletin 36: 321–328. Scottish Home and Health Department, Edinburgh

Barry W J, Kunzel H J 1978 A note on the devoicing of nasals. Journal of the International Phonetic Association vol 8, nos 1–2

Calnan J 1956 Diagnosis, prognosis and treatment of palatopharyngeal incompetence with special reference to radiographic investigations. British Journal of Plastic Surgery 8: 265

Comroe J H 1950 Mouthpieces and masks. In: Comroe J H (ed) Methods in medical research. Yearbook Medical Publishers, Chicago, vol 2

Fleish A 1925 Pneumatochograph: apparatus for recording respiratory flow. Archiv für die gesamte Physiologie 209: 713

Fourcin A J 1974 Laryngographic examination of vocal fold vibration. In: Wyke B (ed) Ventilatory and phonatory control systems. Oxford University Press

House A S, Stevens K N 1956 Analog studies of the nasalization of vowels. Journal of Speech and Hearing Disorders 21: 218–232

Ingram T T S, Anthony A, Bogle D, McIsaac M W 1971 The Edinburgh articulation test. Churchill Livingstone, Edinburgh

Jespersen O 1909 A modern English grammar, part 1. Carl Winter's Universitätsbuchhandling, Heidelberg

Lubker J F, Moll K L 1965 Simultaneous oral–nasal flow measurements and cinefluorographic observations during speech production. Cleft Palate Journal 2: 257–272

Milic-Emili J, Pengelly L D 1970 Ventilatory effects of mechanical loading. In: Campbell E J M, Agostini E, Newson-Davies J M (eds) The respiratory muscles: Mechanics and neurol control, 2nd edn. Lloyd-Luke, London, 271–290

Rothenburg M 1968 The breath-stream dynamics of simple-released plosive production. NJ Bibliotheca Phonetica no 6, Kavgar

ACKNOWLEDGEMENTS

Pneumotachograph heads were supplied by Mercury Electronics (Scotland) Limited, Pollok Industrial Estate, Newton Mearns, Glasgow, Scotland. Pressure and Flow Transducers were supplied by Gaeltec Limited, Dunvegan, Isle of Skye, Scotland. Voiscope was supplied by Laryngograph Limited, 162 Gower Street, London NW1, England.

Secondary surgery

INTRODUCTION

Dr Morley has frequently stressed the importance of the proper sequence in the development of speech in the growing child with a palatal cleft. In the same way, this chapter on secondary surgical problems will consider these matters sequentially and discuss them as they relate to the age of the patient. However, while the public in general and our medical colleagues in particular demand better facial appearance in patients with clefts of the lip, they often assume that the child with a cleft palate will have distorted speech and, indeed, is expected to have distorted speech. Most secondary palatal problems can be improved, and often corrected, through the co-ordinated efforts of the specialists involved. However, the likelihood of success in speech is usually much better when approached at an early age. The acceptance of a poor speech result hinders the possibility of improving speech.

Secondary cleft palate surgery usually involves three defects: velopharyngeal valving, oronasal fistulae, and surgical problems of the dental arch. In the first situation, the surgeon works closely with the speech pathologist and sometimes the prosthodontist; in the second, he usually works alone or with the prosthodontist; and in the third, he works with an orthodontist or oral surgeon and prosthodontist. These specialists must co-ordinate their plans so the appropriate priority is given to specific steps. The most important function to the patient—whether socially, educationally or economically—is good speech. This goal should be kept in mind at all times. The importance of the timely diagnosis and treatment of these defects will be discussed along with possible complications.

DEVELOPMENT

It is interesting to reflect that the first three actions we do on entering this world, apart from flailing arms and legs, are (i) to start breathing, (ii) to start screaming, and (iii) to start swallowing. Each of these actions involves the soft palate and its contiguous musculature in a very special, complicated and co-ordinated way. The 'programming' in the brain for these actions must indeed be exquisite. Furthermore, there is good evidence that two of them (respiratory movements and swallowing) occur normally before birth, and the third, intrauterine vocalization, is also said to occur. It is also interesting that one seldom sees a newborn with a palatal cleft who has not already developed a Passavant's ridge. I would interpret this as a prepartum effort to overcome the functional deficiencies of a mechanism literally rent asunder.

The normal palate, in the process of normal speech, moves with great ease and speed similar to that of a blink. If the palatal tissues are not repaired at each step with the care and precision one would use in operating on an eyelid, the surgically repaired palate is likely to be heavily scarred and sluggish in movement. It may indeed be able to achieve velopharyngeal closure (VPC) and might be able to produce competency for the correct production of single test sounds, but the chances of its working for relaxed conversational speech would be minimal.

The point I wish to make in this discussion is that we should direct our attention to the function of the soft palate shortly after its initial repair, and if inadequate function is found, should plan on doing something about it without delay.

What does this mean? First, the palate repair should be done early, usually at 10 to 14 months of age, though perhaps 3 to 6 months of age will prove to be an advantage. We have operated on a number of children 3 to 6 months of age and though as yet we do not have proof of improved speech, these children are being followed closely. Secondly, these patients should be followed at 6- to 12-month intervals or until their conditions have stabilized.

EXAMINATION

The proper examination of the child with a cleft has been well detailed elsewhere in this text. For this chapter, however, it might be appropriate to mention a few points which, as a plastic surgeon, I have found to be helpful. To me, the most important part of the examination is to listen, perhaps as a bystander, while the child or adult chatters away in a conversational manner. This is not always possible or easy, but a few suggestions might help.

My most valuable tool has been a school lunch box full of small plastic toys. This will usually start a child talking, but there are several additional tricks for its successful use. One is just to give it to the child and let him play, either by himself or with a sibling, friend or parent. The presence of the surgeon in the examination room can easily inhibit conversation, so eavesdropping by the surgeon may be needed. Occasionally, if the surgeon will engage the parent in conversation and ignore the child, the child will insist on being heard, and conversational speech is produced.

I question the parents on how *they* feel the child's speech is progressing. If they have little to say, I ask them what sounds the child says well and which ones are causing difficulties. I ask if they are having trouble understanding the child, and if the child is having difficulty being understood by others. Other questions include whether there is leakage of fluid into the nose such as chocolate milk or chocolate ice cream, and whether they are having trouble with ear infections, all of which would point to possible palatal problems.

Before examining the inside of the mouth, I try to have the child repeat a number of test words and sentences.* While listening to the speech, I first try to get an overall picture. Is it fairly normal speech with good, crisp, easy production of consonants, or are there deficiencies? I evaluate the overall quality, whether there is hypernasality or hyponasality. If abnormal, is this something that is intermittent or present throughout the speech sample? Can the child impound air to produce a plosive sound such as [b], [p], [t]? Can he produce consonants such as [s], [sh], and soft [ch] and [th] sounds? Can he do this consistently and are these sounds accompanied by audible leakage of air into the nose (nasal escape)? Does the child use the accessory muscles of the constrictor nares? Is the child hoarse?

In addition, I make the repeated sentences longer and longer to check the child's memory as a rough test of intelligence, and at times when asking questions, I speak very quietly to obtain some measure of the child's ability to hear. I also use a metal hand mirror (camping equipment) and hold it under the child's nose while he repeats the test words to check for nasal escape (that causes fogging on the mirror). With the nasal consonants [m] and [n] one can test for an obstructed nasal airway.

To examine the palate in infants or relatively young children, simply place their head in the examiner's lap with the mother holding the feet, and they usually will open their mouths. A good examination lamp or flashlight is needed. Often a good child will learn to open his mouth while sitting or standing as soon as you pick up a flashlight. If the child co-operates, I think it is very important not to thrust a tongue blade down his throat and make him gag as the initial step. That might well be the last time the patient allows you near him. Rather, it is better to inspect as much as you can simply by looking with the light, checking the hard palate for fistulae, observing the condition of the teeth and gums, having the child bite, and checking his occlusion. Next, I like to watch the soft palate while the child says 'kah . . . kah . . . kah'. See how much the soft palate moves, how easily and how quickly it moves, and whether it moves symmetrically. Then look at the lateral pharyngeal walls and see how large the tonsils are (the adenoids can be expected to be of comparable size), and again, have the child phonate 'kah . . . kah . . . kah' and watch the lateral and posterior pharyngeal walls. Try to develop an ability to evaluate the amount of motion of these structures as being slight, moderate or excessive. Excessive lateral or posterior pharyngeal wall motion usually indicates that the soft palate is not moving normally. (Usually this evaluation does require the use of the tongue blade.)

This quick screening examination tells me a great deal, and, as will be noted, we have found considerable reliability in being able to place children in four specific groups according to their speech. While I feel it is essential to have the service of a competent speech pathologist, I also feel that the surgeon should be able to assess the function of the structure on which he is operating. As an orthopaedist who operates on a knee joint or a wrist will want to test its function

---

* 'Sun', 'bicycle', 'bus', 'kitty, kitty, kitty', 'chicken', 'rooster', 'chocolate chip cookies', 'car', etc. 'Sue roasted the goose', 'Bessie stayed all summer', 'Jane rang the triangle', 'the angry man came', 'old cars don't go', 'pay for the apples and soap', 'about half a dozen people sat on the sofa', 'judges sometimes live to a very old age', 'chimes rang from all the churches', etc.

himself, so a plastic surgeon should be able to evaluate palatal function. After deciding into which of the four speech groups the child should be placed, I check my examination with that of the speech pathologist and, on the basis of these evaluations, decide what further examination should be done or what plan of treatment to follow.

ASSESSMENT

In assessing soft palate function, we classify the speech of each patient in one of four categories:

1. *Good velopharyngeal competence (VPC)* with crisp, accurate, effortless speech (except for certain errors appropriate for age)
2. *Partial or inconsistent VP competence* consisting of slight or occasional hyper-nasality and/or a patient who has some difficulty with some consonant sounds, particularly the sibilants
3. *Clearcut velopharyngeal incompetence (VPI)*
4. A classification of *'indeterminant'* for the child who is too young or too unco-operative to allow an accurate assessment

In comparing the findings of the speech pathologist and the plastic surgeon with a battery of testing modalities (pressure studies, maximum breathing capacity, lateral static films, cine fluorographic studies, and sound spectro-graphic studies) and using the eventual status of the patient as the determinant factor, two observations were made. First, the clinicians were far more accurate in predicting the eventual outcome even in the very young child of 3 to 5 years of age than any of the testing modalities. Perhaps some of the newer testing techniques comparing nasal sound with oral sound and measuring the nasal air flow, etc. will prove to be more accurate, but these techniques are difficult or impossible to use in the very young child. Secondly, it became clear that neither group 1 (velopharyngeal competence) nor group 3 (severe velopharyngeal in-competence) needed a battery of tests or frequent testing to confirm the diag-nosis. The child with good speech is simply seen at yearly intervals and rarely slips below this classification. Occasionally, a child with *good* VP competence will become incompetent as his pharynx deepens and his adenoids shrink. The child with obvious poor speech needs a better speech mechanism right away and rarely, if ever, was a child in this group elevated to group 1 through either speech therapy alone or the passage of time. Furthermore, when diagnosed as belonging to group 3 (VPI) there was seldom, if ever, any reason to delay treatment.

The patients in group 2 with inconsistent or partial incompetence, in our hands, are much more difficult to handle. These children probably need as much investigation as is available, and as close follow-up as possible with trial speech therapy or a temporary dental palatal lift or possibly a prosthetic obturator. On the other hand, the child with borderline incompetence is much more likely to do well with almost any kind of secondary palatal surgery than the child with a more severe defect, simply because he probably does not need very much to correct the velopharyngeal incompetence.

The child in group 4 whose evaluation is unsatisfactory should be watched closely to determine which group he really belongs to or whether there is some underlying reason such as deafness, mental retardation, or a neurological deficit. Perhaps this child is one of those unusual children who has an incompetent palate and seems to be smart enough to keep his mouth shut even at a very early age because he knows his speech is inadequate. Perhaps this child is just shy and reluctant to speak, but in any case he deserves attention.

In summary, the child in group 1 with good speech should probably be seen yearly, but does not need extensive studies. The child in group 2 with slight or inconsistent incompetence probably needs a great deal of study and definitive treatment when indicated. The child in group 3 with clearcut incompetence needs to have something done without delay, and the child in group 4 whose testing is inconclusive should be seen frequently to determine into which of the first three groups he belongs.

TREATMENT OF VELOPHARYNGEAL INCOMPETENCE

Throughout the world, surgeons and dentists seem to be well aware of a wide variety of ways to treat velopharyngeal incompetence (VPI). Each seems to have his own favourite procedure for treating this condition, which is then used almost to the exclusion of other approaches. Surprisingly, in the vast majority of cases, the results seem to be good, almost regardless of which technique is used. This observation, unfortunately, has a number of fallacies. Probably no area of investigation is subject to more variables. They include how severe the incompetence must be before being treated, the condition of the tissue, the skill of the surgeon, the postoperative care, the home environment of the patient and the evaluation of the speech result.

In Britain and the United States, the superiorly based posterior pharyngeal flap (PPF) is favoured (Owsley et al 1970) (Fig. 17.1), though the inferiorly based posterior pharyngeal flap is used in some cases. In a prospective randomized series of 35 patients, Whitaker et al (1972) were unable to show a significant difference between these two operations. Skoog (1965), in a retrospective study of 82 cases, and Hamlen (1970), in another retrospective study of 91 cases, both came to the same conclusion. The pharyngoplasty of Hynes (1956) (Fig. 17.2) has been popular in the British Isles for minimal insufficiencies and apparently has produced excellent results. In Britain and the South American countries, the operation of Orticochea (1968) has done well. It consists of superiorly based flaps of the posterior tonsillar pillars containing the palatopharyngeus muscles which are sutured to the defect on the posterior pharyngeal wall created by raising a small, inferiorly based flap. Jackson & Silverton (1977) have modified it by using a superiorly based pharyngeal flap (Fig. 17.3) and have also produced good results. Kapetansky (1973) greatly favours two lateral pharyngeal flaps sutured into the palate (Fig. 17.4) and is also enthusiastic about his results. These flaps would appear to preserve the neurovascular supply to the flap better than the vertically oriented flap. However, their insertion into the central part of the soft palate also would appear to disrupt the continuity of the levator muscles.

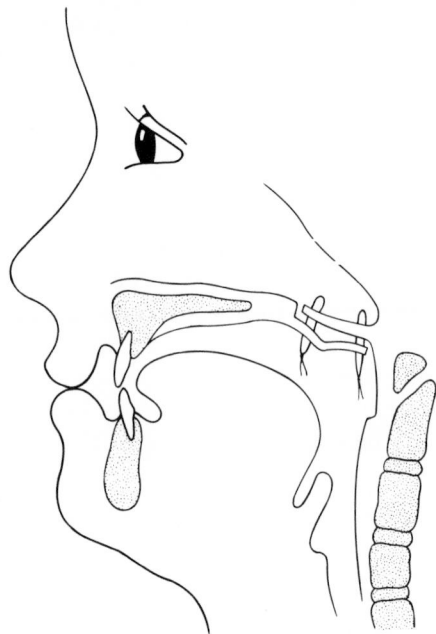

Fig. 17.1 The superiorly based posterior pharyngeal flap seems to be favoured by most surgeons. It consists of a trap-door of mucosa and muscle based (or hinged) at the base of the adenoid tissue and sutured into the nasal side of the soft palate—leaving an air space on either side

Superiorly based lateral pharyngeal wall flaps, similar to those of Hynes but inserted into the nasal side of the soft palate parallel to the levator muscles are favoured by Moore (1960) and Sullivan (1961). Dickson & Dickson (1972) have noted that the salpingo pharyngeus muscle, on which the Hynes pharyngoplasty flaps are theoretically based, is absent in a high percentage of patients with clefts.

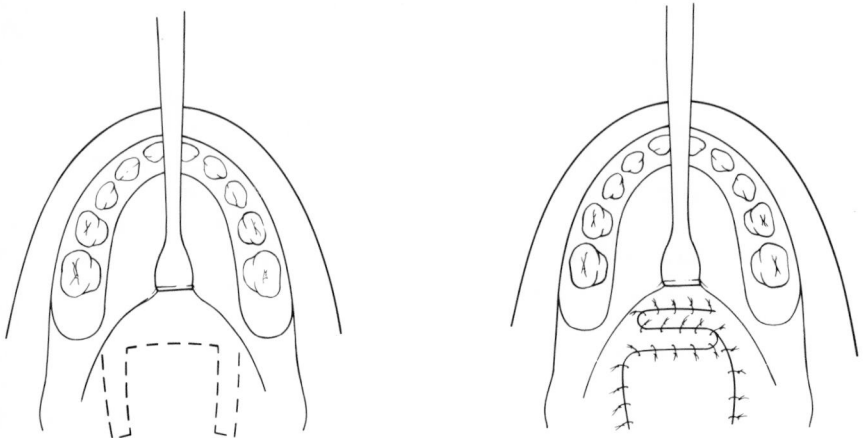

Fig. 17.2 The Hynes pharyngoplasty has been widely used in Britain for cases of slight incompetency. Vertical flaps of mucosa and muscle (salpingo pharyngeus) are raised from the lateral pharyngeal walls and sutured in an overlapping position horizontally in the posterior pharyngeal wall above the arch of the atlas. They are wider than they seem in the illustration, as they are seen from the side

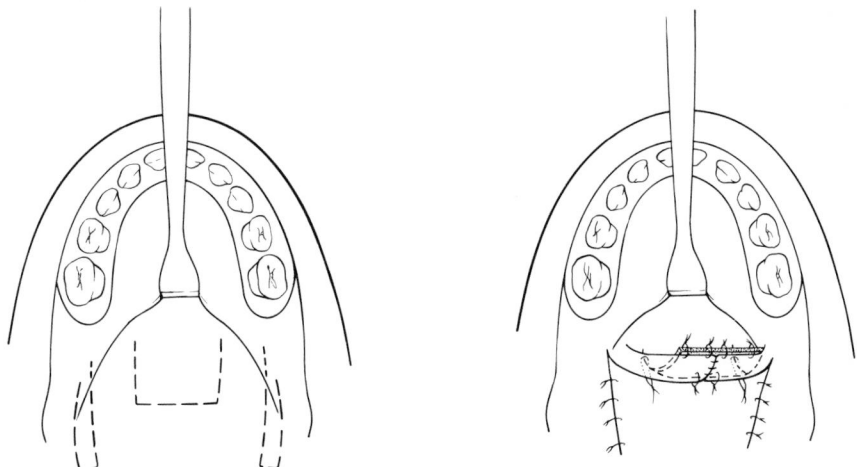

Fig. 17.3 Jackson uses flaps of palato pharyngeus muscle as suggested by Orticochea—suturing them end-to-end on the underneath side of a short superiorly based posterior pharyngeal flap

Those favouring retropharyngeal implants (Blocksma 1963, Bluestone et al 1968), whether they use shredded Teflon (now restricted in the United States), silicone 'pillows', or autogenous tissue, note that these procedures can only overcome small gaps of 2 to 3 mm and can be expected to be successful only if the palate already has good motion. In some patients, the palate is extremely short, scarred and immobile and this greatly limits what can be done. The lateral pharyngeal walls may be excessively active or may seem to be paralysed. Skolnick et al (1973) have stressed the importance of a thorough radiographic evaluation of the patient preoperatively before selecting the operation to be used. Pigott (1975), Shprintzen et al (1979), and others evaluate the situation with a nasopharyngoscope to select the operation depending on what they observe (see

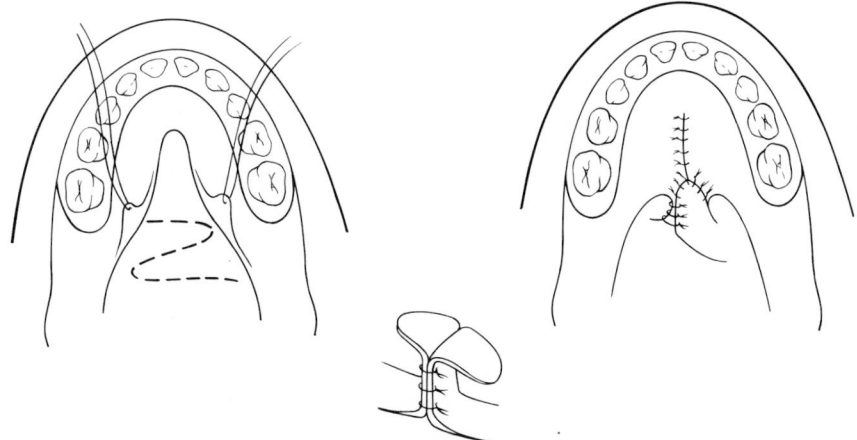

Fig. 17.4 Kapetansky suggests laterally based flaps from the posterior pharyngeal wall sutured first to each other then into an incision made in the posterior edge of the soft palate

Chapter 15). In my opinion, all these factors have a bearing on choosing which secondary procedure to use and in predicting the likelihood of success.

Procedures designed only to lengthen the palate secondarily have not been very impressive. Conceivably, this step alone could overcome a small degree of incompetency, but it is probably advisable to include a posterior pharyngeal flap or some other kind of pharyngoplasty. In any kind of a lengthening procedure, it is felt that the nasal lining should be provided either with mucosa from the floor of the nose or in the form of an island flap, as suggested by Millard (1963), or with a superiorly based posterior pharyngeal flap as suggested by Hönig (1964). Complete levator muscle repositioning (as in an intravelar veloplasty) has been carried out only recently (Braithwaite & Maurice 1968, Kriens 1970). Consequently, in older children and adults, or when the operative note indicates no reconstruction of this muscle, one can expect to find the levator muscle improperly oriented in a longitudinal direction and, perhaps, it might still be attached to the posterior edge of the bony cleft. Under these conditions, it can hardly be expected to function adequately, and should be severed from its bony insertion and reoriented in a secondary operation.

The soft palate should be soft, pliable, and well muscled and one should be able to see it move quickly. If it is not moving well, this may be due to an abnormal position of the levator muscles or simply due to heavy scarring. If heavy scarring is evident, further surgery, such as a lengthening operation, is unlikely to achieve significant improvement.

Good movement in the lateral pharyngeal wall usually indicates that a pharyngoplasty, particularly the posterior pharyngeal flap, is more likely to be successful than when very little movement is seen in this area.

With borderline incompetence, there is considerable difference of opinion about which operation should be advised or whether or not any surgery should be advised at all. Many speech pathologists undoubtedly prefer intensive speech therapy. Dentists often prefer a palatal lift procedure, expecting to hold the palate in an upward and posterior position, and if this is successful, occasionally the 'lift' can be reduced gradually until the entire prosthesis is removed. Most of the time, however, these dental prostheses must be kept in indefinitely. Occasionally, prosthetic obturation of the palatopharyngeal defect is advised.

There are a number of extenuating circumstances which might warn the surgeon of a possible poor result. These include the older child or adult who is so accustomed to his distorted way of speaking that he is more comfortable with this type of speech and subconsciously prefers to continue. Other reasons include patients with severe hearing defects who cannot hear either the errors or good speech, and the patient with a parent or sibling with the same problem, producing a home environment which the child copies. Patients may also have mental retardation or a local neuromuscular weakness. Occasionally, a patient with a seemingly good result will still sound hypernasal and have articulation errors in spite of what seems to be a good speech mechanism, good motion and good environment. Further nasopharyngoscopy and/or video examination in the basal view position can often shed light on the cause, which may be adequate closure on one side but inadequate closure on the other.

When considerable incompetence is present, my preference is a very wide, superiorly based, posterior pharyngeal flap with lining for the underneath side, if at all possible. In older children or adults with VPI, we tend to agree with Hogan (1973) in aiming to 'overcorrect' these cases, even to the point of producing hyponasality, so that the patient can be reoriented towards an oral air stream, even though this may mean going back at a later stage and making the lateral ports larger to improve the nasal airway.

SURGERY

In our clinic the most frequently used operation for velopharyngeal incompetence is the posterior pharyngeal flap. This is a 'trap-door' flap of posterior pharyngeal mucosa and muscle with its base (or hinge) placed either superiorly at the base of the adenoid pad (superiorly based PPF), or inferiorly about 1.5 to 2 cm below the adenoid pad (inferiorly based PPF). Dissection is carried down to the prevertebral fascia and usually the donor site is closed from side to side with three or four catgut sutures. Many prefer to leave the donor site open to heal in secondarily (as in a tonsillectomy).

If a superiorly based PPF is used, it is usually necessary to open the midline of the soft palate so that 'turnover flaps' of nasal mucosa can be raised (with their base placed at the free edge of the palate) to provide not only lining tissue but also a large recipient area for the pharyngeal flap (Fig. 17.5). If the flap is based inferiorly and placed on the oral side of the soft palate, a similar flap of oral mucosa is obtained from the oral side of the soft palate, and again, used for lining of the pharyngeal flap, but the muscle layer can be left undisturbed.

Width. The posterior pharyngeal flap can vary considerably in width. I will usually select the width depending on the age and particular problems of the patient. If the flap is used as a 'primary PPF' (constructed at the time of the primary palate repair) in a child with a very short palate or a palate with a large horseshoe-shaped cleft, or in a child who is found to have very little levator muscle when the muscle is dissected out, then I prefer to use only about half the width of the posterior pharyngeal wall. At the other extreme in the older patient who has a great deal of hypernasality, I prefer to use the entire width of the posterior pharynx, and to snug the lateral ports down around an 18 gauge catheter and virtually overcorrect the problem. This can lead to nasal obstruction, hyponasality, and mouth breathing. If this does occur, the lateral ports can be made larger, but because the flap has a tendency to shrink, this secondary adjustment is not done for at least a year. In moderately severe defects, I use about two-thirds to three-quarters of the pharyngeal wall or the entire posterior pharyngeal wall and avoid making the lateral ports too small.

Great care must be taken in operating secondarily on patients who have had a Pierre Robin anomalad, laryngotracheal malacia, neurological swallowing difficulties, or other similar airway problems because the surgery produces obstruction of the nasopharynx and a pharyngoplasty can lead to acute respiratory obstruction or chronic oxygen lack and sleep anoxia. Under these circumstances, again about half the posterior pharyngeal wall is used. Should severe obstruction occur postoperatively, it must be relieved without delay first by passing

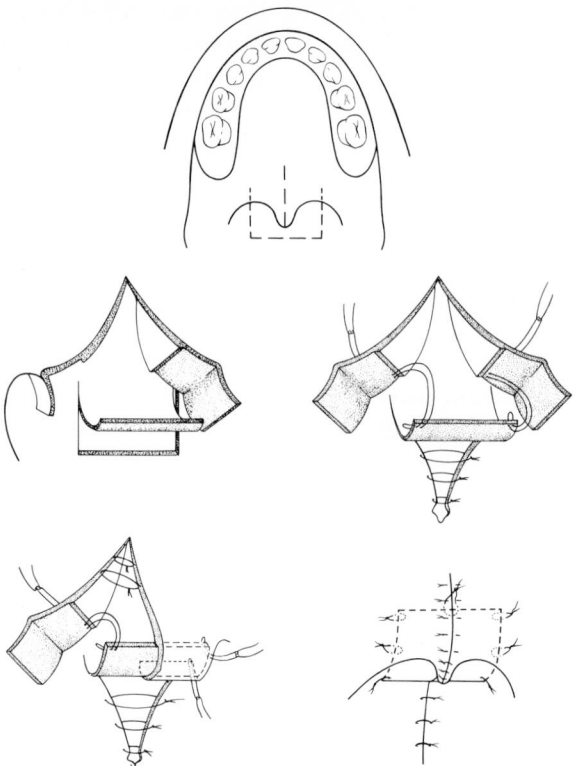

Fig. 17.5 To insert a superiorly based posterior pharyngeal flap into the nasal side of the soft palate, it is usually necessary to incise the soft palate in the mid-line. 'Turnover flaps' of nasal mucosa are raised from each side of the soft palate—based at the free edge of the palate, and used for lining the underneath side of the pharyngeal flap

a nasopharyngeal or oropharyngeal airway and later by opening the lateral ports or by taking down the entire flap.

Superior versus inferior based flaps

Though the superiorly based PPF is by far the most preferred procedure at the present time, it is interesting that three studies previously mentioned have failed to show any significant difference between the results obtained with the superiorly based compared with the inferiorly based flaps. At present, we choose one or the other for a variety of particular reasons (Randall et al 1978). The superiorly based flap seems to have an advantage in being so located that as it contracts, it tends to pull the palate upwards and backwards towards the usual point of contact of the soft palate with the adenoid pad. The inferiorly based flap, on the other hand, tends to pull the palate downward and is more likely to 'tether' the palate and interfere with its usual upward excursion. However, both of these flaps usually contract towards the central part of the donor site and, often, it is difficult in examining a patient to know whether the flap is superiorly or inferiorly based. Both flaps also tend to become narrower. In my hands, it is rare to be able to obtain an anterior insertion (anterior to the levator eminence) with the superiorly based flap without incising through the muscular part of the palate. If a palate has very good motion, I am reluctant to add additional scar in this area. The superiorly based flap can be raised almost to any length. In some patients, the inferiorly based flap simply will not reach a very short palate. The inferiorly based flap operation, on the other hand, is easier and quicker, does not require incising through the muscles of the palate, and can be completed more easily in patients who have poor exposure. In addition, its inferior position may place it in a location where there is greater excursion of the lateral pharyngeal wall and allow it to act as a better 'sounding board', which is desirable in older patients whose primary problem is hypernasality.

In summary, I prefer to use the superiorly based flap most of the time and particularly as a primary flap at the time of the original palate repair, if this is indicated. It is also used in patients who have a very short palate which cannot be reached by the inferiorly based flap and in patients who have little residual motion in the palate. The inferiorly based flap is preferred in those patients who are older and whose primary problem is hypernasality, in palates with very good muscular action, and in those who are poor anaesthetic risks or who have very poor exposure such as the patients with Pierre Robin anomalad or the Treacher Collins syndrome. Often, it is difficult to decide which pharyngoplasty to use until the time of surgery when the area can be examined more closely. However, the surgeon can feel reasonably secure in the efficacy of most of these procedures in view of the good results being reported.

Complications

The posterior pharyngeal flap is not without problems (Graham et al 1973). These include dehiscence, nasorespiratory obstruction and bleeding. The area is quite vascular and though vasoconstrictors are routinely used during surgery (adrenaline 1 : 100 000), postoperative bleeding can be a problem (as it is in routine tonsillectomies). Often, reinjection of the area with a vasoconstrictor can control a minor amount of bleeding. At times, reoperation and ligature or cauterization are necessary. Overobturation or underobturation by a posterior pharyngeal flap usually requires reoperation. I prefer what has been called a 'reverse Z-plasty' (Fig. 17.6) to narrow the lateral ports and an ordinary Z-plasty on the edges to make the lateral ports larger. Nasorespiratory obstruction, if it is not causing serious oxygen lack, can be observed for several years, and often will clear as the posterior pharyngeal flap shrinks and as the child's nasopharynx grows. However, as noted, several cases of severe respiratory obstruction, chronic oxygen lack, sleep apnoea, etc. have been described and should be treated promptly, usually by complete severance of the flap until the child is older. Huge tonsils also can cause serious airway obstruction after a pharyngoplasty. I prefer to remove them at the time of the pharyngoplasty; others plan a tonsillectomy several weeks before. In either case, the adenoid tissue usually should be left undisturbed.

Fistulae

General

There is one cardinal rule to observe when closing fistulae in either the hard or soft palate: the tissue must be closed without tension. This not only means that the edges should be approximated with ease, but also that the sutures should not be tied too tightly. I prefer 5–0 chromic catgut tied just tightly enough to approximate the tissue edges, though occasionally 4–0 and rarely 3–0 chromic in older patients will be needed. If the fine sutures will not hold the flaps in place, the flaps probably have not been relaxed sufficiently to assure success.

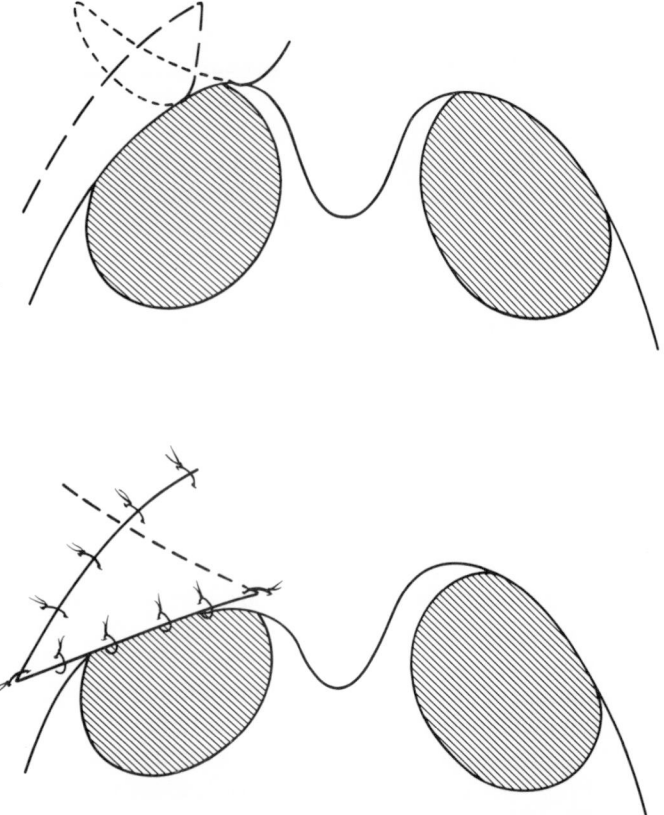

Fig. 17.6 Should the lateral ports on either side of a posterior pharyngeal flap be too large, they can be made smaller with a 'reverse Z-plasty' advancing each flap as far as needed

Soft palate fistulae are usually not so difficult to close. Small fistulae are simply excised or incised and closed in layers. If larger, relaxing incisions may be needed or a large adjacent pedicle flap may be used. It should be placed with the base towards the major blood supply or at least free of previous incisions. The operation is done preferably with nasal closure as well as oral closure, though nasal closure may be impossible. Usually one can assume that if a soft palate has a large surgical defect, it probably was not operated on by a surgeon who had a great deal of experience of cleft palates. It is, thus, unlikely that a good repositioning and reconstruction of the displaced levator muscles was carried out at the initial procedure. Repair of the defect is often enhanced under these conditions by a reconstruction of the levator muscle as well. In addition, the amount of scarring that is seen would probably indicate the desirability of using a posterior pharyngeal flap or some other type of pharyngoplasty as well.

Hard palate fistulae are about the most difficult of all tissue defects to close (Fig. 17.7). Dr James Barrett Brown used to say that closing such a defect was 'like trying to sew up a knot hole in a wooden board'. (Personal communication.)

I have found it virtually impossible to achieve a dependable closure of even the smallest hard palatal fistula by simply sewing the edges together or by creating overlapping turnover flaps. The vomer flap may achieve good closure even when the underside is left raw. More often, however, I have found it necessary to raise a sizeable adjacent flap of oral mucosa and periosteum, even though

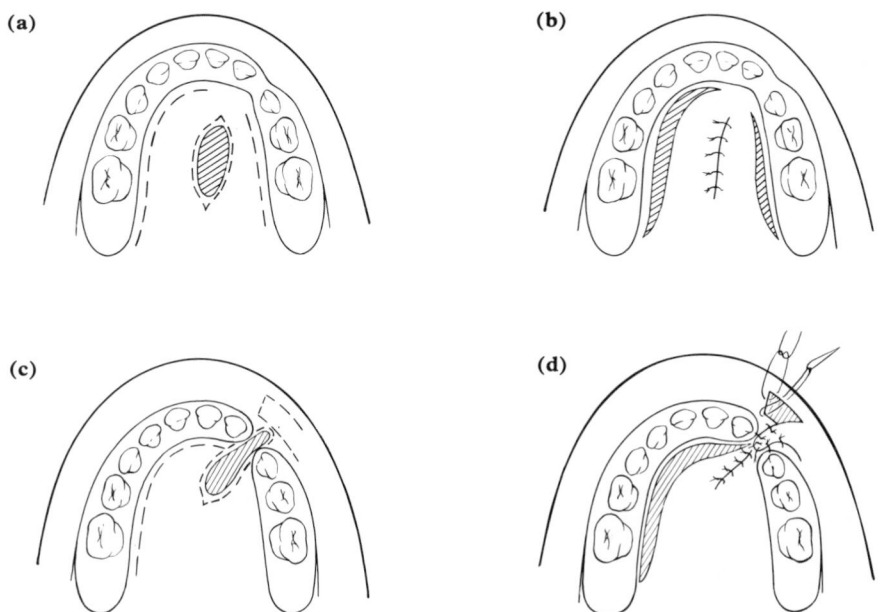

Fig. 17.7 Fistulae in the hard palate can seldom be closed without raising a sizeable flap of adjacent mucosa and periosteum (a & b). A laterally based flap from the buccal sulcus is useful in closing alveolar fistulae and can be used in conjunction with palatal flaps (c & d)

it may slide a matter of only a few millimetres. It is often possible to use tissue that has epithelialized over raw bone at the initial procedure, and if a good oral closure is achieved under these conditions, it is usually not necessary to achieve a nasal closure. The blood supply should be looked at carefully when extensive scarred conditions are present because it may be poor and indicate likely failure.

A very valuable flap of mucosa can be found in the labial mucosa adjacent to the gingival buccal sulcus where a flap based laterally can be used to close alveolar clefts and at times can reach as far as the incisive foramen. The gingival tissue should be reflected to achieve good edge-to-edge closure. This labial mucosa flap does not need to be lined, but if a bone graft is to be used in this area, it is better if a nasal lining is achieved.

Large palatal defects of either the hard or soft palate are usually the result of a sequence of events which probably have produced considerable scarring and shortening of the soft palate. Atrophy of muscles is often seen, and frequently the patient will have very poor oral hygiene. No surgical procedure in the mouth will heal well under these conditions. High bacterial counts have been shown to be harmful in skin graft survival and in wound healing. Healing in the mouth should be no exception. The dental problems should be cleared as much as possible prior to palatal surgery.

In addition, it may be important to include the use of a dental prosthesis as part of the overall plan, and good oral hygiene is essential if this approach is used. Prosthodontists have salvaged many 'surgical cripples' who have had repeated poor surgery in years past. Fortunately, these poor surgical cases have been seen less frequently in recent years.

Surgical repair of large palatal defects may require the use of additional pedicle flap tissue brought in from a distance. Surprising length can be obtained in a superiorly based posterior pharyngeal flap. With good intraoral exposure, or with a lateral cervical pharyngostomy, sufficient length can be obtained to develop a flap that can almost reach to the incisive foramen. Such pedicle flaps should preferably be 'lined' either with adjacent mucosa or with a free skin graft. The dorsum of the tongue can provide considerable pedicle flap tissue (Guerrero Santos et al 1967) and, if necessary, the full thickness of the septum can be turned down based on its inferior attachment (Edgerton & DeVito 1963). This flap provides mucosa on both sides with cartilage in between. A sizeable septal perforation results, but is a good trade-off.

Tube pedicle flaps from a distance are largely a thing of the past because of recent developments for obtaining excellent local and myocutaneous flaps. Sizeable amounts of tissue, however, can be moved into the oral cavity based either on the sternocleidomastoid muscle or superiorly based flaps of platysma muscle. Myocutaneous flaps have recently been used for large defects produced by surgery for malignancies, and it would seem to be only a matter of time before they are adapted to problems of clefts.

Alveolar ridge distortions

Distortions of the alveolar ridge are, strictly speaking, outside the palatal cleft area, but there is no question that they are closely associated and frequently affected by palatal surgery. Accordingly, some time should be spent discussing this area of secondary problems. Furthermore, the dento-alveolar ridge is an important 'articulator' in the production of sounds in most languages. The [s], [sh], [t], and [th] sounds are all recognized as those requiring anterior articulation and frequently they are misarticulated by the child with a cleft.

Secondary surgical problems usually relate to steps taken either to stabilize a 'floating' premaxillary segment in the complete bilateral cleft, or to reposition alveolar segments or the entire maxilla in problems of maxillary collapse or maxillary underdevelopment (Obwegeser 1971). In addition, surgical procedures to correct a relatively prognathic mandible should be considered in those patients (Dingman 1971).

In general, these surgical steps are not taken until the permanent teeth are fully erupted and cleared of caries. For stabilization of the premaxilla in complete bilateral clefts, I prefer to obtain a good closure of the alveolar clefts at one stage and to graft the bony cleft at a seond stage, using rib as a source of autogenous material (Fig. 17.8).

The approach is made through the buccal sulcus and the grafts are used primarily as onlay grafts wired to the nasal process of the maxilla and to the nasal spine. Often, additional layers of split rib can be used to add fullness in the middle one-third of the face, an area which usually shows significant retrusion in these patients. Additional chips of bone can be packed into the alveolar cleft. Good soft tissue coverage is essential.

A variety of ingenious surgical procedures have been described to correct the defects seen in the maxillary segments associated with clefts. In general, these

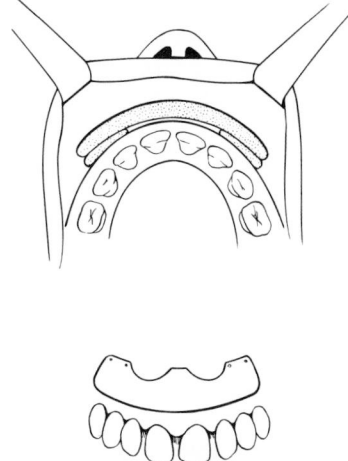

Fig. 17.8 After soft tissue closure in the alveolar area is obtained, split rib onlay grafts can be useful in stabilizing a 'floating' premaxilla in bilateral clefts or in adding bone to a retruded maxilla. Access is obtained through the buccal sulcus and stabilization is with wires to the nasal process of the maxilla and the nasal spine

procedures need careful co-ordination with orthodontic and prosthodontic planning. Relapse has been a discouraging aspect to this type of surgery, but when successful, the benefits are numerous.

Much has been done recently with aggressive orthodontia in moving large segments of alveolus. Though most of such repositioning can also be done in infancy without too much effort, the new position must be held with a retaining shell in place for prolonged periods of time or much of what was gained will be lost. About two-thirds of the patients who have had conservative surgery on their palates will not need such radical orthodontia. For these reasons and because of the problems of prolonged retention, many clinics in the United States have decided to do little or no orthodontic repositioning in the infant or with the deciduous dentition, but rather to confine all the orthodontic efforts to the permanent dentition. Little of this dental care is covered by insurance in the United States and must be paid for privately or through state cleft palate programmes.

Moderate displacements of the alveolar segments in the older child or adult, if not severe, can be overcome orthodontically, thus avoiding surgical repositioning. If the displacements are severe, careful bony surgery with bone grafting and co-ordinated planning with the orthodontist has achieved a great deal. A severely collapsed lateral maxilla, a badly positioned premaxilla, a severe anterior open bite or a badly retruded maxilla can all be approached surgically by selected osteotomies and bone grafts. Many of these deformities are associated with similar mandibular problems, though the most frequently seen mandibular problem is a relative or actual prognathism or protruding mandible. Osteotomies are useful in correcting this problem and must be co-ordinated with the necessary surgery and orthodontia in the maxilla.

Relapse is probably the most frequent complication of this type of surgery and is usually averted by overcorrecting the deformity. Infection leading to osteomyelitis and complete loss of bone grafts or non-union of the segments is not very frequent. Of course, when large segments are moved their blood supply must be maintained, or else the alveolar segment itself will be lost.

More and more it has become evident that if there is no velopharyngeal incompetence prior to maxillary surgery, forward repositioning the entire maxilla is not very likely to produce palatal incompetence. Further, it seems apparent that a tight posterior pharyngeal flap augments the forces leading to relapse of maxillary repositioning so that a lengthening procedure should be carried out on the posterior pharyngeal flap under these circumstances. Alternatively, the PPF can be severed and then replaced if needed after the maxilla is stable. On the other hand, appreciable nasorespiratory obstruction is often a problem in these patients and, if present, the proper positioning of the maxilla can greatly improve the nasal airway.

The greatest problems involve combinations of the above possible palatal problems, alveolar malposition, speech problems missing teeth and palatal fistulae. These cases require the greatest care in diagnosing exactly what the problems are, what steps should be taken to correct them and to co-ordinate the efforts of the specialists involved.

SUMMARY

The secondary surgical problems of cleft palate have been reviewed, emphasizing the importance of speech and discussing velopharyngeal incompetence, soft and hard palatal fistulae, and surgical problems of the alveolus. The co-operative efforts of the specialists involved are needed for proper diagnosis, planning, co-ordination, and completion of the necessary steps.

REFERENCES

Blocksma R 1963 Correction of velopharyngeal insufficiency by Silastic pharyngeal implants. Plastic and Reconstructive Surgery 31: 268

Bluestone C D, Musgrave R H, McWilliams B J, Crozier P A 1968 Teflon injection pharyngoplasty. Cleft Palate Journal 5: 19

Braithwaite F, Maurice D 1968 The importance of the levator palati muscle in cleft palate closure. British Journal of Plastic Surgery 21: 60

Dickson D R, Dickson W M 1972 Velopharyngeal anatomy. Journal of Speech and Hearing Research 15: 372

Dingman R O 1971 Surgical correction of mandibular deformities. In: Grabb W C, Rosenstein S W, Bzoch K W (eds) Cleft lip and palate, Little, Brown, Boston, ch 34

Edgerton M T, DeVito R V 1963 Closure of palatal defects by means of a hinged nasal septum flap. Plastic and Reconstructive Surgery 31: 537

Graham, W P III, Hamilton R, Randall P, Winchester R, Stool S 1973 Complications following posterior pharyngeal flap surgery. Cleft Palate Journal 10: 179

Guerrero Santos J, Garay J, Torres A 1967 Tongue flap with triple fixation in secondary cleft palate surgery. In: Transactions of the fourth international congress of plastic and reconstructive surgery, Excerpta Medica Foundation, Amsterdam, p 396

Hamlen M 1970 Speech results after pharyngeal flap surgery. Plastic and Reconstructive Surgery 46: 437

Hogan M 1973 A clarification of the surgical goals in cleft palate speech and the introduction of Lateral port control (LPC) pharyngeal flaps. Cleft Palate Journal 10: 337

Hönig C A 1964 In: Schuchardt K Treatment of Patients with clefts of lip, alveolus and palate. Thieme, Stuttgart 207

Hynes W 1956 Pharyngoplasty by muscle transplantation. British Journal of Plastic Surgery 3: 128–135

Jackson I T, Silverton J S 1977 The sphincter pharyngoplasty as a secondary procedure in cleft palates. Plastic and Reconstructive Surgery 59: 518

Kapetansky D I 1973 Bilateral transverse pharyngeal flaps for repair of cleft palate. Plastic and Reconstructive Surgery 52: 52

Kriens O B 1970 Fundamental anatomic findings for an intravelar veloplasty. Cleft Palate Journal 7: 27

Millard D R Jr 1963 The island flap in cleft palate surgery. Surgery Gynecology and Obstetrics 116: 297

Moore F T 1960 A new operation to cure nasopharyngeal incompetence. British Journal of Surgery 47: 424

Obwegeser H L 1971 Surgical correction of maxillary deformities. In: Grabb W C, Rosenstein S W, Bzoch K R (eds) Cleft lip and palate. Little, Brown, Boston, ch 35, p 451

Orticochea M 1968 Construction of a dynamic muscle sphincter in cleft palates. Plastic and Reconstructive Surgery 41: 323

Owsley J Q Jr, Lawson L, Miller E R 1970 Speech results from the high attached pharyngeal flap operation. Plastic and Reconstructive Surgery 7: 306

Pigott R W 1975 The results of nasopharyngoscopic assessment of pharyngoplasty. Scandinavian Journal of Plastic and Reconstructive Surgery 8: 148

Randall P 1972 Surgery for cleft palate. In: Goldwyn R (ed) The unfavorable result in plastic surgery. Little Brown, Boston, ch 10, p 125–145

Randall, P, Whitaker, L A, Noone R B, Jones III W D 1978 The case for the inferiorly based posterior pharyngeal flap. Cleft Palate Journal 15: 262

Rees T D 1964 Operations for the correction of palatopharyngeal incompetence. In: Converse J M (ed) Reconstructive Plastic Surgery, W B Saunders, Philadelphia

Shprintzen R J, Lewin M L, Croft C B, Daniller A I, Argamaso R V, Ship A G, Strauch B 1979 A comprehensive study of pharyngeal flap surgery: tailor-made flaps. Cleft Palate Journal 16: 46

Skolnick M L, McCall G N, Barnes M 1973 The sphincter mechanism of velopharyngeal closure. Cleft Palate Journal 10: 286

Skoog T 1965 The pharyngeal flap operation in cleft palate. British Journal of Plastic Surgery 18: 265

Sullivan D E 1961 Bilateral pharyngoplasty as an aid to velopharyngeal closure. Plastic and Reconstructive Surgery 27: 31

Whitaker L A, Randall P, Graham W P III, Hamilton R W, Winchester R 1972 A prospective and randomized series comparing superiorly and inferiorly based posterior pharyngeal flaps. . Cleft Palate Journal 9: 304

18

Prosthodontic considerations in speech management

Modern plastic surgical techniques have eliminated most of the gross facial deformities and the speech and other functional problems associated with the cleft palate anomaly. However, the facial and intra-oral appearance of the surgically treated cleft lip and palate patient is inevitably altered, frequently making prosthodontic treatment essential.

The prosthodontist's role has evolved from one of mere plugging of morphologic defects with suitable materials, to scientifically based techniques which are intricate and ingenious, and involve an understanding of the several morphologic hard and soft tissue variants which are frequently encountered (Table

Table 18.1 Soft and hard tissue variants frequently encountered in cleft palate patients

Soft tissue	Hard tissue
1. Upper lip is thin, short and scarred	1. Skeletal malrelationships
2. Residual fistulae in residual alveolus, mucolabial fold, hard or soft palate	(a) Maxillary retrusion
	(b) Altered mandibular rest position
3. Anatomic disproportion between palate and posterior pharynx	2. Occlusal malrelationships
	(a) Anterior and posterior cross-bites
	(b) Anterior open bite, posterior infra-occlusion
	3. Missing teeth and supernumary teeth
	4. Malformed anomalous teeth
	(a) Hypoplasia
	(b) Peg teeth
	5. Malposed teeth
	(a) Rotated teeth
	(b) Tilted teeth
	(c) Transposed teeth

18.1). The prosthodontist plays a major role in correcting the cosmetic and masticatory problems which result from this anomaly, as well as an important adjunctive role in speech rehabilitation. The modern team approach to treatment ensures that morphologic defects and functional shortcomings can usually be overcome by surgical and/or prosthodontic management. However, the ability of the patient to use the restored mechanism to speak effectively will depend on other behavioural and psychological variables for which the speech pathologist is best qualified to diagnose and recommend treatment.

The role of the prosthodontist on the cleft palate team can begin with the fabrication of a neonatal prosthesis, which is a resilient mouth-guard like, maxillary obturator used as a feeding aid. As the child develops and matures, the role becomes one of ongoing obturator therapy which seeks to reinforce proper speech patterns. During adolescence, orthodontic and routine conservative dental treatment are the major dental initiatives taken. Towards the end of adolescence, the prosthodontic role becomes more prominent, since permanent restorations can then be planned as an integral part of the patient's long-term cosmetic and functional rehabilitation.

This chapter aims at describing some of the prosthodontic considerations in the cleft palate team's effort to help the patient achieve socially acceptable speech.

INDICATIONS AND CONTRAINDICATIONS FOR PROSTHODONTIC TREATMENT

Prosthodontic therapy is prescribed instead of, or else after, surgical therapy has proved unsuccessful. As a result of research in growth and development, biomaterials, and the longitudinal effects of different types of dental and surgical treatments the indications for prosthetic intervention are reasonably explicit. They include:

1. Clefts of the hard and/or soft palate with insufficient local tissue available for a surgical repair (Fig. 18.1)

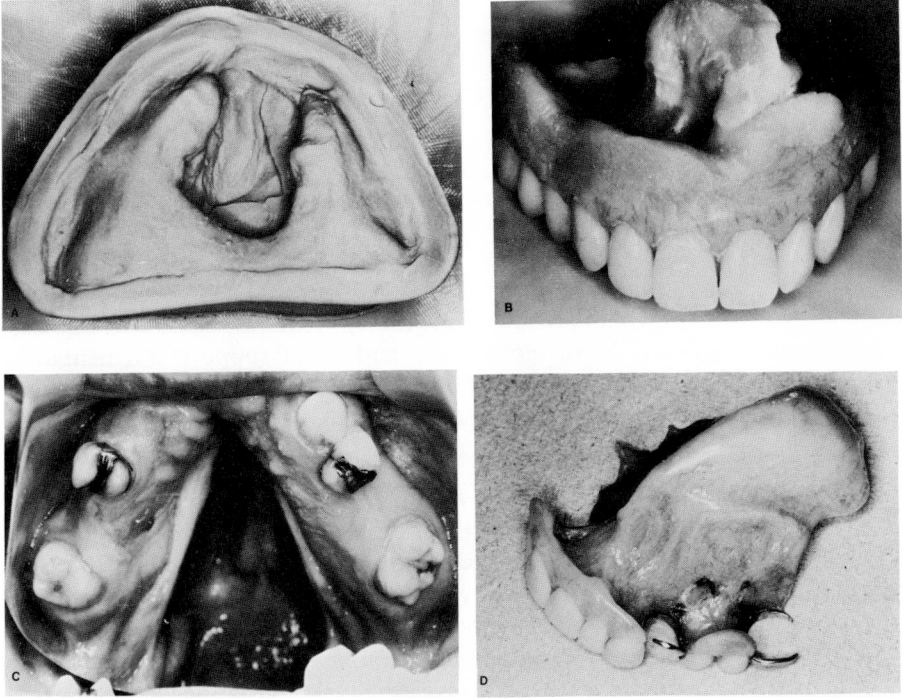

Fig. 18.1 (a) Stone cast of a hard palatal cleft and (c) intra-oral view of both a hard and soft palatal cleft; (b) and (d) show the prostheses fabricated for (a) and (c) respectively

2. Children in whom surgery is contraindicated, or is to be delayed, for systemic health reasons
3. Adult patients
4. Neuromuscular disease or disturbance of the soft palate and pharynx
5. Operated patients in whom one or more of the following conditions is present: velopharyngeal insufficiency resulting from scarring and/or soft palatal immobility, an inadequate pharyngoplasty, residual palatal fistula(e) (Fig. 18.2)

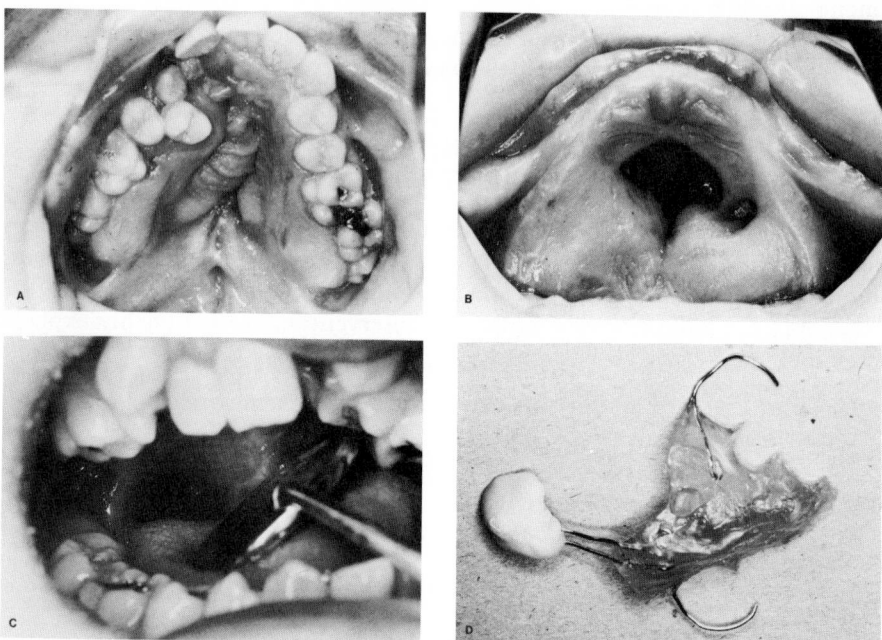

Fig. 18.2 Three postoperative patients needing prosthodontic treatment. In (a) the soft palate is immobile because of excessive scarring. The large residual hard palatal fistula in (b) was obturated with a prosthesis. The prosthesis in (d) was used to obturate the inefficient portal in (c); in this patient cranial nerve involvement interfered with lateral pharyngeal wall movement, with a resultant post-pharyngoplasty hypernasality

6. Those patients for whom prosthodontic therapy is required for cosmetic and functional purposes: tooth replacement and labial support, augmentation or restoration of dental arch morphology, restoration of vertical dimension of occlusion (morphologic face height) (Fig. 18.3)

Contraindications to treatment may be considered as:

1. Intra-oral contraindications. The obvious ones are poor oral hygiene, advanced periodontal disease, and a high caries rate. All three conditions occurring singly or concomitantly militate against prosthodontic treatment. However, compromise treatment is frequently prescribed since non-intervention may lead to worse cosmetic and functional problems.
2. Patient contraindications. A patient may be unco-operative for medical, systemic or psychological reasons (e.g. severe mental retardation). Unmotivated or unco-operative patients will maximize the biologic price exacted by the prosthodontic intervention, and frustrate the prosthodontist's efforts to main-

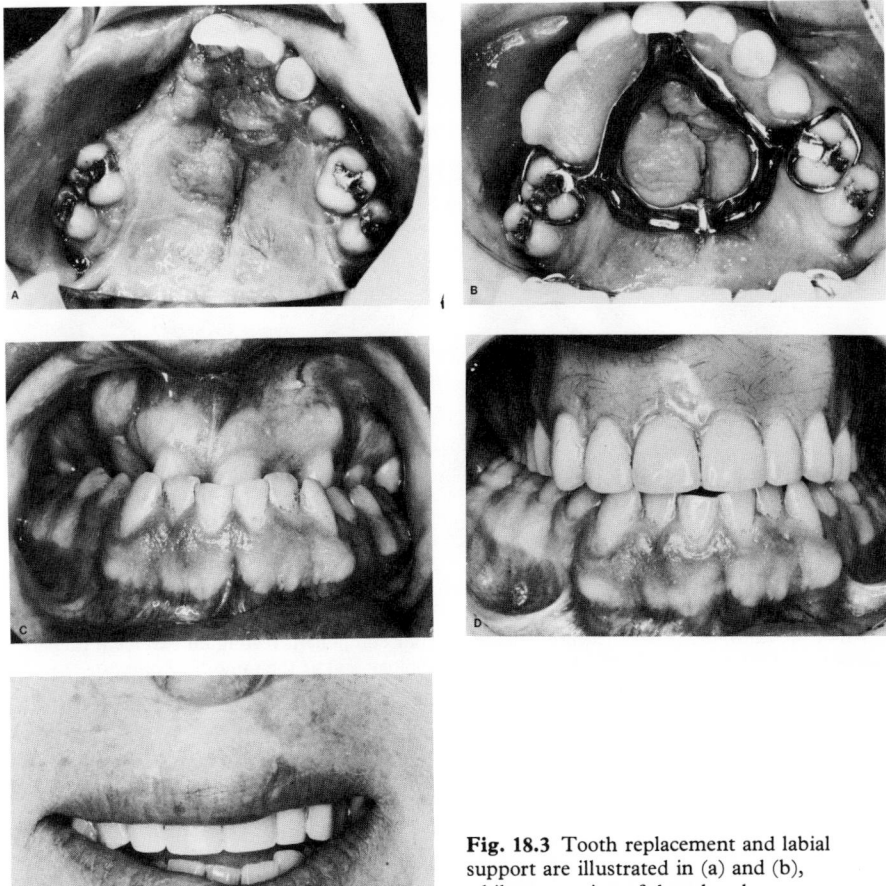

Fig. 18.3 Tooth replacement and labial support are illustrated in (a) and (b), while restoration of dental arch morphology and morphologic free height are clearly evident in (c), (d) and (e)

tain and prolong the integrity of his reconstruction. The poor systemic health of a few patients contraindicates complex dental treatment with its long, arduous procedures. The objective with such patients is a compromise, palliative type of treatment with close monitoring of the masticatory system. The lack of availability of a skilled and qualified dentist is also a contraindication to prosthodontic treatment. Finally, from a practical standpoint, in some circumstances the patient's fiscal commitment may also be considered. The good clinician must be resilient and sensitive, and able to modify treatment plans so as to maintain a balance between a patient's fiscal realities and one or more restorative programmes.

METHODS OF PROSTHODONTIC TREATMENT

These usually consist of removable prostheses which are designed according to the existing palatal function morphology, as well as the age of the patient and the dental structures present.

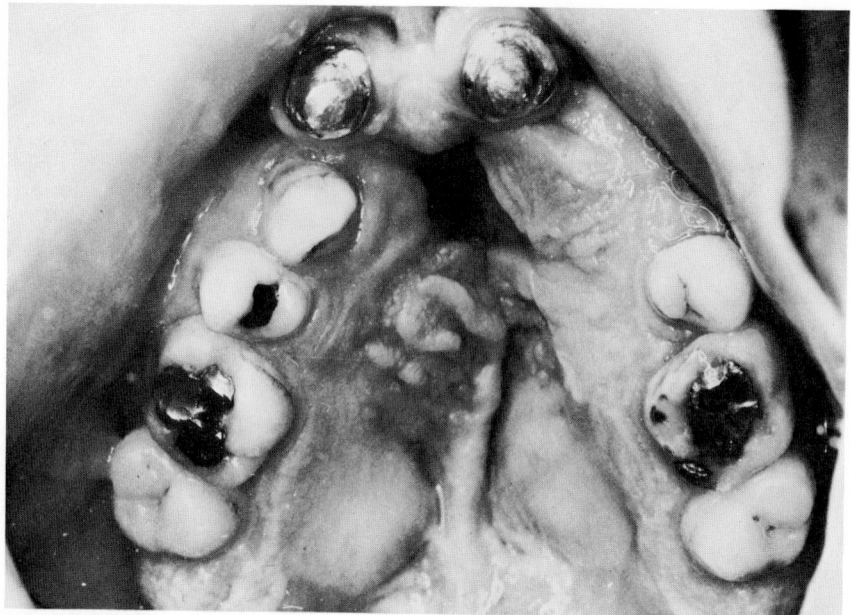

Fig. 18.4 A removable partial denture with an anterior component resting on two teeth prepared with cast-gold crowns will restore dental arch morphology and at the same time obturate the residual fistula

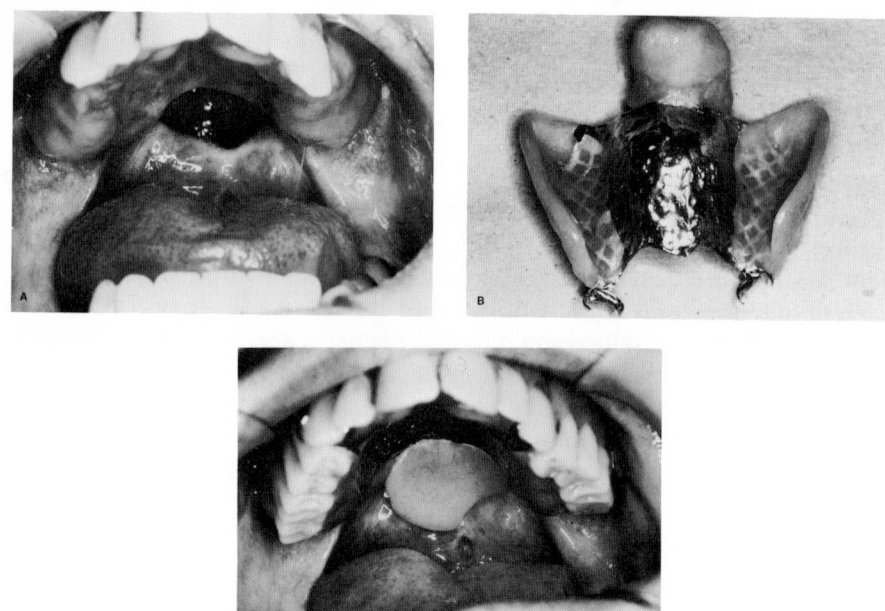

Fig. 18.5 The residual soft palate fistula in (a) is obturated by a prosthesis, as seen in (b) and (c)

Residual fistulae in hard or soft palate, alveolus, mucolabial fold
Some authors believe that most labial and hard palatal fistulae do not affect speech or deglutition and therefore do not require obturation. However, evaluation by a speech pathologist and testing with temporary soft wax obturation should be first carried out. Careful questioning with regard to fluid escape into the nasal cavity during swallowing, will further determine the need for obturation. A new surgical attempt at fistula closure may be successful, but such successes are limited when excessive scar tissue is already present. The patient's prosthesis must then be designed with an obturator component. Either a removable acrylic resin palatal base or labial flange in combination with a fixed partial denture can be used, or a removable partial denture designed to fulfil the dual objectives of hard and soft tissue replacement (Fig. 18.4).

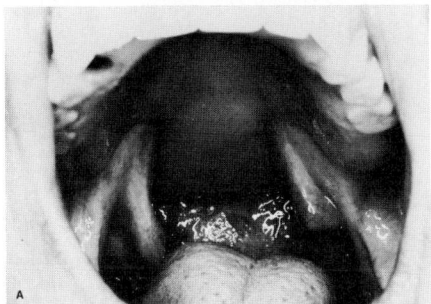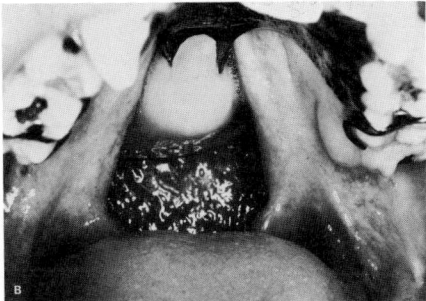

Fig. 18.6 Obturation of unrepaired soft palates in edentulous (a) and dentulous (b) patients

The occasional occurrence of a soft palatal defect can be obturated by an abbreviated strap-and-bulb prosthesis design (Fig. 18.5). If this defect is accompanied by velopharyngeal incompetence, the prosthetic design and fabrication of the speech-aid appliance is facilitated by a pre-prosthetic surgical snipping of the inferior boundary of the fistula. The defect is then treated in a manner identical to that of obturating an unrepaired soft palate (Fig. 18.6).

Velopharyngeal incompetence due to an anatomic disproportion between palate and posterior pharynx
When the repaired soft palate is short, or the pharynx is too deep to ensure adequate valving, a prosthesis design is required which employs the principle of soft palate lift combined with obturation of the residual velopharyngeal lumen (Fig. 18.7). The amount of soft palatal lift obtained is limited by the displacability of the soft palate, which in turn depends upon its rigidity and degree of scarring. The more mobile or displacable the soft palate, the greater will be the lift provided by the strap or palatal extension section of the prosthesis (and this section will also be concomitantly wider on the prosthesis itself), and the pharyngeal section will be correspondingly smaller. If the soft palate is taut and immobile, the pharyngeal part of the prosthesis does the obturating *in toto*, since the strap or palatal extension will serve only as a narrow connector between the pharyngeal and the maxillary sections. In both situations the possible torque which may be exerted on the abutment teeth must be kept in mind. This torque

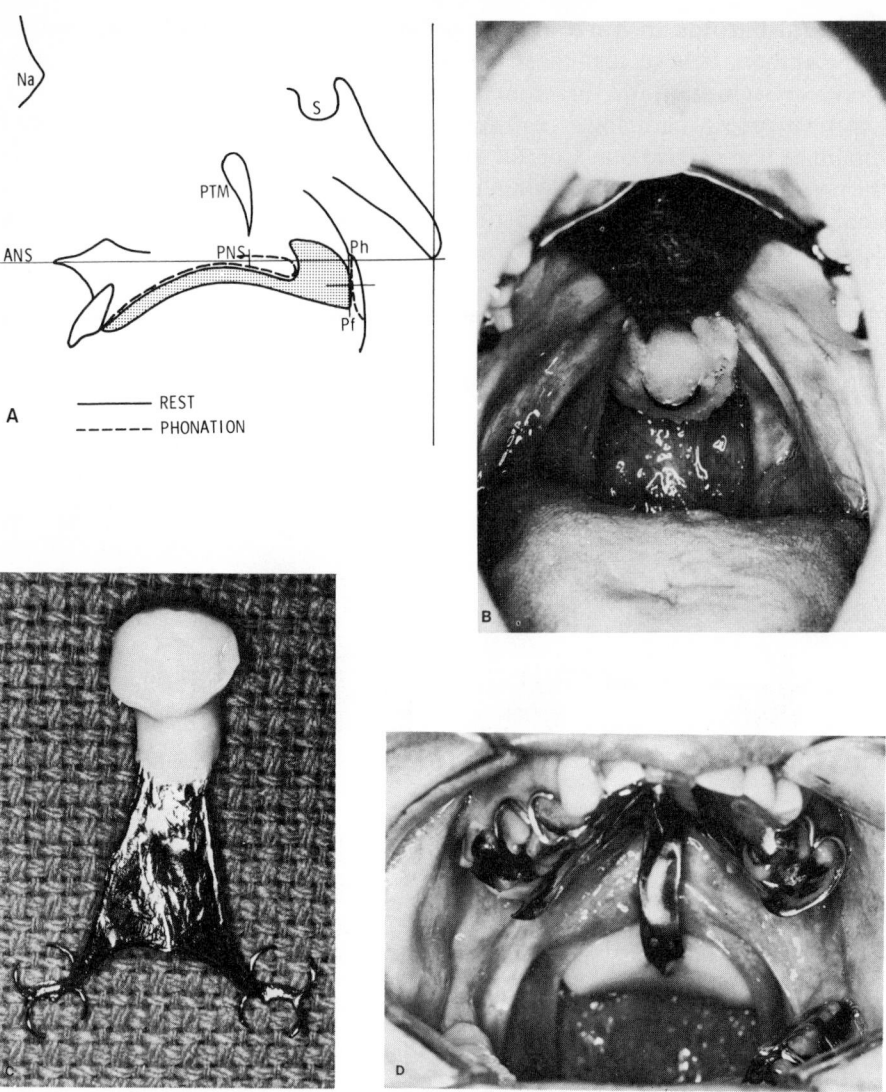

Fig. 18.7 (a) A palatal lift prosthesis is shown in a mid-line cephalometric tracing (ANS = anterior nasal spine, PNS = posterior nasal spine, Ph = posterior pharyngeal wall, Pf = posterior pharyngeal wall during phonation). (b) Intra-oral view of prosthesis (c), which provides lift to the displacable soft palate as well as a prosthetic pharyngeal section. In (d) the strap serves as a connector from the palatal to the pharyngeal sections, without providing a lift for the immobile residual soft palate

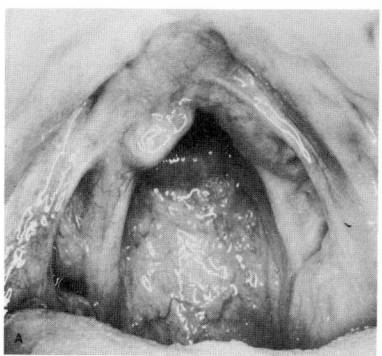
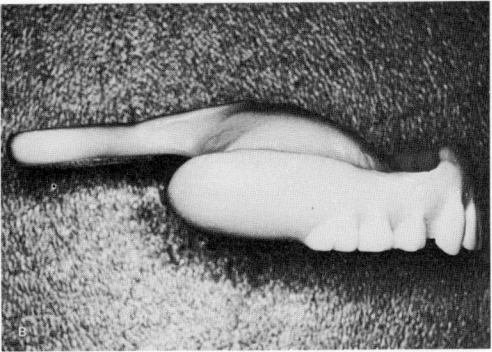

Fig. 18.8 (a) An edentulous maxilla with repaired incompetent soft palate is treated with a complete denture (b), carrying a strap for soft palatal support, combined with a nasopharyngeal section to complete obturation. Denture retention was adequate to withstand the downward tug of the relatively mobile soft palate

is easily countered by careful abutment selection and clasp design in healthy, nearly intact dentitions. This is not always the case in a depleted dentition or edentulous state (Fig. 18.8), and sometimes the objective of optimal palato-pharyngeal valving may be compromised.

Velopharyngeal incompetence due to an immobile palate without disproportion

The objective of the prosthesis here is to elevate the soft palate to a position approximating that of normal retraction, thereby narrowing the nasopharyngeal orifice (Fig. 18.9). The desired closure can be verified on a lateral cephalometric film and fluoroscopy using audio-video tape. This technique is also the one used in treating patients with neuromuscular difficulties and depends on the retentive and stabilizing qualities of the maxillary part of the prosthesis design.

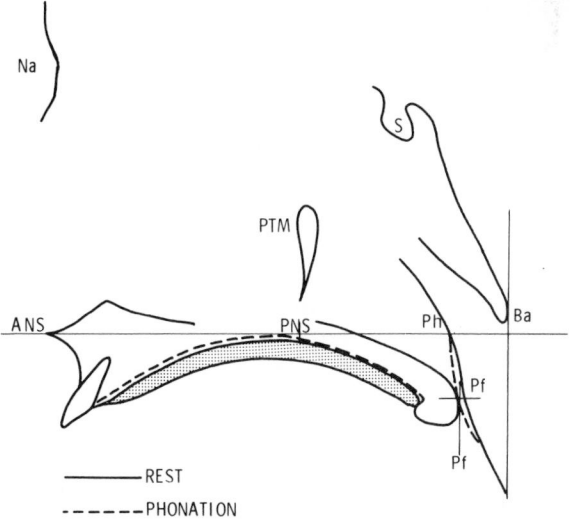

Fig. 18.9 A mid-line cephalometric tracing of a patient with a palatal lift prosthesis elevating the soft palate to the appropriate level

DENTAL AND AGE CONSIDERATIONS

The reader may find it convenient at this stage to have the methods of prosthodontic treatment discussed in the context of the patient's age and state of dental
structures present. Speech prostheses constructed for the child are interim ones,
since anticipated changes in facial, dental and palatal growth and development
will require modifications to the prosthesis. The proposed abutment teeth in
this age group do not usually lend themselves to adequate prosthesis retention.
Therefore orthodontic bands with buccal tubes are fitted to the abutment teeth
to ensure retention of the prosthesis. Wrought-wire clasps are used for retention,

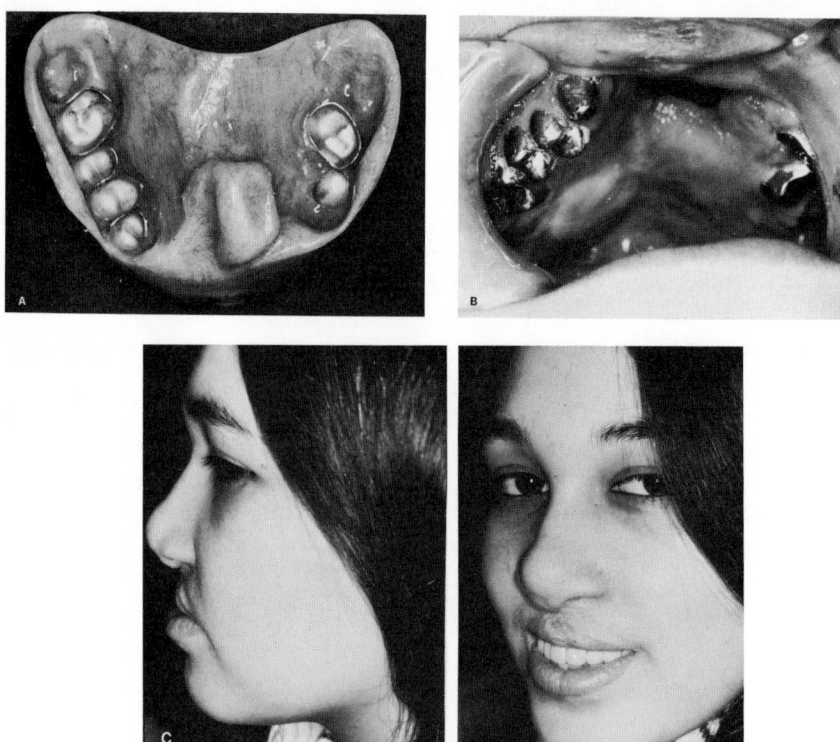

Fig. 18.10 A complete maxillary overdenture (a) alleviates the disharmony in the size and
relationship of the dental arches. Prepared maxillary teeth are restored with cast-gold copings (b).
The result (c)

and the prosthesis is made out of a pink or clear acrylic resin. The palatal part
of the prosthesis is made out of acrylic resin if it is to act as a soft palatal cleft,
or a cast-metal bar if it is to function as a connector of maxillary and pharyngeal
parts. The pharyngeal part of the prosthesis is preferably made out of clear
acrylic resin to facilitate the clinician's ability to determine any areas of soft
tissue impingement. A multistage procedure is used in the fabrication of the
speech component so as to provide the child with enhanced scope for easy
adaptation. Blakeley (1964) reported that obturator use may stimulate muscle
movement as treatment progresses, necessitating a reduction in the size of the
pharyngeal section of the prosthesis. The conditions under which obturator re-

duction will influence pharyngeal wall movements appear to be limited, and are still not identified (Shelton et al 1971).

The late adolescent group has usually completed growth and development and is frequently undergoing or has recently completed orthodontic treatment. This group demands the most meticulous dental/speech pathology treatment planning, since if the speech prognosis depends upon a prosthodontic intervention, the prosthesis design and its implications must be carefully analysed.

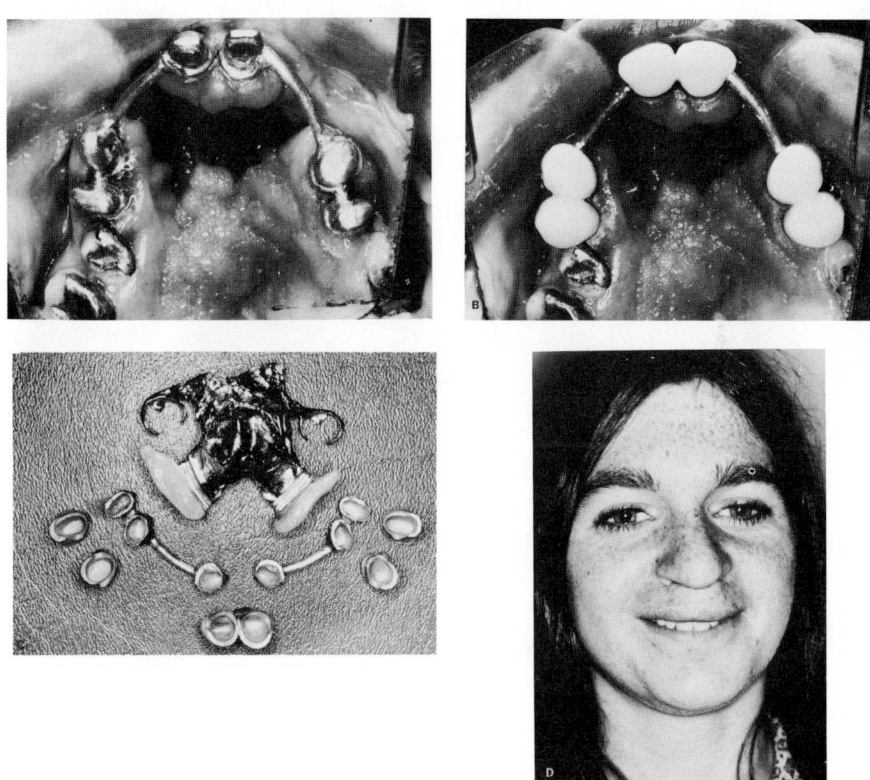

Fig. 18.11 In (a) the mobile premaxillary segment is splinted via cast-gold crowns and bars to other similarly restored teeth (b). A combination of porcelain veneer crowns and a removable partial denture (c) complete the 'jigsaw' treatment puzzle prescribed for this patient with an excellent cosmetic (d) and functional result

Speech prostheses have to be stable and well retained to be effective. This is accomplished by a prosthesis design which is clasped or locked onto healthy natural or prepared teeth. Luckily the vast majority of adolescent patients we treat present with dentitions in a reasonable state of health* and most designs consist of variations on a theme of designing conventional removable partial dentures. Some adolescents present with disharmonies in the size and relationships of the maxillary and mandibular dental arches. These patients require a prosthetic design which not only obturates defects or provides soft palatal support, but which compensates for mid-facial retrusion and inadequate

* This may not be the case universally!

development of vertical dimension of occlusion. Overdentures, of the partial or complete variety, are usually resorted to with excellent clinical results (Fig. 18.10). This type of treatment is most demanding of the patient because of its inherent potential to entrap plaque in intimate contact with vulnerable gingival and enamel tissues. An impeccable plaque-free oral environment is mandatory for success, and both dentist and speech pathologist must do everything possible to motivate these patients in preventive dental care measures.

In the adult, the designed prosthesis is more permanent, and Stellite alloy (chrome cobalt) castings are frequently used. Abutment teeth are frequently restored and/or prepared for optimal retention, with gold or porcelain baked

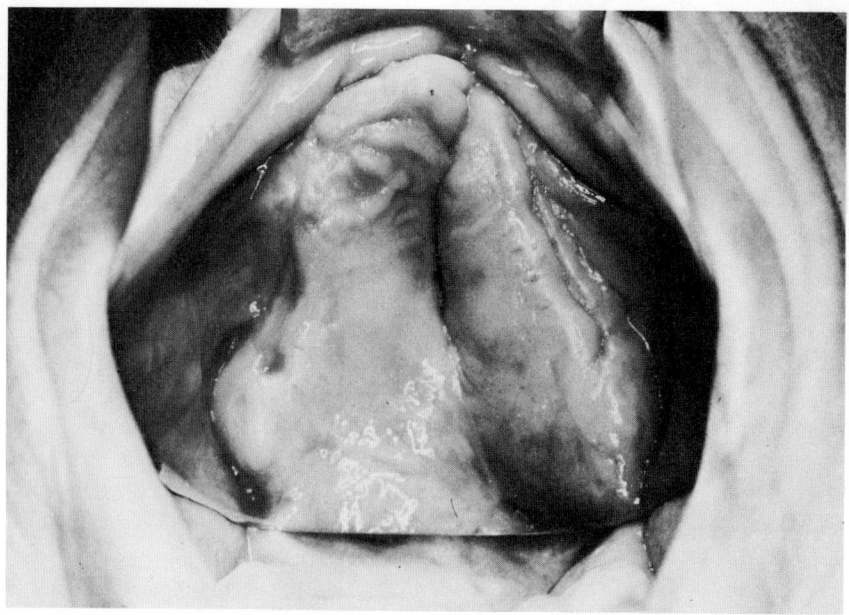

Fig. 18.12 An edentulous maxilla which demonstrates minimal sulcus depth (space between alveolar ridge and labial or cheek mucosa) and poor potential for even conventional prosthesis retention. A cleft palate prosthesis with a speech and extension is probably not feasible unless an increased area of retention is created surgically

to gold crowns (Fig. 18.11). Regrettably, a very large number of our older cleft palate patients are edentulous. The absence of abutment teeth not only presents a threat to the feasibility of a palatal lift or obturator type of design, but frequently the conventional maxillary part of the prosthesis *per se* cannot be retained (Fig. 18.12). Vestibular sulcus deepening procedures (Boucher et al 1975) may provide the prosthodontist with more denture-bearing area for achieving retention, but is still not a very good substitute for the firm retention afforded by an intact or even a depleted dentition. Speech pathologists should be vigilant in encouraging tooth retention, especially in their adult patients.

All patients will need regular follow-up of their prosthetic treatment, not only to ensure optimal oral health, but also to modify the prosthesis where necessary. Muscular changes in the nasopharyngeal area can occur, and the continued efficacy of the prosthesis depends upon the dentist's recognition of such changes and the appropriate modification of the prosthesis.

FABRICATION OF PROSTHESES

For reasons of both description and fabrication convenience, the speech prosthesis consists of three parts: (i) the maxillary section, (ii) the palatal extension, and (iii) the pharyngeal section.

Maxillary section. The principles of construction are similar to those prescribed for conventional partial or complete dentures (Boucher et al 1975, Zarb et al 1978). Impressions are made in stock trays following appropriate mouth preparation. Custom trays are next used for making final impressions which will also record the soft palatal shape. The poured working casts are used for Stellite alloy casting which is tested in the mouth for framework fit, and then tested again with the selected tooth arrangement. The artificial teeth are attached to the metal framework by means of acrylic resin, which is also the material used for the entire maxillary section if a complete denture or a complete overdenture is indicated.

Palatal extension section. This part connects the maxillary and pharyngeal sections and is usually an extension of the metal maxillary section fabricated on the working cast. When constructed out of acrylic resin it is usually reinforced by a metal insert. A metal bar palatal extension extends beyond the soft palate into the nasopharynx where it will support the next section of the prosthesis.

Pharyngeal section. This area is developed in a wax or modelling compound, or a functional impression material, and conforms to pharyngeal muscle activity. The so-called 'muscle trimming' or moulding results from patient swallowing and head rotation, flexion and extension which will reproduce an accurate recording of contact with the surrounding musculature during function. The speech pathologist's guidance at this appointment is of course indispensable. The speech bulb is adjusted until the patient can produce a clear /p/, a sustained /f/ or /s/ without nasal emission (easily determined by asking the patient to produce the required sounds, while holding a mirror under the patient's nose), as well as produce an adequate nasal sound /m/. The correction of the remaining speech differences will depend on the motivation and co-operation of the subject in overcoming misarticulation habits. Millard (1971) asserts that speech therapy is required to produce new speech patterns after the speech prosthesis is completed and describes several subjective as well as objective tests which may be employed to determine velopharyngeal adequacy.

The location of the speech bulb has caused some controversy. At one time it was believed that Passavant's pad identified the vertical locale of the nasopharyngeal portion of the prosthesis. However, the variable occurrence and location of Passavant's pad usurped its employment as a reliable landmark. Currently the bulge of the anterior tubercle of the atlas is used for bulb level orientation, keeping in mind that the area of pharyngeal constriction may occur above this locale. Aram & Subtelny (1959) studied normal subjects, and concluded that the pharyngeal section must be properly designed at the desired level. They acknowledged the existence of individual asymmetries in pharyngeal function which makes it necessary to modify the shape and placement of the pharyngeal section, and concluded that the dentist should design a bulb that is minimal in size, since the span of soft palatal tissue contacting the posterior pharyngeal wall during velopharyngeal closure was not great. A minimal mass to the speech bulb also helps relieve muscular strain and torque on the prosthesis, while contacting both lateral and posterior pharyngeal walls.

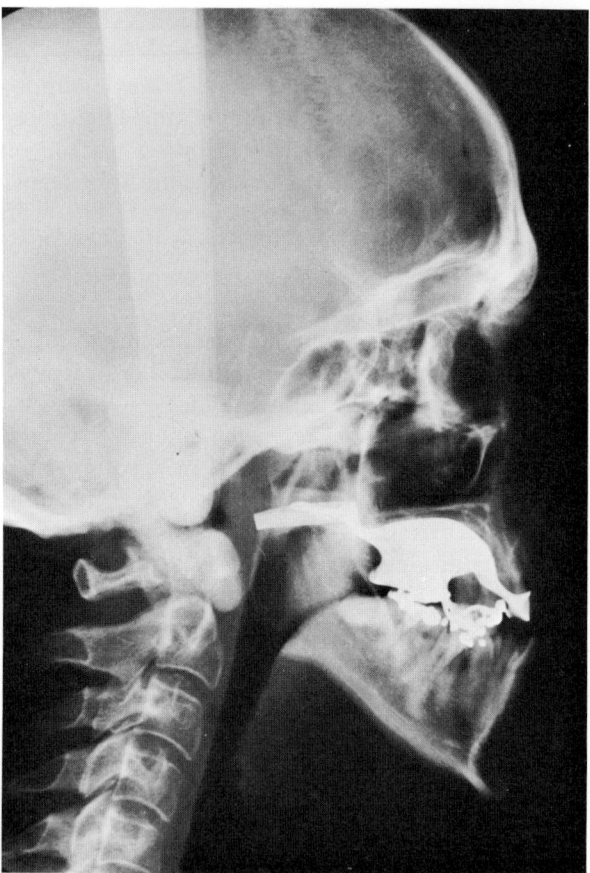

Fig. 18.13 A cephalometric radiograph of a patient with an adequate speech prosthesis. The pharyngeal section is above the palatal plane.

Aram & Subtelny (1959) also concluded from their normative data that the projected level of the hard palate serves as a 'guidepost' in approximating the region of muscular function during speech (Fig. 18.13).

Mazaheri & Millard (1965) attempted to correlate voice quality with location and dimension of the pharyngeal bulb. Their results showed that optimal bulb position varied with each individual patient. Voice quality was judged as best when the bulb was positioned in the area of greatest lateral and posterior pharyngeal wall activity.

ADVANTAGES AND DISADVANTAGES OF PROSTHODONTIC TREATMENT

The major advantage of prosthodontic treatment lies in its relative simplicity. A prosthesis is not an inhibiting factor in the growth and development of pharyngeal tissues, and can be adapted easily to the succeeding stages of the child's growth. Above all, prosthodontic treatment offers the advantage of versatility, since it can be designed to accommodate to a large variety of occlusal and arch form disturbances. A speech prosthesis can eliminate hypernasality and even the distortion of consonant sounds due to audible nasal emission, but cannot of itself correct habits of misarticulation. On the other hand, voice quality may be altered mechanically to the extreme of hyponasality by enlarging the size of the speech bulb. However, this is easily corrected by adjusting the size of the pharyngeal portion.

Some of the disadvantages accompanying treatment include: (i) the risk of undermining dental/oral health and the stability of the maxillary dentition; (ii) the discomfort which may develop from contact of the prosthesis with mucosal tissues; (iii) interference with swallowing and nasal mucus drainage; (iv) the development of mouth breathing; and (v) the obvious necessity for manual coordination and digital dexterity in handling the prosthesis and ensuring a plaque-free environment. Most of these problems can be solved by the prosthodontist's meticulous attention to detail, and by the patient's conscientious efforts to maintain good hygienic measures. When nocturnal difficulties are encountered with mouth breathing or inadequate nasal mucus drainage, the prosthesis can be left out at night. If the obturator is an integral part of an orthodontic retainer, a second bulbless retainer can be made.

Perhaps the most disappointing part of prosthodontic therapy is the recognition of less-intelligible speech following obturator wear. The prosthodontist must appreciate the limits to his adjunctive role, since the speech deficiency in such cases may not only be on a functional or habitual basis (Rosen & Bzoch 1958), but may also be related to overriding psychological factors (Shelton & Lloyd 1963). Patients who receive speech prostheses following cancer surgery, respond predictably, rapidly and almost always successfully to prosthodontic interventions. Patients with cleft palates do not. While the choice of therapy for the cleft palate patient reflects the team's preoccupation with what is best for each patient, there is no one method of predicting the success of speech improvement.

REFERENCES

Aram A, Subtelny J D 1959 Velopharyngeal function and cleft palate prostheses. Joural of Prosthetic Dentistry 9: 149–158

Blakeley R W 1964 The complementary use of speech prostheses and pharyngeal flaps in palatal insufficiency. Cleft Palate Journal 1: 194–198

Boucher C O, Hickey J C, Zarb G A 1975 Prosthodontic treatment for edentulous patients, 7th edn. C V Mosby, St Louis

Mazaheri M, Millard R T 1965 Changes in nasal resonance related to differences in location and dimension of speech bulb. Cleft Palate Journal 2: 167

Millard R T 1971 Training for optimal use of the prosthetic speech appliance. In: Grabb W C, Rosenstein S W, Bzoch K R (eds) Cleft lip and palate. Little Brown, Boston, ch 63, p 861–867

Rosen M S, Bzoch K R 1958 The prosthetic speech appliance in rehabilitation of patients with cleft palate. Journal of the American Dental Association 57: 203–210

Shelton R L, Lindquist A F, Knox A W, Wright V L, Arndt W B, Elbert M, Youngstrom K A 1971 The relationship between pharyngeal wall movements and exchangeable speech appliance sections. Cleft Palate Journal 8: 145–158

Shelton R L, Lloyd R S 1963 Prosthetic facilitation of palatopharyngeal closure. Journal of Speech and Hearing Disorders 28: 58–66

Zarb G A, Bergman B, Clayton J A, MacKay H F 1978 Prosthodontic treatment for partially edentulous patients. C V Mosby, St Louis

19

Future prospects

In this book the authors have attempted to outline current research and to illustrate present practices in the management of the cleft palate deformity. The lists of references at the end of each chapter testify to the volume of research that is being carried out, and yet every contributor has made it clear that many uncertainties persist and that there is a great deal more to learn.

One thing is certain: the subject is so complex that the need for team work is greater than ever. Combined cleft palate clinics have been in existence for many years throughout the world and yet there are still many places where specialists work in isolation, deprived of the benefit of the expertise of their colleagues in other disciplines. Sometimes this isolation is inevitable because of geographical factors, but in other cases it may be self-imposed. Under these circumstances the patients inevitably receive poorer care than they deserve, and it is hoped that the practice of combined care will continue to spread.

Another important trend is the wider recognition of the need for better counselling. The blow to parents of realizing that they have a deformed child can be greatly softened if a member of the team which will be looking after the child can, within a few days of the baby's birth, discuss plans for future treatment. Such counselling must be reinforced during the difficult first months of the child's life, and one very effective way of doing this has been described in detail in this book. The more general introduction of domiciliary supervision would be of great benefit. There is usually a need for continuing support of the family as the child grows. One of the main purposes of the combined cleft palate clinic is to provide such support, but parents often find that it is helpful to discuss their problems with parents of other similarly affected children. Associations formed for this purpose have been in existence in the United States and elsewhere for many years, and a Cleft Palate Association has recently been formed in Britain.

The enormous amount of research into all aspects of the cleft palate problem which has been undertaken in the last decade has led to some very significant advances. Among these are the new methods of investigating velopharyngeal function. The development of EMG techniques, multiview video fluoroscopy, endoscopy and aerodynamic and acoustic analysis has resulted in a far better understanding of the normal physiology of speech and of how this is distorted in the cleft palate patient. Studies using these and other modern techniques to evaluate different types of treatment should, in the next decade, clarify some of the controversies which still exist in the management of speech problems.

Improvement in the surgical treatment of cleft palate has resulted in fewer children with gross hypernasality, and this has highlighted more subtle disturbances, for example in the timing of velopharyngeal closure, in the function of other structures such as the tongue, and in oral sensation and proprioception. The acquisition of language by the child with a cleft is only now being investigated in detail. It seems to be delayed compared with the normal child, and this may be related to the fact that it is in aspects of verbal intelligence that cleft palate children appear to be less favoured, while they hold their own with unaffected children in other aspects of intelligence. Clearly, great advances can be made in the understanding of these problems in the near future.

In surgical management the great advance is in the appreciation of the importance of obtaining proper alignment of the muscles of the soft palate, which must be freed from their abnormal attachment and transposed in the same way as the muscle in the cleft lip. In other respects the recent surgical literature has revealed more areas of uncertainty than it has resolved. The influence of surgery on facial growth remains a subject of bitter contention.

Yet the cleft palate deformity is so complex in its aetiology, in its severity and in the structures that are involved that it is not surprising that investigations on growth and development involving different populations produce conflicting results. Longitudinal studies of the growth of untreated clefts will never be available, but without them the controversies about the effect of surgery on development will continue. Nevertheless, a series of carefully controlled trials comparing different surgical regimes over many years would be of great value. Equal attention would need to be paid to the assessment and reporting of both growth and speech development. Regrettably, in the past, controlled trials have been very uncommon, and while the protagonists of early surgery have concentrated on their good speech results, they have often said little about deformity. On the other hand, their opponents tend to lend more weight to recording and reporting growth, while dealing only cursorily with speech.

Unfortunately the problems involved in the design of a satisfactory trial are enormous and are unlikely to be overcome in the immediate future. One of the difficulties in comparing speech results from different centres is that assessment of speech has, of necessity, been subjective, so that it is most uncommon for one group's results to be generally accepted as better than another's. Until an objective, preferably quantitative, method of reporting cleft palate speech can be devised and find acceptance, there is little chance of ending the arguments over which regime produces the best speech. Attempts have been made to produce such a quantitative method of assessment, but are a long way from being generally satisfactory. A great deal still has to be learned about how normal speech can vary with age, sex, accent and language before a start can be made on quantifying the abnormal. However, as knowledge of speech production increases, so will the chance of more objective assessment.

Another problem is the great variation in the underlying deformity. In an attempt to introduce some degree of consistency in their reports, most authors have grouped their series into patients with unilateral and bilateral clefts of lip and palate and those with clefts of palate alone. Yet the severity of deformity can vary widely within these groups, and if some of the apparent inconsistencies in our present knowledge are to be clarified, it will be necessary to split these groups up into small subgroups for analysis. In addition, more attention needs to be paid to deformity and distortion of the soft tissues. The lack of a generally accepted classification for such detailed recording adds to the problem. Smaller subgroups imply the need for very large series, and although there is evidence that cleft lip and palate is increasing in frequency, the falling birth rate in Western countries makes it difficult for any one centre to treat enough patients for a satisfactory trial. There is, therefore, a need for large-scale, multicentre trials. Here too, of course, many problems stand in the way. Not the least of these is the need to persuade a disparate collection of enthusiasts to agree to any one plan of treatment. However, a practical first step would be for a number of centres to adopt a generally agreed way of recording the deformity, for methods of assessment and for the age at which they are carried out to be standardized, and for treatment to be recorded in an accepted manner. The adoption of such a protocol would allow a better comparison of results than at present, and might lead to a greater acceptability for a claim that one method of treatment is better than another.

Among all the uncertainties of the management of cleft palate, one rather depressing fact stands out clearly: no method of treatment has succeeded in avoiding a stubborn residue of 20 to 30 per cent of bad results. Many reasons can be suggested for this—they include those children with gross tissue deficiency, deafness, low intelligence and uninterested families, and it will be fascinating to find out, as knowledge increases, whether these results can be improved significantly.

Whatever improvements in management that continuing research may bring, differing social circumstances throughout the world will prevent any single regime of treatment from proving to be universally acceptable or appropriate. There are wide differences from place to place in the availability of resources and of the various professionals who should ideally be involved in the care of the patient with a cleft palate. These differences, and a healthy scepticism and individuality, will provide a continuing stimulus for lively discussion among those working in this fascinating field. This will lead to an ever greater understanding of the many problems affecting the child born with a cleft of the palate, who will benefit from the resulting improvement in care.

Appendix

Construction of modified Burston nursing frame for the Pierre Robin syndrome

Basic frame

A and B are the side and end pieces, C, D and E are the cross members. These are lengths of slotted angle iron—British trade name 'Handy Angle'—1.5 × 1.5 inches cross-section. (Manufacturers: Handy Angle, Uxbridge Road, Hayes, Middlesex, England.)

A is 60 cm long, B is 30 cm long, C, D and E are all 30 cm long.

1. Sections A and B are joined together with Handy Angle anchor plates.
2. The cross member C is placed 6.5 cm from rear end B.
3. The cross member D is placed 25 cm from cross member C.
4. The cross member E is placed 3 cm from the cross member D.

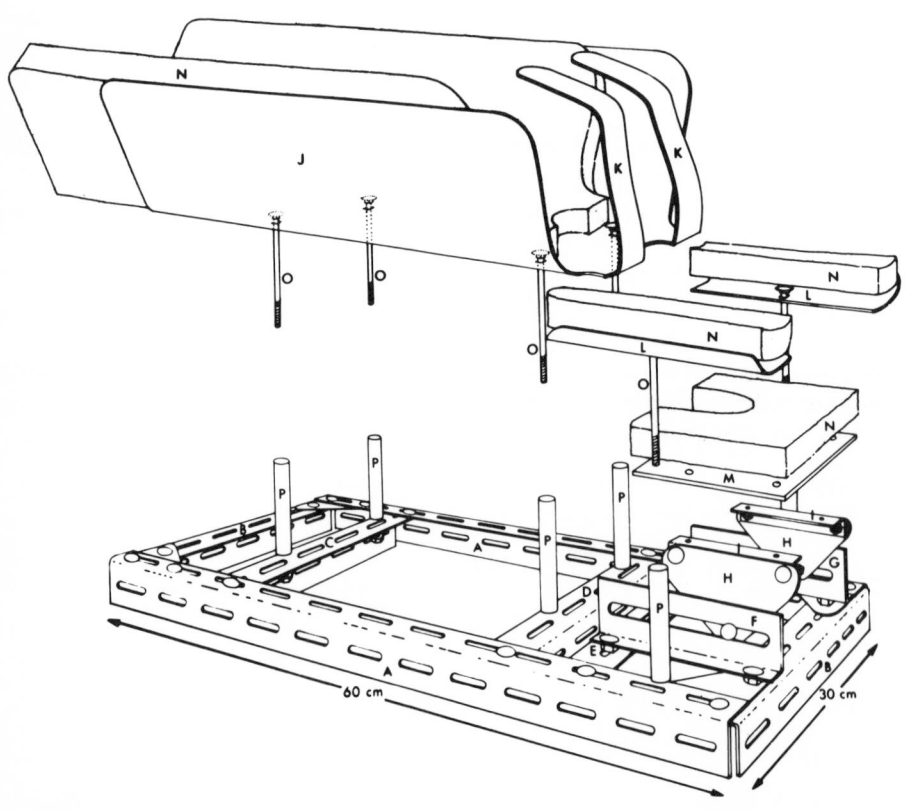

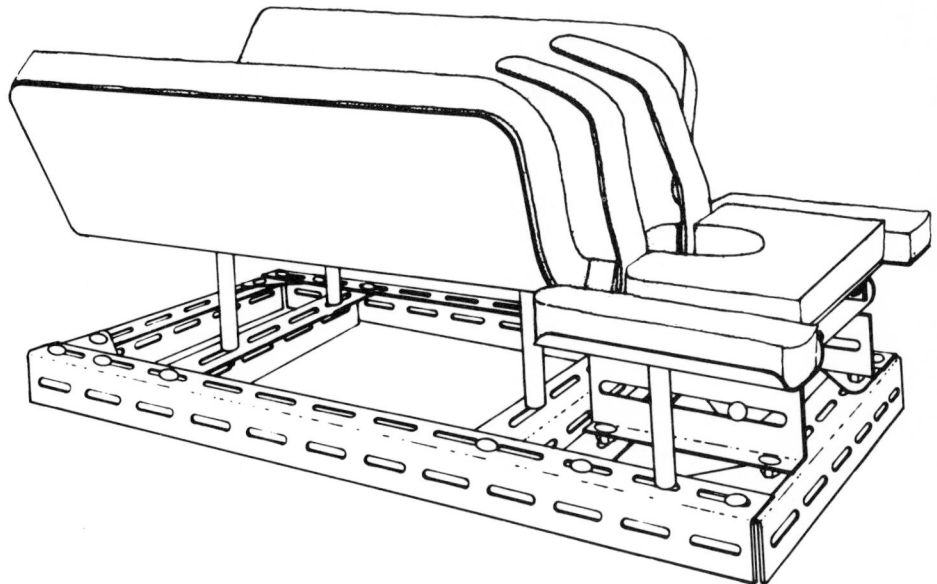

5. The supports for the head rest, parts F and G are modified slotted angle iron. These are 15 cm long; there are three slots in this length—which are made continuous to make the head rest adjustable. The distance between pieces F and G is governed by where the anchor plate joins A and B at the front end. It may be found that packers are needed under F and G to get them to the correct height, and hanger nuts as supplied with Handy Angle will serve this purpose.
6. Parts H are Handy Angle anchor plates and are attached to parts F and G.
7. I parts are modified slotted angle iron, 10 cm long. Each side of the slotted angle iron is trimmed, leaving 1.5 cm on each side; these pieces are attached to parts H.

Bed, arm and head rest parts

Parts J, K, L, M and N are all made from aluminium sheet 2 mm thick. J is 47 cm long × 38 cm broad—the metal is shaped so that the sides are 13 cm high, width of wall at top 30 cm. K shoulder stops—21 cm long × 2.5 cm broad. These pieces can be either a continuous part of part J or separated pieces riveted to part J..

Arm rests

L is 17.5 cm long, 7 cm wide at rear, 6 cm wide at front; the outer edge is bent upwards making flange 1 cm high.

Head rest

M is 22 cm × 13 cm semicircular piece cut out with 8 cm diameter for the face to be kept free.

Padding

N is foam plastic, 2.5 cm thick; this is cut to shape and stuck to parts J, K, L and M with adhesive after assembly.

Parts O: these are coach bolts, 6 mm in diameter and 10 cm long. Holes are drilled in floor of J 6 mm in diameter—14 cm apart and 13 cm from the rear and 6.5 cm from the front of part J; these will line up with slots in cross members C and D. The holes in parts L are based midway along its length to line up with slots in the sides of the basic frame

A. The bolts having a square base under the head are put through the holes and hammered home, making a square hole in the sheet aluminium preventing the bolts rotating.

Before assembly the coach bolts O are covered with lengths of suitable diameter aluminium tubing, 8 cm lengths for the coach bolts joining J to the basic frame, and 7 cm lengths for the coach bolts joining the arm rests L to the basic frame.

The padding N is upholstered with white leatherette or plastic material. Legs can now be attached to the basic frame if desired; these can be bought ready to assemble.

All other nuts and bolts are the type supplied when purchasing the slotted angle iron Handy Angle.

Author Index

Subject Index